Techniques in Vascular Surgery

DENTON A. COOLEY, M.D.

Surgeon-in-Chief
Clinical Professor of Surgery

DON C. WUKASCH, M.D.

Attending Surgeon
Clinical Associate Professor of Surgery

The Texas Heart Institute
of St. Luke's Episcopal and Texas Children's Hospitals
Houston, Texas
and
Department of Surgery, The University of Texas Health Science Center at Houston

Foreword by HARRIS B. SHUMACKER, JR., M.D.

Illustrated by
TIMOTHY C. HENGST, M.A., BARBARA E. HYAMS, M.A., and RUSSELL G. JONES, M.A.

W. B. SAUNDERS COMPANY / Philadelphia / London / Toronto

W. B. Saunders Company: West Washington Square
Philadelphia, Pa. 19105

1 St. Anne's Road
Eastbourne, East Sussex BN21 3UN, England

1 Goldthorne Avenue
Toronto, Ontario M8Z 5T9, Canada

Library of Congress Cataloging in Publication Data

Cooley, Denton A   1920–

Techniques in vascular surgery.

Includes bibliographies and index.

1. Blood-vessels—Surgery.   I. Wukasch, Don C., joint
author.   II. Title.

RD598.5.C66   617'.413   78–64705

ISBN 0–7216–2700–5

Techniques in Vascular Surgery   ISBN 0-7216-2700-5

Last digit is the print number: 9   8   7   6   5   4   3

To our wives, Louise and Linda,
and to our fine colleagues and trainees who provided inspiration

Foreword

Techniques in Vascular Surgery by Denton A. Cooley and Don C. Wukasch is a valuable companion to Cooley and Norman's *Techniques in Cardiac Surgery,* which was published in 1975. Written by two outstanding physicians in their field, the book should prove valuable not only to those just entering into cardiovascular surgery but also to those with considerable background in this area of surgery. It has several extremely desirable characteristics: The subject matter is presented concisely, in an easily understood manner, accompanied by clear, to-the-point illustrations; and the references are pertinent yet limited, as they should be in a work of this kind. Also, the suggestions are based upon two very important prerequisites — wide background experience and long-term observation.

In a field progressing as rapidly as vascular surgery, change and expansion are as certain for the future as in the past. Surgeons who do not agree completely with all of the recommendations made here must, nevertheless, give them careful consideration, since they are based upon long-term follow-up studies and a considerable volume of work essential for proper evaluation. Success in a few cases with one method may be followed by failure when the same method is applied on a broader basis. There is no guarantee that good results a few months after operation will be long-lasting, but the large number of patients treated by the authors and the long periods of follow-up observation lend special weight to the procedures advocated here.

This book should be on the desk of every surgeon working in the arterial field. It should also be available as a ready reference for medical students, surgical trainees, and paramedical personnel.

HARRIS B. SHUMACKER, JR.
Distinguished Professor of Surgery
Indiana University Medical Center and
Chief, Section of Cardiovascular-Thoracic Surgery
St. Vincent Hospital and Health Care Center

Preface

*He that will not apply new remedies
must expect new evils.*
— Bacon

Since the practice of vascular surgery changes so rapidly, a book describing current techniques will be obsolete within a few years; nevertheless, such a manual or atlas should be valuable as a summary of the state-of-the-art, and also as a reference for surgeons in training. This book is not intended as a comprehensive reference detailing the evolving techniques throughout the history of vascular surgery; nor is it meant to demonstrate those employed in other institutions. Its basic purpose is to provide a convenient source for surgeons in training — residents and fellows — who wish to review the methods currently used in our surgical program. If others are interested, we are pleased that they consider our approach. Obviously, we could not cover in depth every aspect of vascular surgery, since the field is expanding and already encompasses a vast number of surgical procedures. There are vascular surgeons, for example, who are entering the cranium to attack lesions in the distal carotid circulation. We are not yet involved in such efforts. Some vascular surgeons are also performing myocardial revascularization. Since we consider this technique to be a task for the cardiothoracic surgeon, it was not included, but has been discussed in a companion text.*

Because the authors prepared chapters individually, certain discrepancies in this book may be apparent. The reader will probably recognize a difference in style. We have tried to place some emphasis on clarity and simplicity and sincerely hope that the material is presented clearly enough to have important practical value.

We were fortunate to be joined in this endeavor by two talented medical illustrators, Timothy Hengst and Barbara Hyams, both holding Master of Science degrees from the Department of Medical Illustration of the Johns Hopkins School of Medicine. Most of the illustrations were developed from sketches made in the operating rooms of the Texas Heart Institute. Since both of these artists had commitments elsewhere when final manuscripts were being prepared, Russell G. Jones, another fine medical illustrator from the University of Texas Health Science Center at Dallas, prepared the supplementary art work that was necessary to update our material. The authors are indebted to these artists for the high quality of their work.

Finally, we must acknowledge our deepest debt to Evelyn Lawrence, who brought order out of the chaos which resulted when two overworked surgeons decided that writing a book of this type would be an enjoyable and stimulating spare-time task. When the situation appeared almost hopeless, she coordinated the

---

Techniques in Cardiac Surgery by Denton A. Cooley and John C. Norman, Texas Medical Press, 6600 South Main Street, Houston, Texas 77030.

material into book form. Others who contributed were Eugenia Campbell, Virginia Fairchild, Martha Moseley, Joan Rabinowitz, and Joyce Staton.

This book is humbly submitted to other members of the medical profession as a summary of conclusions which we have drawn from that greatest of teachers— personal experience.

DENTON A. COOLEY, M.D.
DON C. WUKASCH, M.D.

Contents

CHAPTER 1

Introduction

The rapid progress of vascular surgery during the first half of the twentieth century exceeded the expectations of even the most imaginative surgeons and investigators.[1, 2] Availability of aseptic technique, anticoagulants, antibiotics, blood transfusion, and general anesthesia was fundamental to this development, but the major impetus came as surgeons first accepted the practicality of a direct rather than an indirect attack upon vascular diseases. Emphasis upon restoration of normal circulatory dynamics, or, more simplistically, upon restoration of normal pulsatile flow distal to the lesion, has stimulated remarkable improvement of the surgical approach. New diagnostic techniques such as arteriography and venography, vascular substitutes of various types, and improvement of the fundamentals of surgical technique have enormously expanded the field of vascular surgery during the past few decades.[3, 4, 5]

LIGHTING AND SURGICAL EXPOSURE

Essential to good vascular surgical technique is adequate illumination and anatomic exposure. The standard fixed surgical lamps may provide acceptable lighting for most surgical procedures, but the vascular surgeon often needs intense lighting to perform a small, tedious anastomosis, e.g., one located deep in the supraclavicular space or in the pelvis of the patient. We have found the fiberoptic headlamp* to be the most satisfactory device for lighting the surgical field in all types of vascular surgery. Optical loupes** with a three-power magnification can also greatly enhance the ability of the surgeon to perform an accurate and precise vascular repair (Fig. 1–1). Attention to detail and exact technique are surgical requisites to obtain the best results and to prevent hemorrhage and thrombosis after operation.[6]

VASCULAR ANASTOMOSIS

Restoration of vascular continuity may be accomplished by a variety of techniques. For example, the anastomosis may be end-to-end, end-to-side, or side-to-side, depending upon local conditions and anatomic and pathologic features. In almost all instances, the suture technique may be simple and continuous around the entire circumference of the opening. The suture must be inserted properly, by using the correct tension, to prevent leakage and to avoid stenosis, which can be caused by puckering or "purse-stringing" the anastomosis. The intima-to-intima anastomosis with the use of everting sutures, as advocated by Alexis Carrel more than 50 years

---

*Available from Texas Medical Products, Inc., P.O. Box 20663, Houston, Texas 77025.
**Obtainable from Designs for Vision, 40 E. 21st Street, New York City 10003.

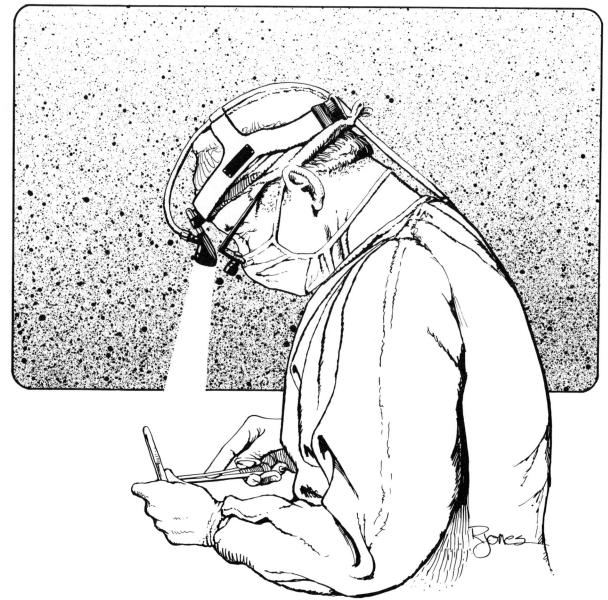

Figure 1–1   The fiberoptic headlamp is a most satisfactory device for lighting the surgical field in all types of vascular surgery.

ago,[1] has been generally discarded, although it may still be useful in venous anastomoses. An anastomosis should be carefully and precisely performed in an attempt to produce accurate approximation of intima and adventitia, particularly in vessels of small caliber. When a vascular substitute such as a fabric graft is used in an anastomosis to an atherosclerotic artery, some surgeons insist that the needle and suture be passed from the lumen to the outside to prevent dislodgement, or the lifting of an atherosclerotic plaque, which may occur if the opposite technique is used; however, we suture in both directions, depending upon which can be done most conveniently. With practice, the surgeon can prevent the technical problem of plaque dislodgement and can facilitate and expedite the performance of an anastomosis (Fig. 1–2).

Reinforcement of an anastomotic suture line is often necessary, particularly in aortic replacement when the aorta has a dissecting process adjacent to the suture line, or if there is an aneurysmal or degenerative condition locally. For such patients,

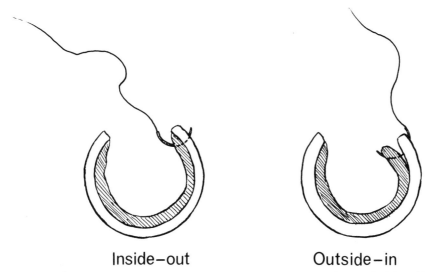

Inside-out   Outside-in

Figure 1–2 Two techniques of inserting an arterial suture into an arteriotomy incision. Usually the sugeon may use whichever method is the most convenient and least awkward. If the intimal and medial layers are diseased, they may separate from the adventitia in the "outside-in" technique; in that case, the "inside-out" technique is used.

a collar composed of a knitted Dacron tube may be placed around the distal vessel contiguous to the suture line. This reduces pulsatile expansion of the adjacent aorta and provides immediate hemostasis; it also prevents late complications, such as suture disruption or formation of a false aneurysm. This technique is applicable in other situations, such as reinforcement of an aortocoronary site in the aorta, when cannulation is performed for perfusion after standard repair of the opening. A collar wrap of Dacron tube graft controls hemorrhage and prevents late disruption. (See Fig. 10–2).

SUTURE TECHNIQUES

END-TO-END ANASTOMOSES (LARGE VESSELS)

Running suture is the preferred technique for all anastomoses except in children, whose vessels have not yet attained maximum diameter. In such instances, at least half of the suture line should consist of interrupted sutures to allow for future vessel growth. Our technique for anastomosing vessels 1.0 cm or larger in diameter is illustrated in Figure 1–3, a–e. It is unnecessary to tie the first stitch (Fig. 1–3, a). Note that both the posterior and anterior suture lines are made in the most convenient fashion, regardless of whether the needle enters the arterial wall from inside or out (Fig. 1–3, b–d). Air and debris are allowed to escape prior to tying the final stitches (Fig. 1–3, e).

END-TO-SIDE ANASTOMOSES (LARGE VESSELS)

This type of anastomosis is also made with running sutures (Fig. 1–4). The end of the graft or vessel should be tailored, however, so that there are rounded contours at both ventricle aspects of the arteriotomy (Fig. 1–4, a). This is accomplished by cutting the graft in an S-shaped fashion rather than in a straight line, which would result in a V-shaped contour at both vertical aspects.

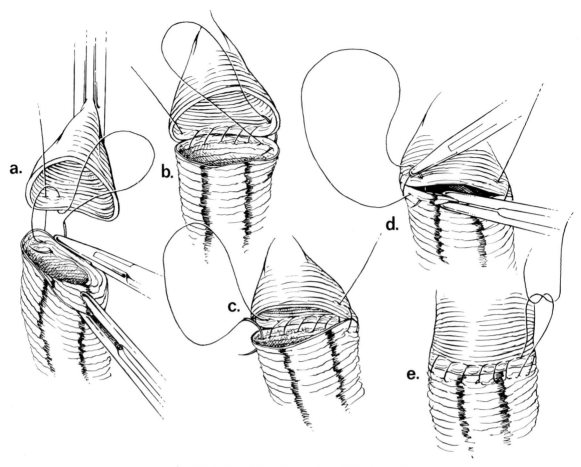

Figure 1–3   End-to-end large-vessel anastomosis.

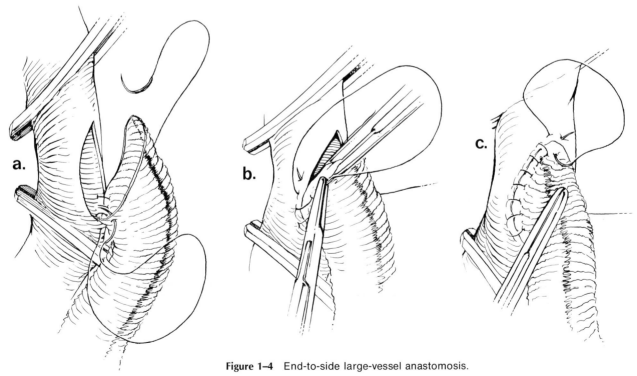

Figure 1–4   End-to-side large-vessel anastomosis.

Illustration continued on opposite page.

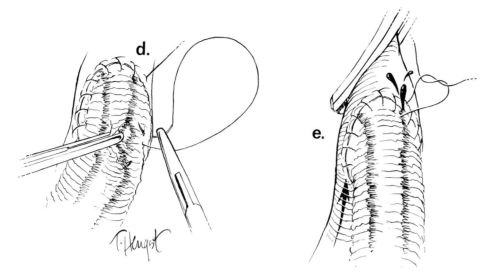

Figure 1–4 *Continued.*

END-TO-END ANASTOMOSES (SMALL VESSELS)

The only difference in anastomosing smaller vessels (less than 1.0 cm) is that both vessels should be transected obliquely in an S-shaped fashion rather than transversely at a 45° angle (Fig. 1–5, *a*). This results in a full lumen anastomosis without concentric constriction. The suture technique is otherwise similar to that used in larger vessels (Fig. 1–5, *b–e*).

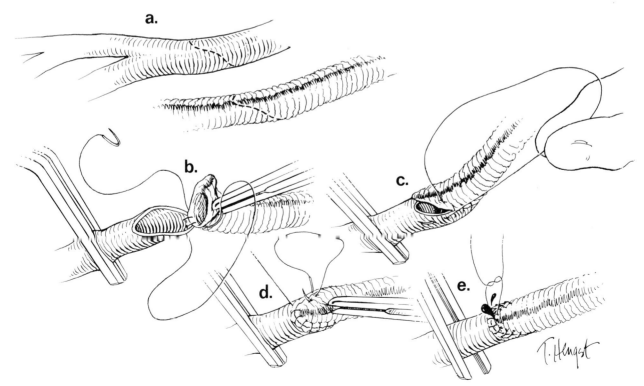

Figure 1–5 End-to-end small-vessel anastomosis.

VASCULAR INSTRUMENTS

Special instruments adapted to large and small vessels should be available.[6] Vascular thumb forceps without teeth on the holding surface should be used. The serrations should not be exceedingly deep because they may cause trauma to the intima. On the holding surface of the vascular forceps and clamps we use, there is a double row of low serrations that provide optimum holding ability without undue trauma (Fig. 1–6). Forceps without serrations should be available for the smallest and most delicate vessels. Vessel scissors that have a 45° angle and those with a 135° angle are useful when the incision is made in a forward and reverse direction.

Clamps for occluding arteries and veins should be designed to hold securely without excessive trauma. The ideal vascular clamp has moderately flexible shafts and jaws so that the proper amount of force may be applied; most important is a long ratchet with six or more teeth that allows the surgeon to estimate by "feel" the extent to which the clamp should be closed. This feature has several important aspects. For example, when a clamp is released on the abdominal or, particularly, the descending thoracic aorta, it may be removed stepwise by setting the ratchet at different levels of release. There are two advantages to this: first, redistribution of blood into the lower body may be accomplished gradually without producing hypotension; and second, bleeding through the interstices of a fabric vascular graft can be controlled so that the graft will seal itself, preventing excessive blood loss. These design features should be incorporated into vascular clamps of all sizes. If the clamps are similar in design, in the semblance of a matched set, the

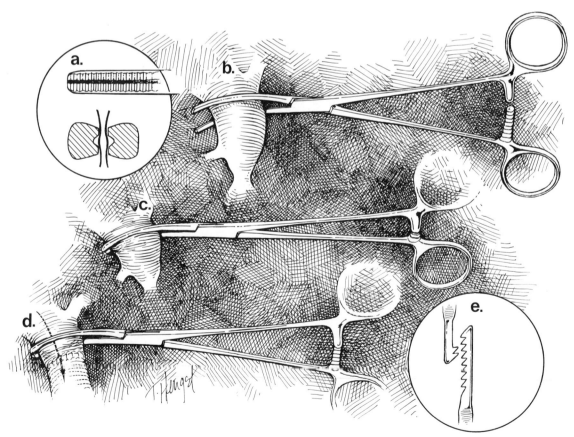

Figure 1–6 Vascular clamps: With the longer ratchets (*e*), a clamp may be released gradually, stop by stop, a factor of considerable importance when releasing the clamp after resection of an aortic aneurysm or coarctation, particularly when a somewhat porous fabric graft is used (*a* to *d*).

surgeon has the responsibility, and, with experience, should be able to apply the desired amount of pressure to meet the requirements of a particular situation.

In some circumstances vascular clamps may not be satisfactory for occluding an artery or vein. When previously performed anastomoses, such as that accompanying carotid endarterectomy or repair of a false aneurysm in the groin, require revision, dissection of the vessel may be impossible because it has become imbedded in scar tissue. For these situations the inflatable balloon-tipped catheter inserted into the arterial lumen may solve the problem without causing arterial damage. This technique and principle of arterial control has practical usefulness in complicated vascular cases.[7]

FABRIC GRAFTS AS VASCULAR SUBSTITUTES

Vascular surgery has been revolutionized by the introduction and improvement of fabric grafts.[8-10] Earlier in this era the vascular substitutes were mostly homografts. Homografts are now used only rarely, and in general they are inferior to synthetic materials, which have more durability, better resistance to infection, and greater ease of handling. A possible exception may be the recently introduced umbilical vessel grafts for femoral and popliteal revascularizations.[11] Polyester, manufactured under the trade name of Dacron, is presently the optimum synthetic fiber for fabrication of grafts. This fiber causes minimal or no tissue reaction, does not absorb fluid, has strength and dependable durability, and can be fabricated into a variety of forms, as introduced by modern textile technology. Some fabric grafts of other materials (Nylon) have displayed late degeneration, but fabric grafts of Dacron have never shown evidence of failure from wear. Grafts fabricated from Teflon do not incorporate well into surrounding tissues, and thereby retard the healing process.

Textile experts have answered most of the needs for vascular substitutes in the use of polyester fiber, except for special circumstances involving areas of the systemic venous system or arteries of small caliber. The various types of fabric should be familiar to the vascular surgeon, who must select the best graft for the requirements of a particular operation.

The two types of available fabrics for grafts are *woven* and *knitted*.[8] The principal advantage of the woven graft over the knitted one is its provision for low porosity. Unfortunately, the lower the porosity, the less the tendency for surrounding tissues to grow firmly into the graft. This tendency can be tested in the experimental animal by implanting several types of grafts into the aorta and, at specified intervals, removing the graft and determining the amount of force necessary to "peel" off the surrounding tissue and fibrous ingrowth.[9] The greater the peeling force required to separate the graft from the tissues, the greater is the degree of healing between graft and tissue. In general, tissues peel most easily from woven grafts, whereas more force is required to peel tissues from knitted grafts. Velour grafts that have small tufts or hooklets on the surface require the largest peeling forces and therefore heal best.

Neointimas forming on the luminal surface are nourished by tissues that have grown through the graft wall; thus, the woven grafts are less satisfactory with small caliber vessels because of the reduced tissue ingrowth from the outside. Since loosely adherent neointimas break off, the woven grafts in the femoral and popliteal regions tend to cause embolization. Moreover, woven grafts in the extremities behave in the manner of impervious foreign bodies and are less resistant to infection than knitted grafts. Thus, we have used the woven grafts only for replacement of large caliber arteries, usually the aorta and its major tributaries, and in patients whose blood loss must be strictly controlled.

Knitted Dacron grafts are available in the form of the jersey knit, warp knit, and velour.[9] The principal differences in the three knits are related to porosity and ease of handling. Weaving and knitting processes may vary to such extremes that the graft may be excessively porous, causing an intolerable amount of bleeding when arterial blood is introduced. Likewise, the weave of the graft may be so tight that the surgeon has difficulty passing a needle through the graft. The optimum graft should have porosity and flexibility somewhere between these extremes. Another point of practical importance is that knitted grafts have almost no tendency to fray along the margins as sutures are inserted. Woven grafts will fray, however, particularly if the edges are soaked with blood. To prevent the fraying, a disposable hot cautery may be used to seal the threads. This is somewhat impractical if the graft is already wet.

As this book goes to press, our experience with the relatively new graft made from expanded microporous polytetrafluoroethylene (PTFE) (Gore-Tex®) suggests that this material may be as good if not better than fabric grafts for reconstruction of small caliber arteries and large veins. We have used Gore-Tex for reconstruction of the superficial femoral, popliteal, and renal arteries, the venae cavae, pulmonary aortic anastomosis, and for other vessels.[36]

PRECLOTTING

To prevent excessive bleeding when arterial circulation is resumed, preclotting is an important aspect in the preparation of fabric grafts. The need for preclotting Dacron grafts primarily depends upon the porosity of the grafts, which may vary widely.

A unique feature of the surface of the velour grafts deserves mention. Laboratory or bench testing for porosity with the use of saline as a medium reveals that velour grafts may have greater porosity than the jersey and warp knit grafts.[8, 9] After being preclotted, however, the velour graft has considerably lower porosity than preclotted jersey and warp knit grafts. Fibrin and other blood elements are entrapped by the hooklets of the velour fabric and provide a low porosity graft that permits optimal conditions for tissue ingrowth. Thus, the velour grafts, particularly those of double velour (internal and external surfaces), are superior in controlling blood loss. They tend to be more pliable and easier to handle than the standard knit and woven grafts. As already stated, the woven grafts have lower porosity than knitted grafts. In the so-called tightly woven or low porosity grafts, preclotting is unnecessary, but the close weave causes them to be stiffer and more difficult to handle.[8]

All knitted grafts should be preclotted. Before the patient receives systemic heparin, about 20 to 30 ml of blood is withdrawn in a syringe from an artery or vein. The selected graft is placed in a shallow basin and blood is applied to the graft. The surgeon or instrument nurse stretches and massages the graft to ensure that the blood has permeated into all interstices. Excess blood is wiped away and the basin is placed on a side table where it will be ready for use in five or ten minutes. Systemic heparinization is then accomplished.

GRAFT DESIGN

A wide range of sizes, diameters, and configurations should be available. Most fabric grafts are crimped to prevent kinking, since they must be bent or curved according to anatomic formations, or as they cross flexion areas in the extremities. The graft manufacturer produces the crimping by setting indentations mechanically and placing the graft in a heat-controlled oven. The crimps are permanently set and remain even after stretching of the graft.[12]

Fabric grafts are often passed through both body cavities into the extremities.

When the graft is passed through tissue tunnels, twisting the graft can cause a technical problem by kinking and obstructing the lumen. Addition of a guideline or stripe down the graft effectively prevents this complication (Fig. 1–7).[10]

Diameter of the tube grafts may vary from 4 mm to 36 mm. In general, fabric grafts now available are not practical in diameters of less than 4 mm because thrombosis occurs frequently in small caliber grafts — even if the patient is receiving anticoagulants.[13]

Bifurcation grafts are available in a range of sizes (Fig. 1–8).* Most have limbs with diameters half the diameter of the proximal end. This configuration may be acceptable for replacement of an abdominal aneurysm in which the proximal aorta or neck of the aneurysm is dilated and destroys the more normal anastomotic relationship. For abdominal aneurysms, therefore, standard bifurcation grafts measuring 14 × 6, 16 × 8, 18 × 9, and 20 × 10 mm in diameter may be satisfactory, and ends conform well to the proximal aorta and iliac arteries. For patients with aortoiliac occlusive disease, the diameters of the aorta and iliac and femoral vessels tend to follow the normal anatomy. In cadavers, we determined that the aorta-to-iliac-vessel size correlation was related to the cross-sectional area of the

*Available from Meadox Medicals, Oakland, New Jersey.

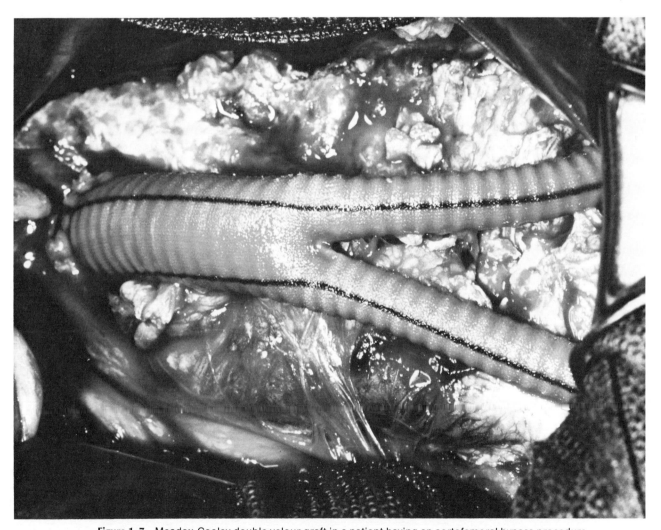

Figure 1–7 Meadox-Cooley double velour graft in a patient having an aortofemoral bypass procedure for occlusive disease. The guideline stripe facilitates proper orientation of the graft in the retroperitoneal tunnel. (From Buxton et al: Am J Surg 125:288, 1973.)

IDEAL DIAMETER OF BIFURCATION $A = \pi r^2$

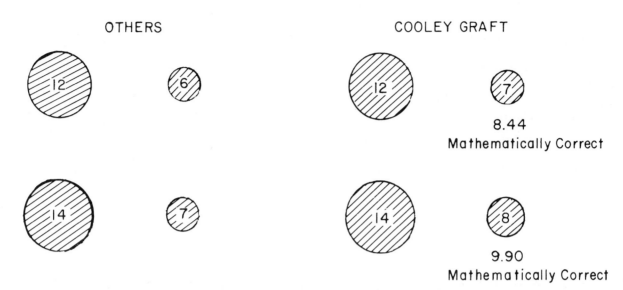

Figure 1–8   Diagram showing the basic difference in size relationships between Cooley bifurcated grafts and standard grafts. The ideal diameter of bifurcation is A = πr^2. (From Cooley et al: Vascular Grafts, edited by Sawyer PN and Kaplitt MJ, New York, Appleton-Century-Crofts, 1978, pp 197–208.)

lumen rather than to the diameter of these arteries.[13] Thus, each of the iliac limbs of a bifurcation graft should be half the *area* of the proximal aortic end, and this relationship can be determined by using the equation:

$$\text{Area} = \pi \times \text{radius}^2.$$

Working with the graft manufacturers, we developed a bifurcation graft that approximated this relationship, and grafts are available in 10 × 6, 12 × 7, and 14 × 8 mm. These grafts are used mostly for patients, often women, who are undergoing bypass grafting for aortoiliac occlusive disease. The small proximal abdominal aorta may have a diameter of only 10 mm, yet the distal branches of 6 mm provide optimum flow without threat of thrombosis.[9]

BIOLOGICAL TISSUE GRAFTS

Most surgeons are of the opinion that grafts of autologous tissue provide the ideal vascular substitute; the saphenous vein has proved to be the most practical and successful autologous tissue graft available. Other autologous vessels still used are the cephalic vein (arm), internal iliac arteries for short arterial grafts, external jugular vein, and occasionally the internal mammary artery for coronary substitution. Of these autologous grafts, the cephalic vein is used most frequently, but usually only for myocardial revascularization in a patient who has undergone previous coronary artery or saphenous vein stripping for varicosities, or when the saphenous vein is unsuitable because of previous inflammatory disease or varicose changes.[14-16]

DIAGNOSTIC TECHNIQUES: ARTERIOGRAPHY

INTRODUCTION

Accurate visualization of the arterial circulation is essential to almost all vascular surgical procedures. Various techniques of arteriography were developed in the 1920's: the upper extremity by Berberich in 1923,[17] the femoral by Brooks in 1924,[18] the carotid by Moniz in 1928,[19] and the translumbar by dos Santos in 1929.[20] Refinement and widespread utilization of these techniques, however, awaited a special need for their use, which was created by the innovation of vascular surgical techniques in the 1950's.

In many centers, arteriography is routinely performed by radiologists. Because the techniques used in our center were frequently developed by surgeons during initial revascularization attempts, however, most of our arteriography is still performed by the responsible surgeon. This arrangement allows the surgeon making the operative decisions an opportunity to obtain visualization required for competent surgical determinations. Complications are better handled by the surgeon who performs the arteriogram than by a third person who has not been involved previously. Despite these advantages, the trend is for such procedures to be performed by vascular radiologists. Nevertheless, the vascular surgeon should be experienced in arteriography, since it is he who is ultimately responsible for obtaining adequate delineation of the anatomic lesions to be evaluated and for resolving complications when they occur.

ANESTHESIA, EQUIPMENT, AND CONTRAST MEDIA

Local anesthesia is preferred in most instances, because it is best to avoid the use of more than one general anesthetic within a two-day period. Also, arteriography is expedited by the cooperation of an awake patient. On occasion, a procedure (usually carotid arteriography) attempted under local anesthesia will require conversion to general anesthesia, because the patient is uncooperative, or because of complications, such as hematoma formation around the vessel. It is imperative that the room in which arteriography is performed be well equipped for general anesthesia induction on a standby basis. Anaphylactic shock reactions to contrast media may require emergency intubation and controlled ventilation, again emphasizing the importance of having personnel and equipment ready at all times for use with general anesthesia.

In addition to the capability for emergency conversion to general anesthesia, the basic equipment necessary for arteriography includes: (1) a rapid film changer capable of making cerebral films at a rate of two per second and long films at a rate of every other second, (2) a pressure injector adjustable in measuring the rate of pressure and the rate of ingestion, and (3) a fluoroscopic unit for selective catheter techniques if they are to be used.

All commonly used contrast materials are iodinated benzene ring compounds combined with sodium or methylglucamine salt solutions. While the sodium salt solutions are less viscous[21] and are associated with less histamine[22] than the methylglucamine compounds, they have been shown to be more neurotoxic.[22-26] Therefore, we prefer those contrast media containing primarily methylglucamine salts. Hypaque 60, which contains only 60 percent methylglucamine diatrizoate and no sodium salts, or Conray 60 is used for carotid arteriography. Aortic or femoral injections are made with Hypaque 75, Renografin 76, or Conray 80, which contain methylglucamine diatrizoate primarily and a smaller amount of sodium diatrizoate.

Reactions to contrast material are of two types: hypersensitive and chemotoxic. Hypersensitivity reactions are apparently related to histamine release.[27, 28] Because these allergic reactions are more frequent with intravenous than with intra-arterial injections,[29] the lung is suspected of being the organ primarily responsible for the histamine release. The manifestations of these allergic reactions range from sneezing, skin rash, bronchospasm, and shock to cardiac arrest. Pretesting by conjunctional or oral methods is not useful in identifying sensitive individuals.[30]

Our technique is to inject several cc's of contrast material via the arterial needle to preclude subintimal placement of the needle, and to satisfy the medical-legal requirements for pretesting the contrast material. From a practical standpoint, however, this serves little purpose. The rare patient who shows mild allergic symptoms or who has a history of severe anaphylactic shock reaction during a previous study should receive 100 mg Solu-Cortef and 25 mg Benadryl intravenously immediately prior to injection of the contrast material. Additionally, aminophylline and epinephrine are drawn into a syringe for immediate intravenous administration, should they be required. Among several hundred patients who have undergone arteriography in our institution and have been known to have previous allergic reactions to iodinated compounds, no fatalities have occurred with the use of this regimen.

Chemotoxic reactions are a result of injury to sensitive organs, primarily the kidney and brain, and are dose-related. Injection of contrast material into the cerebral circulation produces a "hot-flush" sensation that the patient should be told to anticipate, along with reassurance of its transience. Other toxic effects may include headache, altered consciousness and, occasionally, convulsions, which appear to be a result of altering the blood-brain barrier, causing increased endothelial permeability and diffusion of the contrast material into the brain tissue.[31] These symptoms are best minimized by limiting the amount of contrast material and by using methylglucamine compounds, which are less neurotoxic than sodium-containing salts.[23-26] Prevention of nephrotoxic effects is achieved by assuring adequate hydration of the patient, by placing the aortography needle above rather than adjacent to the renal artery ostia, and by limiting the volume of contrast material presented to the kidneys.

PERCUTANEOUS CAROTID ARTERIOGRAPHY

Premedication is kept light to avoid hypotension, which causes difficulty in palpating the carotid arteries and increases the risk of neurological complications. Demerol (25 mg) and atropine (0.4 mg), given intramuscularly 30 minutes prior to the study, or Valium (10 mg), given intravenously just prior to dye injection, usually provides satisfactory short-term analgesia. Dehydration may cause difficulty in palpating the carotid arteries; this problem can be alleviated by intravenous fluid administration.

Visualization of the carotid arteries is enhanced by placing a roll beneath the supine patient's shoulders. The patient's head is arched backward and placed on a rubber doughnut for comfort. The common carotid artery is palpated with the finger of the left hand, and, after injection of local anesthesia, a small nick is made with a No. 11 blade. A Cournand-Potts disposable 17-gauge needle is inserted over the common carotid artery approximately 2 cm above the clavicle and directed through the anterior carotid wall (Fig. 1–9, a). The stylet is removed and the needle threaded up the artery. Prior to injection, visualization of the carotid bifurcation is enhanced by having the patient reach as far as possible toward his feet to displace the shoulder in a caudad direction out of the x-ray beam. Hypaque 60 percent (8 cc) is hand-injected after first withdrawing the syringe to ascertain free flow and to preclude subintimal placement of the needle.

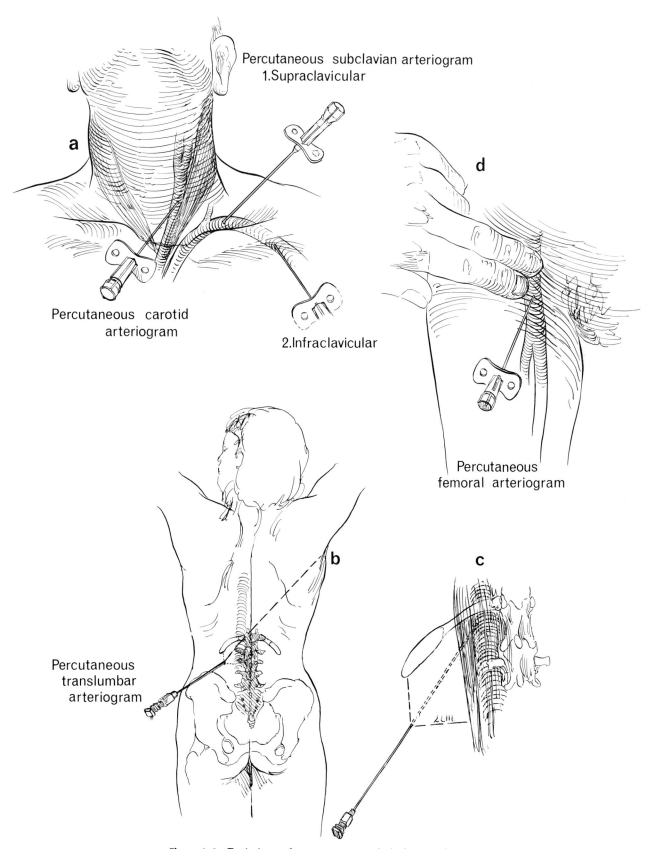

Percutaneous subclavian arteriogram
1.Supraclavicular

a

d

Percutaneous carotid
arteriogram

2.Infraclavicular

Percutaneous
femoral arteriogram

Percutaneous
translumbar
arteriogram

b

c

Figure 1–9 Technique of percutaneous subclavian arteriography.

Usually the presence or absence of significant stenosis in the extracranial carotid artery can be determined with a lateral projection film by a single injection. Occasionally the external carotid artery will overlie and obscure the internal carotid artery in the lateral projection. Separation of these vessels can be facilitated by turning the head toward the side of the vessel being studied. When the extent of an extracranial carotid lesion cannot be determined by a lateral film alone, an anterior-posterior view should be obtained. When intracranial pathology is suspected, sequential views of the intracranial circulation are indicated.

The most frequent serious complication of percutaneous carotid arteriography is hemiparesis resulting from air embolism. This can be prevented by carefully evacuating all air from the tubing and syringe prior to injection.

The most severe complication is subintimal dissection caused by the needle or dye injection. This can be avoided by ascertaining free flow retrograde before using hand-controlled injection, which can be terminated at any time if undue resistance is encountered. It should be emphasized that the use of pressure injectors is contraindicated in percutaneous carotid arteriography; the damaged artery can produce a cerebrovascular accident by causing complete thrombosis at the injection site, extending up the entire internal carotid artery.

The surgeon can evaluate the patency of the internal carotid artery postoperatively by placing the middle finger of his gloved hand into the patient's mouth and palpating the internal carotid artery pulse just posterior to the tonsillar pillar. Absence of a pulse associated with hemiplegia is an indication for emergency exploration, repair, and thrombectomy of the artery. The incidence of complications following cerebral angiography has been reported by Allen et al to be 3.9 percent, and death or severe complications to be 0.4 percent.[32]

PERCUTANEOUS SUBCLAVIAN (VERTEBRAL) ARTERIOGRAPHY

Four-vessel arteriography was formerly considered necessary for complete evaluation of all patients undergoing work-ups for symptoms of cerebrovascular insufficiency, whether or not there were indications of vertebral-basilar insufficiency. Because of frequent unsatisfactory results of vertebral artery surgery and the trend toward more rigid indications for operating upon patients with vertebral lesions, however, we no longer recommend routine four-vessel studies.

Visualization of the vertebral arteries, which is readily accomplished by percutaneous subclavian arteriograms, is indicated in patients who have definite vertebral-basilar symptoms and an absence of carotid circulatory symptoms, or normal extracranial carotid arteries demonstrated arteriographically. In our experience, most patients with both carotid circulatory symptoms and vertebral-basilar lesions have responded favorably to revascularization of the carotid circulation alone; vertebral-basilar symptoms will most often be relieved by restoring normal carotid circulation, leaving the vertebral lesions in place. For these reasons, subclavian (vertebral) arteriography is now less commonly performed than formerly.

The subclavian artery may be entered with an 8-inch Cournand-Potts 17-gauge needle from either above or below the clavicle (Fig. 1–9, a). The supraclavicular approach, which is most frequently used, consists of first injecting a local anesthetic and then directing the needle medially through the supraclavicular notch at approximately a 45° angle (Fig. 1–9, a–1.).

The infraclavicular approach is useful in obese patients. The needle is inserted at the midclavicular line and directed in a cephalad direction just below the inferior border of the clavicle (Fig. 1–9, a–2.). A useful trick is to find the resistance of the clavicle with the needle point and then "walk" the needle beneath the inferior border of the clavicle. Following insertion and threading of the needle via either approach, 20 cc of Hypaque 60 percent is *hand*-injected. Anterior-posterior films will adequately visualize the extracranial vertebral arteries. Determination that either one of the vertebral arteries is patent, without stenosis or kinking, precludes the necessity of visualizing the opposite vertebral artery.

This technique will allow satisfactory visualization of the entire subclavian, axillary, and brachial arteries for evaluating such conditions as axillary artery thrombosis.[33]

Because of the proximity of the lung apex to the arch of the subclavian artery (Fig. 1–9, a), the most frequent complication of subclavian arteriography is pneumothorax. Use of the infraclavicular approach lessens the likelihood of this occurrence, because the needle is directed away from the pleura rather than down into it, as in the supraclavicular approach. Air embolism must be avoided by careful evacuation of air bubbles from the tubing. Subintimal dissection and possible thrombosis of the artery can be prevented by ascertaining free flow before injection to assure proper needle placement.

PERCUTANEOUS BRACHIAL ARTERIOGRAPHY

Lesions of the brachial, radial, or ulnar arteries may be easily visualized via the brachial artery. The artery is palpated and held firm against the medial aspect of the humerus posterior to the biceps muscle. A plastic 17-gauge intracath needle is threaded into the artery in a proximal direction.

TRANSLUMBAR AORTOGRAPHY

Translumbar aortography (TLA) is the preferred technique in our institution for visualization of the aorta and distal circulation in aortoiliac occlusive disease, and of the renal arteries in patients with hypertension associated with abdominal aortic aneurysm (AAA). Using lateral films, the celiac and superior mesenteric arteries may also be adequately visualized in patients with suspected abdominal angina and associated severe disease in the femoral and iliac arteries. Aortography is not necessary or indicated in patients with AAA without hypertension. The diagnosis of AAA may be made by palpation of a pulsating abdominal mass, one plain lateral x-ray film of the abdomen, and sonography.

To prevent aspiration resulting from the nausea that commonly occurs after the injection of contrast material, the patient is fed only liquids the morning of the test. Premedication consists of 50 mg Demerol, 25 mg Nembutal, and 0.4 mg atropine. The patient is placed in a prone position with the arms above the head. Following injection of local anesthesia, a 9-inch, 17-gauge needle containing a stylet is inserted at a point 2 cm below the tip of the left twelfth rib and 2 cm lateral to the edge of the paraspinous muscles (Fig. 1–9, b). The needle is directed toward the apex of the right axilla, which is at an angle 45° to three planes — the dorsal surface of the back, the AP midline of the spine, and the transverse waistline (Fig. 1–9, c). This course will usually afford direct entry to the aorta. If difficulty is encountered, the needle may be "walked" along the lateral-anterior aspect of the spine. When the pulsation of the aorta is sensed by the operator's fingers, injection of several cc's of additional local anesthetic prior to penetrating the aorta will alleviate the discomfort of puncture of the aorta, which is surrounded by a sensitive nerve plexus.

Free flow is ascertained by twisting the needle 360°. Fifty cc of Conray 80 is introduced, using a power injector at a rate of 10 to 12 cc per second under 200 pounds per square inch of pressure. Filming is carried out for at least 12 seconds, by which time the contrast material is visualized in the branches of the popliteal arteries. Our method is to use long films that cover the area from the diaphragm to below the knees. The patient is requested to hold his breath and refrain from moving during the filming period, as he may experience a sensation of heat produced by the contrast material.

The complication of renal shutdown can be prevented by several important considerations: First, the tip of the needle should be at least 2 inches cephalad to the origins of the renal arteries to preclude the introduction of an undiluted concentration of contrast material. Needle placement may be ascertained by filming a test injection of 10 cc of contrast material. Second, if possible, only one injection should be made within a 24-hour period, but if a second injection is essential within that time, 25 gm mannitol and 1000 cc of intravenous hydration should follow the contrast material injection. Third, the patient should be adequately hydrated prior to aortography.

A less serious but more frequent complication of TLA is extravasation or extramural injection. Although this complication is rarely serious, hematoma formation of up to 500 cc around the injection site is not infrequently encountered at operation following TLA. Such an occurrence is best prevented by penetrating only one wall of the aorta; penetration can be controlled by sensing the aortic pulsation transmitted through the needle. Subintimal dissection can result in fatal retrograde dissection and may be prevented by assuring free flow from the needle prior to injection and by limiting the pressure of injection to 200 pounds per square inch. Should subintimal placement of the needle be suspected, a test dose of 10 cc of contrast material may be injected under hand pressure; if the patient experiences pain, the needle should be repositioned. Finally, postinjection hemorrhage from the needle site in the aorta may be prevented by assuring an adequate prothrombin time. Patients demonstrating prothrombin times of less than 70 percent are given 50 mg of AquaMephyton in 100 cc of saline intravenously the evening prior to aortography.

PERCUTANEOUS FEMORAL ARTERIOGRAPHY

Bilateral femoral arteriography is indicated for the evaluation of femoral popliteal occlusive disease (FPOD). We prefer bilateral needle insertion into each common femoral artery rather than insertion of a catheter through one femoral artery into the aorta by the Seldinger technique, because the latter method increases the likelihood of thrombosis or embolization. The single insertion of a sharp disposable needle or a 17-gauge Cournand-Potts needle is much less likely to dislodge the friable plaque commonly seen in the femoral arteries of patients being evaluated for FPOD than is a larger bore catheter requiring extensive manipulation of the catheter.

It is essential that all patients who undergo femoral popliteal bypass have no significant proximal occlusive disease in the aorta or iliac arteries. The presence of proximal disease is best excluded by aortography, even in the presence of full femoral pulses. Although 50 percent stenosis of a common iliac artery may not diminish pulses or flow at the time of preoperative evaluation, it may become a hemodynamically significant lesion during the year following operation, and may result in graft failure.[34, 35] Therefore, we recommend that all proximal aortoiliac lesions with an occlusion of the lumen area of 50 percent or greater be bypassed prior to femoral-popliteal revascularization.[35] Quite frequently revascularization of these proximal lesions will relieve symptoms of claudication to the extent that femoral popliteal bypass becomes unnecessary.

Percutaneous femoral artery arteriograms are the simplest of all arteriography techniques. With the patient in the supine position, a local anesthetic is injected over the common artery pulse. A Cournand-Potts 17-gauge disposable needle is advanced at a 45° angle into the anterior wall of the artery and threaded into the lumen (Fig. 1–9, d). Needles are inserted into both arteries, and 60 cc of Conray 60 is injected simultaneously with a pressure injector at 100 pounds per square inch. Four long films are made midway during injection, and at 2, 5, and 7 seconds thereafter. Quite frequently retrograde visualization of the iliac arteries to the level of the aortic bifurcation can be achieved; if not, translumbar aortography should be performed.

Complications such as thrombosis or plaque dislodgement are rare with the needle technique, but not uncommon when the Seldinger catheter method is used. Occasional hematoma formation or extravasation is usually inconsequential. Previously inserted femoral Dacron grafts may be safely injected by the needle technique, with firm but non-occluding pressure applied over the graft for approximately 10 minutes after removing the needle.

SELECTIVE ARTERIOGRAPHY BY SELDINGER CATHETER TECHNIQUE

Although percutaneous arteriography by the techniques described above is preferred by our surgical staff, many vascular radiologists prefer the catheter technique. Selective catheter arteriography does have certain advantages, particularly in selectively demonstrating the renal, celiac, and superior mesenteric arteries. The vascular surgeon should be able to perform his own arteriography, however, in the case of emergencies.

Use of the catheter technique requires complex equipment, including a fluoroscopic unit, rapid film changer, and pressure injector with adjustable rates of pressure and injection. After the administration of local anesthesia, a Seldinger needle is percutaneously introduced into the femoral artery. In patients with extensive aortoiliac or femoral artery disease, the axillary or brachial arteries may be used. The stylet of the needle is removed, and a flexible guide wire is maneuvered through the needle into the aorta. A catheter is then threaded over the guide wire into the lumen of the vessel and directed under fluoroscopic control into the vessel for study.

The major disadvantage and most frequent complication of the Seldinger technique is thrombosis of the artery at the site of entry. This may be caused by multiple attempts to penetrate the artery or by excessive catheter manipulation, which can be eliminated only by experience and practice. Emboli may result from the stripping of thrombotic material from the outer surfaces of the catheter during its removal.[36, 37] This can be prevented by heparinization;[38] we advocate frequent intermittent irrigation of the catheter with a 1000-cc saline solution containing 10,000 units of heparin.

DECISIONS

The many decisions required of the vascular surgeon call for a wide latitude of judgment and experience. Whereas in other fields of surgery the indications for operation and the choice of procedure are relatively well established, this is not true of vascular surgery. Good judgment can be attained only in a supervised clinical environment, where experience will not be gained at the patient's expense.

As the field of vascular surgery continues to expand, the surgeon who does only an occasional vascular operation may discover that he is incapable of staying abreast of newer developments. Under these circumstances, he should not attempt an operation that could be better handled by a more experienced surgeon performing at a major center. Whether or not operative intervention is indicated, the decisions that must be made in considering an operation require sound judgment. The Golden Rule is a good principle to follow — "If I had this patient's condition, would I want the proposed procedure to be performed on me?" Our philosophy in recommending operation generally requires that the condition either present a threat to life or limb, as would be the case with an abdominal aortic or popliteal aneurysm, or interfere with the patient's livelihood or quality of life, as would disabling claudication in a mailman or golfer. For less threatening conditions, serious consideration is given to conservative management; the patient should be allowed to make his own decision based on the question, "Are my symptoms interfering with the quality of my life to the extent that I am willing to undergo the risk, inconvenience, and expense of this operation?"

At the operating table, complex technical problems may arise which, if not skillfully solved, may result in loss of a lower extremity, or even in death. Although less experienced surgeons may consider so-called peripheral vascular surgery, such as that undertaken for femoropopliteal occlusive disease, to be simple and safe, disastrous results may follow a faulty decision. Such errors in judgment and decision-making are inexcusable, and the surgeon may suffer professionally. *Liberal use of consultants and advice from knowledgeable or more experienced colleagues may save both the patient and surgeon from pain and loss.*

REFERENCES

1. Carrel A: The surgery of blood vessels. Bull Johns Hopkins Hosp 18:18, 1907.
2. Blalock A: The expanding scope of cardiovascular surgery. Br J Surg 43:3, 1954.
3. Blalock A: Cardiovascular surgery, past and present. J Thorac Cardiovasc Surg 51:2, 1966.
4. Baker NH, Ewy HG, Moore PJ: Vascular surgery: A decade of progress. Ohio State Med J 67:907, 1971.
5. Rob CG: A history of arterial surgery. Arch Surg 105:821, 1972.
6. Cooley, DA, Norman, JC: *Techniques in Cardiac Surgery.* Houston, Texas, Medical Press, 1975, pp 2–5.
7. Bangash M: Improved design of cardiovascular instruments. Cardiovascular Diseases, Bulletin of the Texas Heart Institute 2(#3):346, 1975.
8. Bennett JG, Trono R, Norman JC, Cooley DA: Experimental comparisons of vascular grafts. Cardiovascular Diseases. Bulletin of the Texas Heart Institute 4(#1):18, 1977.
9. Cooley DA, Wukasch DC, Bennett JG, Trono R: Double velour knitted Dacron grafts for aortoiliac vascular replacements. In *Vascular Grafts* (edited by Sawyer PN and Kaplitt MJ). New York, Appleton-Century-Crofts, 1978, pp 197–208.
10. Buxton BF, Wukasch DC, Martin C, Liebig WJ, Hallman GL, Cooley DA: Practical considerations in fabric vascular grafts: Introduction of a new bifurcated graft. Am J Surg 125:288, 1973.
11. Dardik I, Ibrahim I, Dardik H: Femoral popliteal bypass employing modified human umbilical cord vein: An assessment of early clinical results. Cardiovascular Diseases, Bulletin of the Texas Heart Institute 3(#3):314, 1976.
12. Crawford ES, DeBakey ME, Cooley DA, Morris GC Jr: Use of crimped knitted Dacron grafts in patients with occlusive disease of the aorta and of the iliac femoral and popliteal arteries. In *Fundamentals of Vascular Grafting* (edited by Wesolowski SA and Dennis C). New York, McGraw-Hill Book Co., Inc., 1963, pp 356–366.
13. Buxton BF, Wukasch DC, Cooley DA: Dimensions of the aorto-ilio-femoral arterial segment. Austr NZ J Surg 42:204, 1972.
14. Baier RE, DePalma VA, Goupil D, Perlmutter S, Gott VL: Interfascial biophysics of materials in contact with blood. Annual Report, Contract No N01-BH-3-2953, Division of Blood Diseases and Resources. National Institutes of Health, February 1975, 246 pages. Available from National Technical Information Service, 5285 Port Royal Road, Springfield, Virginia 22151.
15. Darling RC: Autogenous saphenous vein bypass grafts for femoropopliteal occlusive disease. In *Vascular Grafts* (edited by Sawyer PN and Kaplitt MJ). New York, Appleton-Century-Crofts, 1978, pp 237–242.
16. Vollmar JF, Loeprecht H, Hamann H. The experiences at Ulm with grafts of different origin. In *Vascular Grafts* (edited by Sawyer PN and Kaplitt MJ). New York, Appleton-Century-Crofts, 1978, pp 273–278.
17. Berberich J, Hirsch S: Die röntgenographische Darstellung der Arterien und Venen am Lebenden. Münch Klin Wochenschr 49:2226, 1923.
18. Brooks, B: Intra-arterial injection of sodium iodide. JAMA 82:1016, 1924.
19. Moniz E, Diaz A, Lima A: La radioartériographie et la topographie cranioencéphalique. J Radiol Electrol 12:72, 1928.

20. Dos Santos R, Lamas AC, Pereira-Caldas J: Arteriografia da aorta e dos vasos abdominais. Med Contemp 47:93, 1929.
21. Fischer HW: Viscosity, solubility and toxicity in the choice of an angiographic contrast medium. Angiology 16:759, 1965.
22. Lasser EC: Metabolic basis of contrast material toxicity status, 1971. Am J Roentgenol Radium Ther Nucl Med 113:415, 1971.
23. Fisher HW, Cornell SH: The toxicity of sodium and methylglucamine salts of diatrizoate, Iothal and Metrizoate. Radiology 85:1013, 1965.
24. Melartin EP, Tuohimaa J, Daab R: Neurotoxicity of iothalamates and diatrizoates. I. Significance of concentration and cation. Invest Radiol 5:13, 1970.
25. Fischer WH, Eckstein JW: Comparison of cerebral angiographic media by their circulatory effects — an experimental study. Am J Roentgenol Radium Ther Nucl Med 86:166, 1961.
26. Hilal SK: Trends in preparation of new angiographic contrast media with special emphasis on polymeric derivatives. Invest Radiol 5:458, 1970.
27. Mann MR: The pharmacology of contrast media. Proc R Soc Med 54:473, 1961.
28. Lasser EC, Walters A, Reuter SR, Lang J: Histamine release by contrast media. Radiology 200:683, 1971.
29. Lang EK: Clinical evaluation of side effects of radiopaque contrast media administered via intravenous and intra-arterial routes in the same patients—a preliminary report. Radiology 85:665, 1965.
30. McClenahan JL, Klotz KL, Wilson BW: Relationship of iodide toxicity to a history of hypersensitivity. Radiology 80:96, 1962.
31. Harrington G, Michie C, Lunch PR, Russell MA, Oppenheimer MJ: Blood-brain barrier changes associated with unilateral cerebral angiography. Invest Radiol 1:431, 1966.
32. Allen JH, Parera C, Potts DG: The relation of arterial trauma to complications of cerebral angiography. Am J Roentgenol Radium Ther Nucl Med 95:845, 1965.
33. Tullos HS, Erwin WD, Woods GW, Wukasch DC, Cooley DA, King JW: Unusual lesions of the pitching arm. Clin Orthop 88:169, 1972.
34. Crawford ES, Wukasch DC, DeBakey ME: Hemodynamic changes associated with carotid artery occlusion: An experimental and clinical study. Cardiovasc Res Cent Bull 1:3, 1962.
35. Wukasch DC, Toscano M, Cooley DA, Reul GJ Jr, Sandiford FM, Kyger ER III, Hallman GL: Reoperation following direct myocardial revascularization. Circulation (Suppl 2) 56:11(3), Sept, 1977.
36. Siegelman SS, Caplan LH, Annes GP: Complications of catheter angiography: Study with oscillometry and "pullout" angiograms. Radiology 91:251, 1968.
37. Nejad MS, Klaper MA, Stefferda, FR, Gianturco C: Clotting on outer surfaces of vascular catheters. Radiology 91:248, 1968.
38. Wallace S, Medellin H, DeJongh D, Gianturco C: Systemic heparinization for angiography. Am J Roentgenol Radium Ther Nucl Med 116:204, 1972.
39. Campbell CD, Brooks DH, Bahnson, HT: Expanded microporous polytetrafluoroethylene (Gore-Tex) as a vascular conduit. In *Vascular Grafts*, edited by Sawyer PN and Kaplitt MJ. New York, Appleton-Century-Crofts, 1978, pp 335–348.

CHAPTER 2

Revascularization of the Extracranial Cerebral Circulation

INTRODUCTION

Interest in direct surgical removal of atherosclerotic occlusions of the extracranial cerebral circulation was aroused in our center during 1953 and 1954, and since that time the treatment of cerebrovascular insufficiency (CVI) has received increasingly widespread application.[1-3] Despite the fact that the role of the extracranial cerebral circulation in the etiology of cerebral ischemia was described by Gowers as early as 1875,[4] and again by Hunt in 1914,[5] and that cerebral arteriography was developed by Moniz as early as 1927,[6] successful surgical attack on this problem awaited the development of modern cardiovascular surgical techniques. Even today, the concepts of cerebrovascular insufficiency are unsettled; for example, many neurologists believe that the majority of transient ischemic attacks (TIA) are caused by microemboli that result from ulceration of plaque within the carotid arteries rather than by diminished flow from obstructing lesions.

The four principal mechanisms that produce cerebrovascular insufficiency in the major arteries supplying the brain are (1) ulceration producing microemboli (probably the most frequent mechanism, as noted above); (2) reduction of the total flow produced by lesions (depending upon both the diameter of stenosis and length of the obstruction); (3) the "steal syndromes," whereby blood is diverted from the brain by collateral channels; and (4) emboli from distant sites, primarily the heart.

Clinically, cerebrovascular accidents may be considered in three categories: (1) transient ischemic attacks (TIA), (2) the progressive stroke in evolution, and (3) the completed stroke, which may or may not result in residual neurologic deficits. The first two of these categories are amenable to surgical therapy. Transient ischemic attacks are clearly one of the most successfully treated clinical syndromes in vascular surgery. In our experience, the progressive stroke associated with acute complete occlusion of the internal carotid artery and operated upon within four to six hours can be dramatically reversed in approximately 50 percent of patients. On the other hand, some patients of this type have unsatisfactory and sometimes disastrous results from revascularization of the acutely ischemic cerebral hemisphere. Management of patients of this category remains an unsettled issue. To avoid revascularization of a fresh infarction of the brain with resultant intracerebral hemorrhage, the patient who demonstrates a completed stroke should *not* be operated upon during the acute stage. Arteriography within four to six weeks is recommended. If the internal carotid artery is completely occluded, surgery should be deferred. If an ulcerating plaque is found, operation may then be performed to prevent recurrent embolization.

ANESTHESIA FOR CAROTID SURGERY

General anesthesia is used for carotid artery surgery because it provides better oxygenation and more complete control of respiration during operation than local anesthesia.[7] If a patient undergoing operation under local anesthesia develops acute cerebrovascular insufficiency with concomitant convulsion, little can be done to control the patient's status, and the operative procedure may be severely compromised. Adequate monitoring of the electrocardiogram and intra-arterial blood pressure is essential, and there must be assurance that the artery used is not also obstructed by occlusive disease.

Moderate premedication is used in order to facilitate early postoperative awakening and early evaluation of possible postoperative neurologic deficits. Induction is achieved with thiopental, as this agent appears to provide a protective effect against damage from cerebral ischemia. Endotracheal controlled anesthesia is achieved by muscle relaxants to provide maximum respiratory regulation of oxygen and CO_2 tension. Our preference of anesthetic agents is either halothane or enflurane plus nitrous oxide, which, in combination, are effective in maintaining the patient's blood pressure at a desirable level, slightly above his resting blood pressure. Halothane and enflurane are useful in decreasing blood pressure when the patient becomes hypertensive during anesthesia. Narcotic nitrous oxide anesthesia tends to increase blood pressure.

Experimental evidence does not support the use of deliberate hyper- or hypocarbia during the operative interruption of the cerebral circulation; therefore, we advocate maintenance of arterial CO_2 tension between 35 and 40 mm Hg. Heparin, 1 to 2 mg/kg of body weight, is administered before clamping the carotid artery, and is reversed by protamine sulfate (1 mg for each mg of heparin) after declamping. Hypotension and bradycardia during manipulation of the carotid sinus is best treated with intravenous atropine. Hypotension resulting from general anesthetic agents should be treated with intravenous ephedrine or phenylephrine.

Anesthesia should be designed so that the patient awakens within two hours of arrival in the recovery room. Postoperative hypertension, which may be secondary to denervation of the carotid sinus or to increased intracranial pressure, is best treated with small doses of chlorpromazine intravenously or, if unsuccessful, with a dilute infusion of trimethaphan (Arfonad) or nitroprusside.

CAROTID ENDARTERECTOMY

Under general endotracheal anesthesia, the patient is placed in a supine position with the head turned to a 45° angle away from the side of operation. A vertical incision is made parallel to the anterior border of the sternomastoid muscle through the platysma muscle to the anterior border of the sternomastoid muscle (Fig. 2–1, a). The common carotid artery is exposed by reflecting the sternomastoid muscle laterally, with care being taken to leave the internal jugular vein attached to the posterior aspect of the sternomastoid muscle. If the internal jugular vein, which lies anterior to the carotid artery, is separated from the sternomastoid muscle, it will overlie the carotid artery and prevent optimum exposure of the operative field (Fig. 2–1, b).

The facial vein and other medial branches of the internal jugular vein are divided, exposing the common carotid artery and its bifurcation. The ansa hypoglossi nerve is reflected laterally and preserved if possible, but may be transected if necessary for distal exposure of the internal carotid artery. The common carotid, internal carotid, and external carotid arteries are dissected free and retracted with tapes or silicone vessel loops, with care being taken to avoid injury to the hypoglossal and vagus

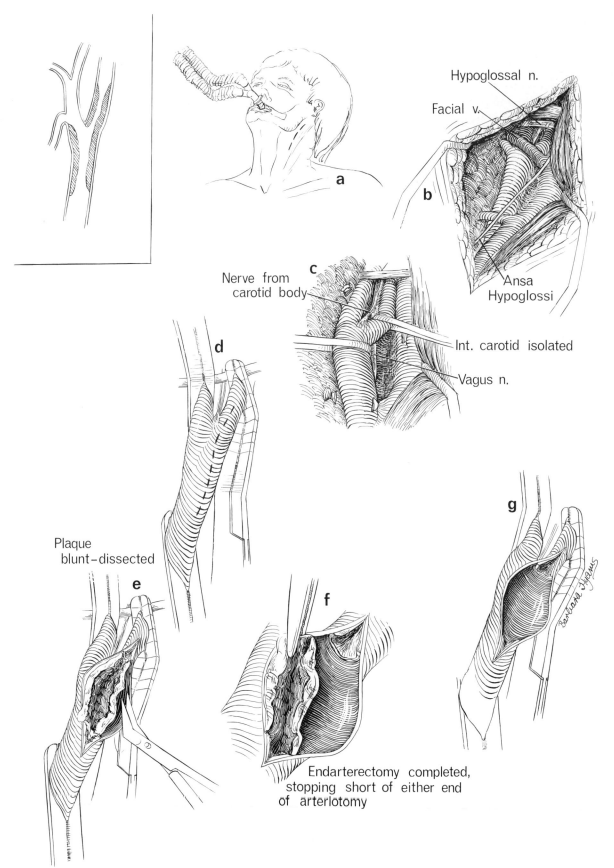

Figure 2–1 Technique of carotid endarterectomy.

Illustration continued on opposite page.

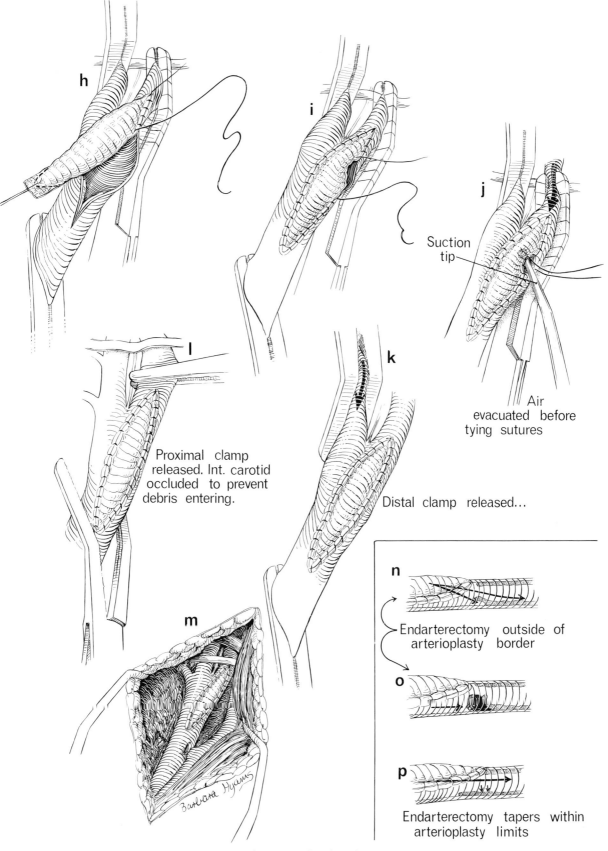

h

i

j

Suction
tip

Air
evacuated before
tying sutures

l

k

Proximal clamp
released. Int. carotid
occluded to prevent
debris entering.

Distal clamp released...

m

n

Endarterectomy outside of
arterioplasty border

o

p

Endarterectomy tapers within
arterioplasty limits

Barbara Hyams

Figure 2–1 *Continued.*

nerves, and the mandibular branch of the facial nerve (Fig. 2–1, c). Stretching or compressing the hypoglossal nerve by excessive retraction can produce serious paresis of the tongue, resulting in dysphasia and dysphagia. To preclude the dislodgment of emboli into the intracranial circulation, excessive manipulation of the artery must be avoided. For a high or distal lesion, freeing of the hypoglossal nerve is facilitated by dividing a small branch of the external carotid artery that forms a sling around the hypoglossal nerve. Both the accompanying vein and the nerve should be ligated. The nerve from the carotid body (carotid sinus plexus) should be preserved, but occasionally must be transected to facilitate exposure of the distal internal carotid artery.

Following systemic heparinization (2 mg/kg of body weight), the common carotid, internal carotid, and external carotid arteries are occluded with vascular clamps (Fig. 2–1, d). A special internal carotid artery clamp is used to occlude the vessel. The clamp is designed to retract the hypoglossal nerve cephalad out of the operative field. The internal carotid artery is clamped first, followed by the common carotid, thus allowing diversion to the external carotid artery of any debris produced by clamping of the common carotid.

Although others have advocated the use of internal shunts during carotid artery occlusion, particularly if the "stump" pressure in the artery distal to clamping is less than 50 mm Hg, we no longer use internal shunts. In our experience, temporary shunts interfere with precise arterial repair and do not prevent neurologic complications. Thus we rely upon an expeditious repair and strive to reduce the clamp time to between 15 and 20 minutes. The brain is relatively "protected" if the patient is under adequate general anesthesia, is heparinized, and has a normal or moderately elevated blood pressure.

A vertical arteriotomy is made in the common carotid artery with a No. 15 scalpel blade, and extended up the internal carotid artery with Potts' scissors (Fig. 2–1, e). The plaque is removed by blunt dissection, with the endarterectomy extending only for the length of the visual field provided by the arteriotomy (Fig. 2–1, f). The critical maneuver in the endarterectomy is in obtaining a smooth transitional plane between the endarterectomized internal carotid arterial wall and the distal intima. This maneuver is executed by first freeing the proximal plaque, and then by grasping the plaque with a hemostat and applying both lateral and caudad traction. Usually a smooth transitional plane can be obtained; if not, several interrupted sutures of 6–0 polypropylene can be placed to tack down the distal intima (Fig. 2–1, g). Plaque within the external carotid artery is removed by the "blind" endarterectomy technique of passing a hemostat up the external carotid artery, grasping the plaque, and removing it. The practice of removing a distal plaque by "blind" retraction and withdrawal should be avoided on the internal carotid artery.

A knitted, preclotted Dacron patch is used almost routinely to close the arteriotomy, since this prevents late stenosis or thrombosis in small-caliber arteries. The patch is applied by using running 4–0 polyester sutures, the first stitch being placed in the distal angle of the arteriotomy (Fig. 2–1, h and i). The patch should be of an appropriate width (usually about 1 cm) to restore the normal circumference of the artery. We routinely use a Dacron patch for closure of an arteriotomy because previous experience revealed late stenosis of the arteriotomy in some patients. Prior to tying the final suture, the internal and external carotid artery clamps are released and a small suction tip is inserted into the artery, thus evacuating air and any debris present (Fig. 2–1, j to l). Before releasing the proximal common carotid clamp, the internal carotid artery is reoccluded for a few sections with vascular forceps to direct the initial flow up the external carotid artery; this prevents debris from entering the internal carotid artery (Fig. 2–1, l). Systemic heparinization is reversed by intravenous protamine sulfate in a ratio of 1.5 protamine/1.0 heparin, and the wound is closed in layers (Fig. 2–1, m). The important technical point regarding the completion of the distal end of the endarterectomy is illustrated (Fig. 2–1, *n* to *p*). This simple maneuver prevents the circulatory flow from lifting a loose flap and causing stenosis and thrombosis.

DESIDERATA

Bilateral carotid endarterectomy should not be performed simultaneously. An interval of four to five days is advisable to lessen cerebral edema. Increased pressure in previously ischemic vessels may lead to increased intracranial pressure with complications similar to those encountered in the "postcoarctation syndrome." Use of a tissue drain is unnecessary and usually contraindicated in the presence of a Dacron patch. Finally, there is no advantage in the use of a vein patch rather than a Dacron patch in the carotid position.

Recurrent stenosis has been described by Cossman et al[8] as resulting primarily from "rapid, exuberant myointimal proliferation." However, we believe that most cases of restenosis following carotid endarterectomy are due to the use of primary closure and subsequent fibrous contracture of the thin residual arterial wall. Thus, we strongly advocate the routine use of a Dacron patch to close the carotid arteriotomy.

The technique for performing carotid endarterectomy for recurrent stenosis deserves special mention because scar tissue hampers dissection and exposure of the distal internal carotid artery. The internal carotid artery should not be dissected; instead, after proximal control and clamping of the common carotid artery, internal occlusion of the artery is obtained by inserting and distending a Fogarty balloon catheter. This controls retrograde bleeding from the artery without interfering with the repair.

Some patients with complete occlusion of the internal carotid artery who also have stenosis of the ipsilateral carotid vessel may be benefited by endarterectomy of the external artery.[9-11] Significant collateral flow to the intracranial circulation may result.

DILATATION IN CAROTID FIBROMUSCULAR HYPERPLASIA

Fibromuscular hyperplasia of the internal carotid arteries can produce symptoms of cerebrovascular insufficiency identical to those associated with atherosclerotic occlusive disease. The condition is caused by a congenital defect in the media and muscularis layers of the arterial wall and is usually seen in the 30-to-40 age group, most often in women. It is commonly associated with fibromuscular hyperplasia of the renal arteries, which results in hypertension. Symptomatic patients demonstrating characteristic arteriographic findings are usually relieved of their symptoms by dilatation of the internal carotid arteries. The procedure is a simple one and is seldom associated with morbidity.

The pathologic process is confined to the extracranial portion of the internal carotid artery and usually extends from the origin of the artery to near the base of the skull (Fig. 2–2, *a*). Exposure of the common and internal carotid arteries is accomplished as described earlier for carotid endarterectomy (Fig. 2–2, *b*). A 1–cm transverse incision is made in the common carotid artery just proximal to the bifurcation (Fig. 2–2, *c*). With the use of progressively sized dilators passed through the arteriotomy to the base of the skull, the artery is gently dilated with several passes of the dilator (Fig. 2–2, *d*). An alternative and, in our opinion, a preferable dilator is the No. 4 Fogarty catheter. It is passed distally, and the catheter balloon is inflated as

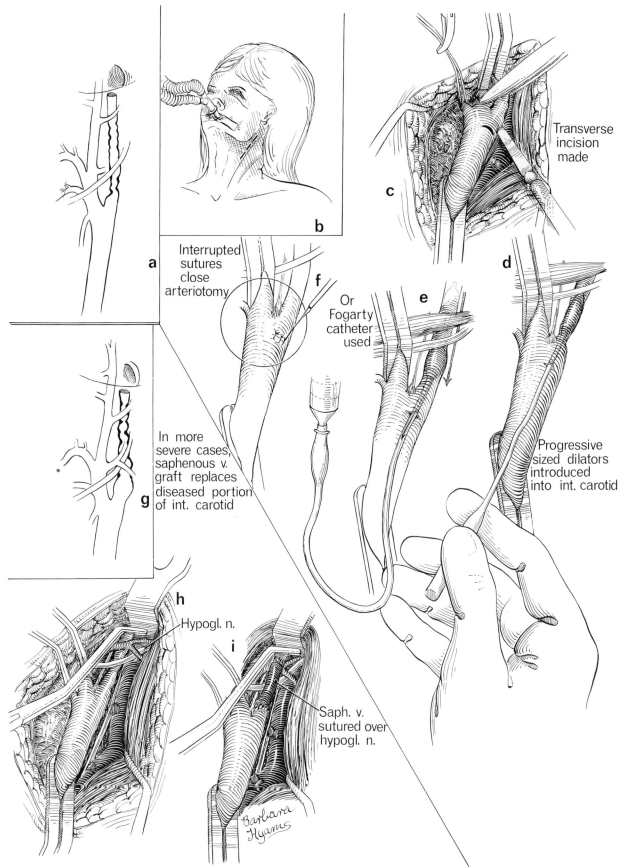

a

b

c Transverse incision made

d

Interrupted sutures close arteriotomy

f

Or Fogarty catheter used

e

In more severe cases, saphenous v. graft replaces diseased portion of int. carotid

g

Progressive sized dilators introduced into int. carotid

h

Hypogl. n.

i

Saph. v. sutured over hypogl. n.

Barbara Hyams

Figure 2–2 Dilatation of internal carotid artery and saphenous vein graft in fibromuscular hyperplasia.

it is gently withdrawn. This is done carefully to prevent rupture of the artery (Fig. 2–2, e). An important technical consideration in avoiding injury to the artery during dilatation with the Fogarty catheter is to begin withdrawal of the catheter *before* inflating the balloon. One can then "feel" the resistance of the balloon, thereby avoiding excessive distension and rupture of the artery.

The arteriotomy is closed with interrupted sutures of 6–0 polypropylene before releasing the distal clamps (Fig. 2–2, f). The wound is closed in layers, and a drain is not required. In patients with severe disease of the artery, the involved segment of the internal carotid artery may be replaced with an autogenous saphenous vein graft (Fig. 2–2, g). For vein replacement in high lesions, exposure and avoidance of injury to the hypoglossal nerve is facilitated by placing the vein graft anterior to the hypoglossal nerve (Fig. 2–2, h and i).

KINKED CAROTID ARTERY SYNDROME

Elongation and kinking of the internal carotid artery, a condition that results from either a congenital abnormality or, more frequently, arteriosclerotic tortuosity, has become recognized as a cause of cerebrovascular insufficiency, usually manifested by transient ischemic attacks. This syndrome may or may not be associated with occlusive disease in the carotid bifurcation but may produce symptoms in the absence of atherosclerotic occlusive disease. Symptoms are frequently initiated by movement of the head or flexion of the neck, and in such cases arterioplasty is indicated. Looped carotid arteries usually cause no obstruction to flow and are asymptomatic. The vessel with a definite kink, however, *does* cause symptoms and is an indication for surgery.

The internal carotid may be elongated, may be kinked, or may form a complete loop (Fig. 2–3, a). Depending upon the anatomic abnormality, the obstruction may be removed by one of three techniques.

Usually the internal carotid artery is merely tortuous, and associated plaque is present at the bifurcation; this requires an endarterectomy and patch graft angioplasty. In such cases, distal freeing of the internal carotid artery and endarterectomy are accomplished first. The tortuous internal carotid artery is then shortened and straightened by insertion of a Dacron patch, taking more widely spaced bites in the artery (approximately 3 mm) than in the patch (approximately 1.5 mm) (Fig. 2–3, b). This maneuver will effectively shorten the internal carotid artery and, in most cases, relieve the kinking (Fig. 2–3, c).

In situations of severe tortuosity or complete looping of the internal carotid artery, it may be necessary to resect a segment of internal carotid artery and perform an end-to-end anastomosis (Fig. 2–3, d and e). If the internal carotid artery is of small diameter, an alternate approach is to detach the origin of the vessel with a cuff of tissue at the carotid bulb, oversew the opening in the bulb, and implant the distal end into the common carotid artery in a more proximal location (Fig. 2–3, f and g). This technique is particularly applicable when a concomitant endarterectomy is required, and in such instances the distal end of the internal carotid artery may be reanastomosed end-to-side into the Dacron patch (Fig. 2–3, h).

EXTRACRANIAL CAROTID ARTERY ANEURYSMS

Although aneurysms of the extracranial carotid arteries are rare,[12] they result in death from rupture, thrombosis, or embolism in approximately 70 percent of pa-

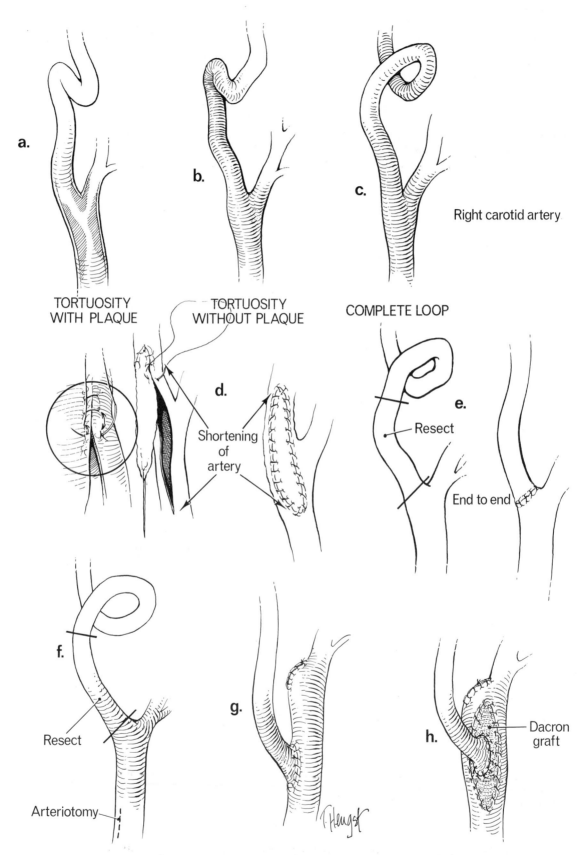

a. TORTUOSITY WITH PLAQUE

b. TORTUOSITY WITHOUT PLAQUE

c. COMPLETE LOOP

Right carotid artery

d. Shortening of artery

e. Resect End to end

f. Resect Arteriotomy

g.

h. Dacron graft

Figure 2–3 Correction of tortuous or kinked carotid artery.

tients.[13] In order to prevent the neurologic sequelae that are the major risks of these lesions, all extracranial carotid aneurysms should be excised.[14-16]

Our preferred technique is resection and replacement with an autogenous saphenous vein graft (see technique for Kinked Carotid Artery Syndrome).

CAROTID-SUBCLAVIAN ARTERY BYPASS

Occlusion of the subclavian artery proximal to the origin of the vertebral artery may produce ischemic symptoms of the upper extremities. Of interest is the effect such lesions have upon the cerebral circulation, particularly the vertebral-basilar system (Fig. 2–4, a). Bypass from the carotid to the subclavian arteries by way of a cervical approach is indicated for symptomatic lesions originating from either of the subclavian arteries when the ipsilateral innominate or common carotid artery is patent. Symptoms may include vertebral-basilar insufficiency that results from the "subclavian steal" syndrome and from claudication in the upper extremity (Fig. 2–4, a). In such instances, although the remainder of the intracranial circulation is normal, the ischemic subclavian artery "steals" blood from the normal contralateral subclavian artery via the vertebral and basilar arteries, thus the term "subclavian steal syndrome."[17, 18] Symptoms of dizziness, facial weakness, numbness, and even syncope may occur, particularly with vigorous exercise of the ischemic arm.

A less common syndrome is ischemia of the hand, caused by recurrent emboli from an ulcerating subclavian plaque. In these cases, the subclavian artery should be ligated proximal to the subclavian anastomosis at the time of bypass operation. Revascularization is not indicated for asymptomatic subclavian lesions. Less commonly, subclavian-to-carotid bypass is indicated for symptomatic lesions in either common carotid artery when the ipsilateral subclavian artery is patent.

Although animal experiments at our center have demonstrated approximately 20 percent diversion of carotid flow following carotid subclavian bypass for experimentally produced subclavian occlusion, no symptoms of carotid insufficiency have been observed in our clinical series. When both subclavian and carotid bifurcation lesions are present on the same side, carotid endarterectomy should be performed in conjunction with the carotid-subclavian bypass as described below.[11]

Under general endotracheal anesthesia, with blood pressure monitored via an arterial line in the arm opposite the involved side, the patient is placed in a supine position with a roll elevating the shoulders, and the arm of the involved side placed next to the body. A 5 cm incision is made 2 cm above and parallel to the clavicle, extending laterally from the posterior border of the sternocleidomastoid muscle (Fig. 2–4, b). Dissection is extended through the subcutaneous tissue, platysma muscle, and superficial cervical fascia; the external jugular vein may be divided or retracted laterally. The thoracic duct is preserved but should be ligated if injured during dissection. The phrenic nerve coursing down the anterior medial aspect of the anterior scalene muscle is retracted medially, and the anterior scalene muscle divided, thus exposing the subclavian artery. Care must be taken to avoid injury to the brachial plexus, which lies immediately lateral to the anterior scalene muscle. The subclavian artery is dissected free, and silicone vessel loops are placed proximally and distally (Fig. 2–4, c). Exposure may be facilitated by dividing the clavicular head of the sternocleidomastoid muscle. If necessary for adequate exposure, the thyrocervical, posterior scapular, and internal mammary arteries may be ligated without consequence.

The common carotid artery is exposed medial and posterior to the sternocleidomastoid muscle and internal jugular vein, avoiding injury to the vagus nerve along the posterior lateral aspect of the artery. If the clavicular head of the sternocleidomastoid muscle has not been divided, a tunnel is made posterior to the muscle and anterior to the internal jugular vein (Fig. 2–4, c). The common carotid artery is

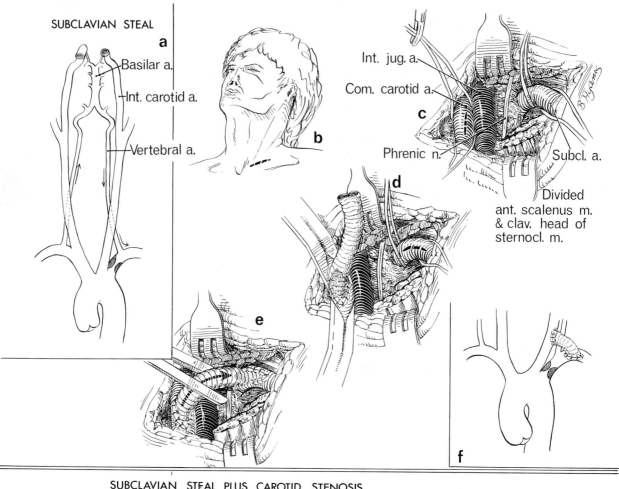

SUBCLAVIAN STEAL

Basilar a.

Int. carotid a.

Vertebral a.

Int. jug. a.

Com. carotid a.

Phrenic n.

Subcl. a.

Divided
ant. scalenus m.
& clav. head of
sternocl. m.

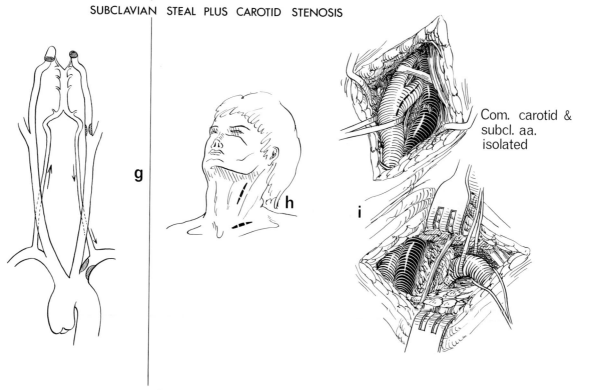

SUBCLAVIAN STEAL PLUS CAROTID STENOSIS

Com. carotid &
subcl. aa.
isolated

Figure 2–4   Technique of carotid-subclavian artery bypass

Illustration continued on opposite page.

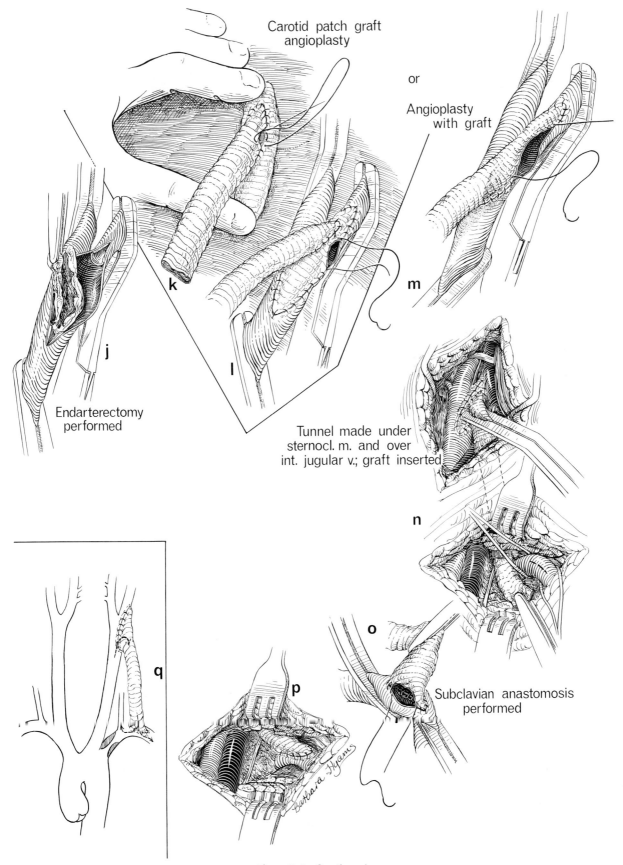

Carotid patch graft
angioplasty

or

Angioplasty
with graft

k

m

l

j

Endarterectomy
performed

Tunnel made under
sternocl. m. and over
int. jugular v.; graft inserted

n

q

o

p

Subclavian anastomosis
performed

Figure 2–4 *Continued.*

double-clamped, the distal clamp being first applied to avoid embolization during clamping of the common carotid artery. A longitudinal arteriotomy is made and a 7 mm preclotted knitted Dacron graft is anastomosed end-to-side, using 4–0 braided polyester suture (Fig. 2–4, d). Before tying the final suture, air and any debris in the artery are removed by releasing the distal carotid clamp, with the graft having been clamped adjacent to the anastomosis. The proximal clamp is then released, restoring flow. The period of carotid occlusion should not exceed 5 to 7 minutes and a shunt is not required.

The graft is passed behind the sternocleidomastoid muscle and similarly anastomosed end-to-side to the subclavian artery (Fig. 2–4, e). Before allowing flow through the graft, air is evacuated via the final sutures and the distal common carotid is temporarily occluded to prevent any residual air or debris from entering the cerebral circulation (Fig. 2–4, f).

When concomitant bifurcation stenosis or ulcerating plaque and ipsilateral symptomatic artery lesions are present, both lesions should be corrected simultaneously (Fig. 2–4, g). The patient is positioned and the subclavian artery exposed as described above (Fig. 2–4, h). The carotid bifurcation is exposed in the manner of the carotid endarterectomy (Fig. 2–4, i). A tunnel is made by sharp and blunt finger dissection posterior to the sternocleidomastoid muscle and anterior to the internal jugular vein, avoiding injury to the vein.

Before clamping the carotid artery, a 7 mm Dacron graft is sutured end-to-side into a Dacron patch using 4–0 polyester suture (Fig. 2–4, k). Carotid endarterectomy is performed as shown previously (Fig. 2–4, j).

The carotid arteriotomy is then closed by applying the patch, using 4–0 polyester suture; the graft is clamped, and air and any debris are evacuated before tying the final suture (Fig. 2–4, l). If the carotid plaque does not extend far up the internal carotid artery as visualized arteriographically, an alternate and simplified technique is to anastomose the tube graft end-to-side directly to the carotid artery as above (Fig. 2–4, m). Prior to tying the last suture, air is evacuated from the graft by releasing the clamps on the graft and allowing flow from the carotid. A tunnel is then made under the sternocleidomastoid muscle and over the internal jugular vein to the level of the subclavian artery. The proximal end of the tube graft is then inserted through the tunnel and is tailored for end-to-side anastomosis to the subclavian artery (Fig. 2–4, n and o). The completed subclavian anastomosis and final graft are shown (Fig. 2–4, p and q).

AORTO-CAROTID-SUBCLAVIAN BYPASS (AORTIC ARCH SYNDROME — TAKAYASU'S DISEASE)

Occlusive lesions of the brachiocephalic system occurring at or near the origin of major tributaries of the aortic arch may require an intrathoracic approach. In symptomatic patients with lesions involving both common carotid (or innominate) and subclavian arteries, bypass grafts from the ascending aorta to the appropriate distal vessel are indicated. Alternatively, a cervical approach may be used, as described subsequently. In our experience, the bypass principle is preferable to endarterectomy and provides better long-term results. The ascending aorta may be exposed either through a median sternotomy or an anterior right second intercostal incision. If the latter incision is utilized, the right internal mammary artery and vein may require ligation. As the median sternotomy incision is becoming more popular with cardiovascular surgeons, the midline full length sternotomy has been the incision of choice for arch lesions. Numerous variations of the revascularization of major branches of the arch are possible, depending upon the locations of the lesions. An example of revascularization of the right subclavian and common carotid arteries for a lesion of the innominate artery is described (Fig. 2–5, a), and various cervical approaches are subsequently shown in this chapter.

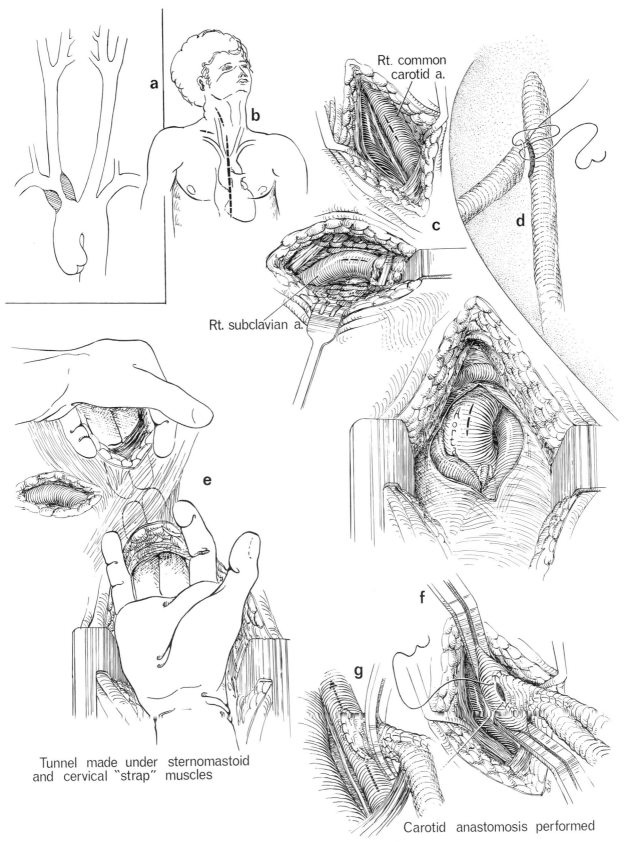

Rt. common carotid a.

Rt. subclavian a.

Tunnel made under sternomastoid and cervical "strap" muscles

Carotid anastomosis performed

Figure 2–5 Technique of aorto-carotid-subclavian bypass.

Illustration continued on following page.

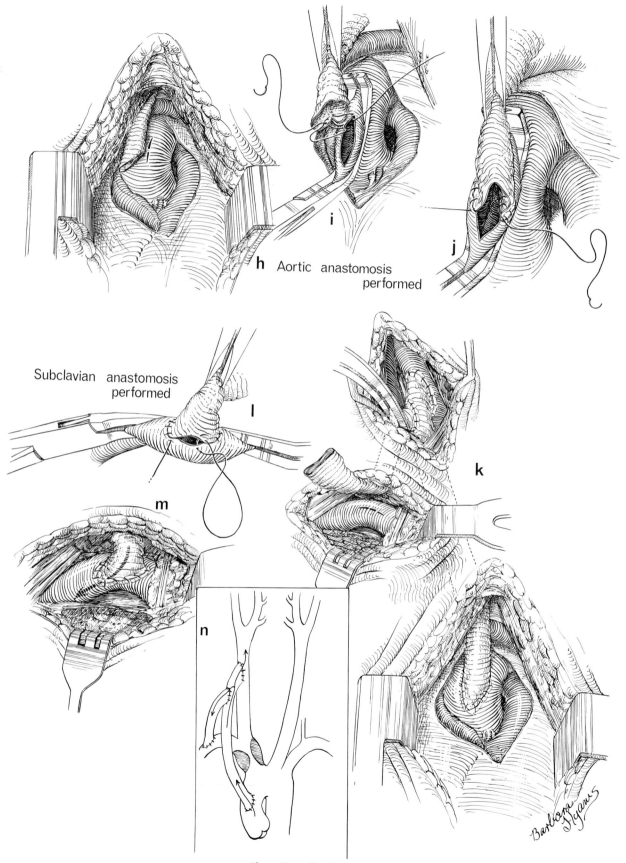

h Aortic anastomosis
performed

Subclavian anastomosis
performed

Figure 2–5 *Continued.*

The patient is placed in the supine position with a roll beneath the right scapula, and the head turned to the left. A median sternal splitting incision is made, the pericardium opened, and the ascending aorta exposed. The more distal right subclavian and common carotid arteries are exposed through separate cervical incisions as described previously (Fig. 2–5, b and c). Following systemic heparinization with intravenous heparin, 2 mg/kg of body weight, the right common carotid artery is clamped and a 7 mm knitted Dacron graft, to which a second similar graft has been previously anastomosed end-to-side, is anastomosed end-to-side via the carotid arteriotomy (Fig. 2–5. d). Air is evacuated from the site of anastomosis by releasing the distal carotid clamp prior to tying the final suture (Fig. 2–5, e). The graft is clamped and flow is restored through the carotid artery (Fig. 2–5, f).

A tunnel is made through the thoracic outlet along the course of the innominate artery, posterior to the right sternocleidomastoid muscle and "strap" muscles, but anterior to the left innominate vein, thus preventing compromise of the vein against the sternum by the graft (Sabathie's sign) (Fig. 2–5, g). The tunnel must be made large enough to permit two fingers and preclude constriction of the graft; some "strap" muscles may be divided if necessary. Bifurcated grafts may cause substernal compression of the innominate vein. For this reason we use a tube graft, 7 or 8 mm in diameter, as the "source" graft and attach side branches to revascularize other arteries as required.

The graft is passed proximally through the tunnel and trimmed obliquely to approximate the size of the aortotomy site (Fig. 2–5, h). A partial occluding clamp is placed on the ascending aorta with the handle directed cephalad if space permits, or directed caudad as shown if the handle will not fit above, thus facilitating exposure (Fig. 2–5, i). Prior to and during partial clamping of the aorta, the systemic blood pressure, if elevated, must be lowered by the anesthesiologist to prevent the clamp from injuring the aortic wall or slipping off the aorta. Before making the aortotomy, the clamp should be left in place a minute or two to ascertain that blood pressure is adequate and that the cardiac output has not been compromised by a bite that is too large in the aorta. The proximal anastomosis is performed by using 4–0 or 3–0 polyester suture, evacuating air before tying the last suture (Fig. 2–5, j). The free end of the side arm graft is passed posterior to the sternocleidomastoid muscle, anterior to the internal jugular vein, and anastomosed end-to-side to the right subclavian artery (Fig. 2–5, k to n).

AORTO-INNOMINATE-SUBCLAVIAN BYPASS

Because the distribution of lesions in the brachiocephalic system is variable, revascularization allows creativity in planning the surgical approach. This and the following two sections describe approaches we have utilized for typical lesions in the origins of the great vessels arising from the aortic arch.

A patient with lesions at the origin of the innominate and left subclavian arteries (Fig. 2–6, a) requires restoration of circulation to both vessels; this may be effected by a single graft egressing the thoracic outlet. A significant point to remember is that the limited space within the thoracic outlet can accommodate only one graft of limited diameter; otherwise, the left innominate vein will be compressed against the sternum.[19] This size limitation precludes the use of two separate grafts from the ascending aorta or the use of a large diameter bifurcation graft. Therefore, the utilization of a single graft from the ascending aorta with side-to-side anastomosis is necessary.

Figure 2–6 depicts our technique for constructing a single 7 mm Dacron graft from the ascending aorta with a side-to-side anastomosis to the innominate artery and a terminal end-to-side anastomosis to the left subclavian artery. The ascending

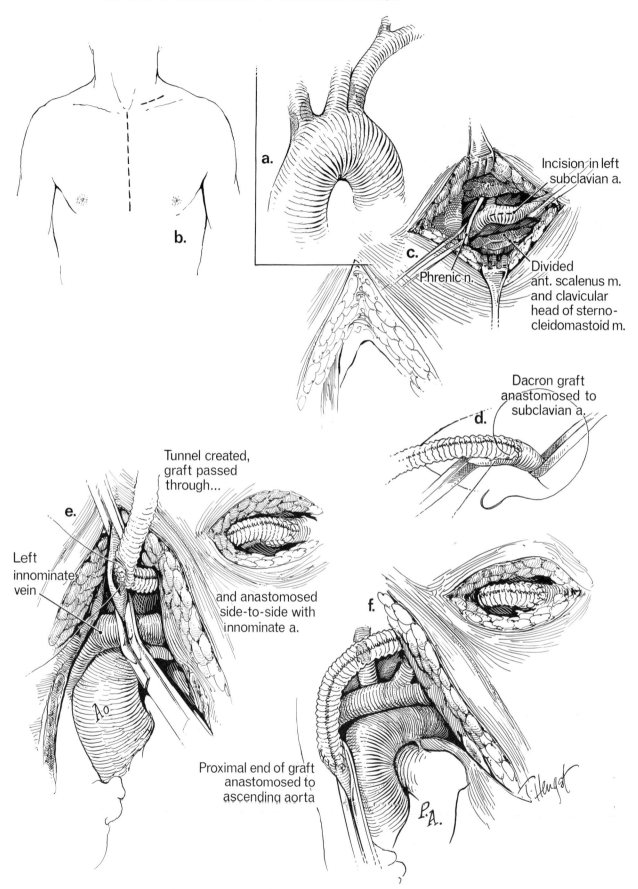

Figure 2–6 Technique of aorto-innominate-subclavian bypass.

aorta and innominate artery are exposed through a median sternotomy (Fig. 2–6, b), and the left subclavian artery is exposed by dividing the anterior scalenus and medial head of the sternocleidomastoid muscles, taking care to preserve and retract medially the phrenic nerve (Fig. 2–6, c). After systemic heparinization (2 mg/kg of body weight) and cross-clamping of the left subclavian artery, a 7 mm Dacron double velour graft is anastomosed end-to-side to the subclavian artery, using 4–0 braided polyester suture (Fig. 2–6, d). The graft is passed medially through a tunnel made by gentle finger dissection through the thoracic outlet. The innominate artery is mobilized cephalad to the left innominate vein, and the graft is anastomosed side-to-side (Fig. 2–6, e). The graft is coursed anterior to the left innominate vein, taking care to prevent kinking, and anastomosed end-to-side to the anterior-right lateral aspect of the ascending aorta (Fig. 2–6, f). When applying the partial occluding clamp to the ascending aorta, it is important to wait approximately two minutes before making the aortotomy incision to assure that the bite of the clamp will not restrict the cardiac output and produce hypotension. The mediastinal tissues and pericardium are reapproximated over the graft and ascending aorta, and a mediastinal drainage tube is placed before closing the chest.

SUBCLAVIAN-SUBCLAVIAN-CAROTID BYPASS

The subclavian steal syndrome, produced by proximal subclavian occlusion with an associated ipsilateral common carotid lesion (Fig. 2–7, a), may be revascularized either by an aorto-subclavian approach, as described previously, or entirely through a cervical approach by subclavian-subclavian bypass (Fig. 2–7, f). Both subclavian arteries are exposed through separate supraclavicular incisions approximately 5 cm in length, extending laterally from the posterior border of the sternocleidomastoid muscle and 2 cm above and parallel to the clavicle (Fig. 2–7, b). As previously described in greater detail, the anterior scalene muscle is divided, taking care to preserve the phrenic nerve coursing along its anterior medial border. By gentle finger dissection, a tunnel is made posterior to the sternocleidomastoid muscle and anterior to the common carotid artery, internal jugular vein, and strap muscles (Fig. 2–7, c). After the tunnel has been made with finger dissection, a 7 mm Dacron velour graft is passed through the tunnel with a ring forceps (Fig. 2–7, c) and anastomosed to both subclavian arteries, using a 4–0 braided polyester suture (Fig. 2–7, d to f). Systemic heparinization (2 mg/kg of body weight) is given prior to clamping the arteries and is later reversed with protamine sulfate. Drains are not required.

Associated common carotid artery lesions (Fig. 2–7, g) may be revascularized by extending a side arm graft to the common or internal carotid artery. A separate incision is made over the carotid bifurcation along the anterior border of the sternocleidomastoid muscle (Fig. 2–7, h), and the carotid artery is exposed as previously described for carotid endarterectomy. A 7 mm Dacron graft is anastomosed to the appropriate site in the common or internal carotid artery (Fig. 2–7, i). A tunnel is then made by gentle finger dissection anterior to the internal jugular vein and posterior to the sternocleidomastoid muscle, and the graft is passed through the tunnel (Fig. 2–7, i). The proximal end of the graft is then anastomosed to the previous subclavian-subclavian graft, using 4–0 braided polyester suture (Fig. 2–7, i). Before tying down the last stitch of the anastomosis, the carotid clamp is released to flush retrograde air within the carotid graft. After the suture line is tied, the carotid graft is again clamped, and the subclavian-subclavian graft is opened to direct any air in this graft to the arm rather than into the cerebral circulation.

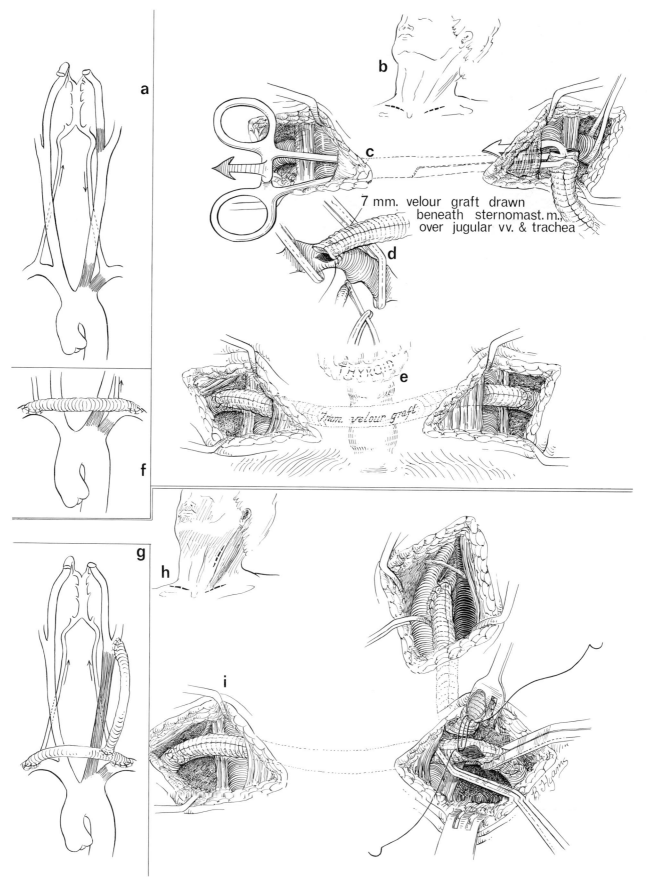

7 mm. velour graft drawn beneath sternomast. m. over jugular vv. & trachea

Figure 2–7 Technique of subclavian-subclavian-carotid bypass.

SUBCLAVIAN-CAROTID-CAROTID BYPASS

If the left subclavian artery is patent, obstructions of both the innominate and left common carotid arteries may be revascularized entirely via a cervical approach (Fig. 2–8, a). A collar incision is made 2 cm above the clavicles, extending from the anterior border of the right sternocleidomastoid muscle to the lateral aspect of the left supraclavicular fossa (Fig. 2–8, b). The right and common carotid and left subclavian arteries are exposed, as previously described (Fig. 2–8, c). Care is taken to avoid injury to the right vagus nerve, which lies posterior-medial to the common carotid artery. A 7 mm Dacron double velour graft is anastomosed end-to-side to the right common carotid artery (Fig. 2–8, d). A clamp is applied to the graft and flow is restored through the right common carotid artery. The graft is then passed posterior to the strap muscles and anastomosed side-to-side to the left common carotid artery (Fig. 2–8, e). Flow is restored through the left common carotid artery, and the graft is passed beneath the left sternocleidomastoid muscle and anastomosed end-to-side to the left subclavian artery (Fig. 2–8, f). Reversal of systemic heparinization with protamine sulfate is effected. After completion of the reconstruction, the graft lies comfortably beneath the strap and left sternocleidomastoid muscles (Fig. 2–8, g), and satisfactory circulation is restored to both carotid arteries without the necessity of a thoracotomy (Fig. 2–8, h).

VERTEBRAL ARTERY RECONSTRUCTION

Lesions in the vertebral arteries that result in reduced flow to the brain stem and circle of Willis through the basilar artery may produce symptoms of vertebral-basilar insufficiency, characterized primarily by vertigo, facial numbness or weakness, and syncope. Many patients with such arteriographically demonstrated lesions, however, remain asymptomatic and do not require operation. A lesion in one vertebral artery with a patent opposite vertebral artery usually does not produce symptoms and should not be surgically treated. Surgical reconstruction of the vertebral arteries is done less frequently than formerly, primarily because revascularization of commonly associated carotid lesions will usually relieve symptoms of cerebrovascular insufficiency by increasing total cerebral flow. Therefore, vertebral artery reconstruction is now seldom performed in our center. Vertebral reconstruction is indicated in patients with (1) bilateral vertebral artery lesions or stenosis of a single vertebral vessel associated with complete occlusion of both internal carotid arteries, and (2) persistent vertebral-basilar symptoms following corrective procedures on all significant carotid lesions.

Exposure of the vertebral artery is obtained as described previously for subclavian carotid bypass (Fig. 2–9, a and b). Mobilization of the subclavian and vertebral arteries can be facilitated by ligating the thyrocervical trunk and internal mammary arteries; this results in no sequelae (Fig. 2–9, c and d).

Following systemic heparinization with 2 mg/kg of body weight, reconstruction of the vertebral artery can be accomplished most simply by ligating the vessel at its origin, resecting the stenotic segment, and reanastomosing the artery end-to-side into the subclavian artery in the most accessibly normal location (Fig. 2–9, e to h). Air is evacuated prior to tying the suture by releasing the vertebral clamp (Fig. 2–9, i). Alternate techniques are patch graft enlargement with the use of a Dacron or vein patch and arterioplasty, as shown (Fig. 2–9, j).

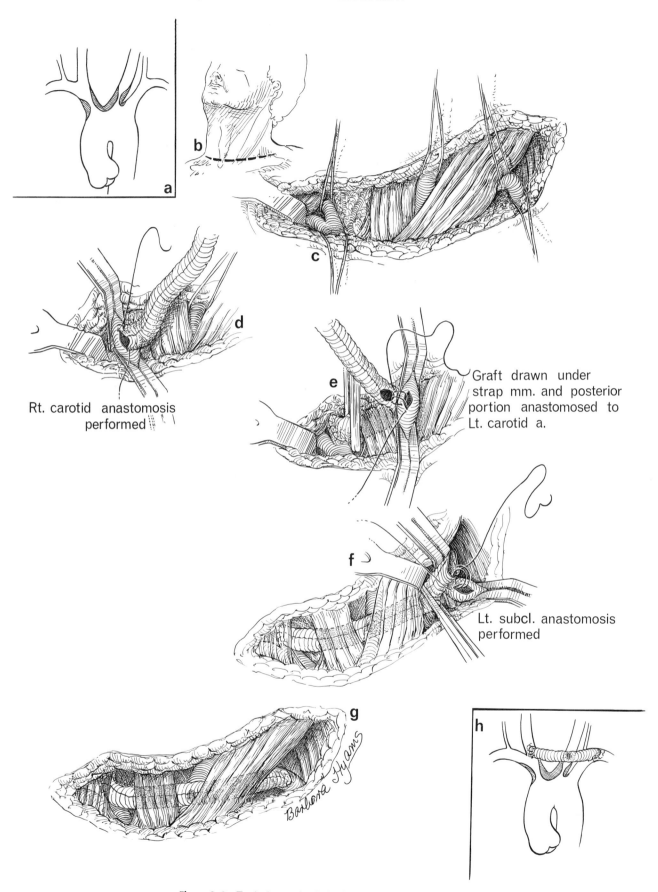

Rt. carotid anastomosis
performed

Graft drawn under
strap mm. and posterior
portion anastomosed to
Lt. carotid a.

Lt. subcl. anastomosis
performed

Figure 2–8   Technique of subclavian-carotid-carotid bypass.

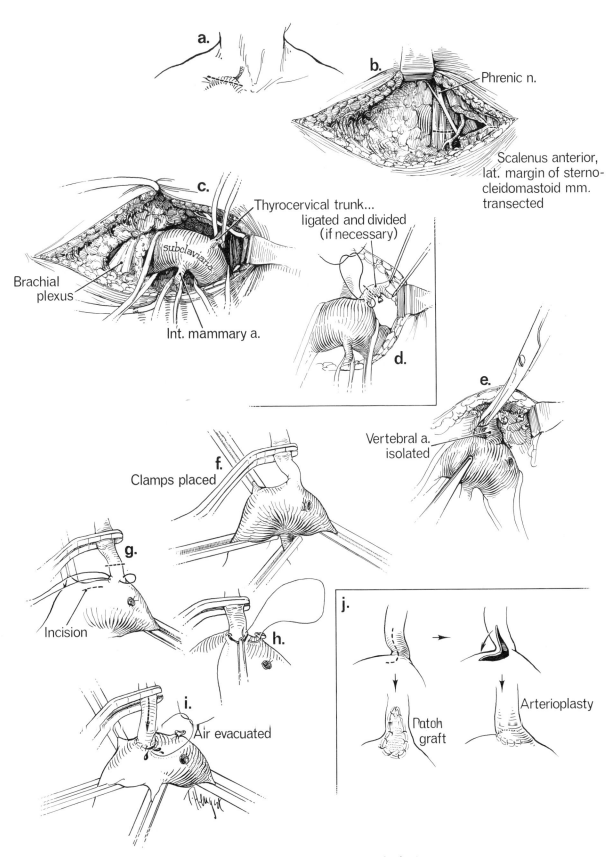

a.

b.

Phrenic n.

Scalenus anterior, lat. margin of sterno-cleidomastoid mm. transected

c.

Thyrocervical trunk... ligated and divided (if necessary)

subclavian

Brachial plexus

Int. mammary a.

d.

e.

Vertebral a. isolated

f.

Clamps placed

g.

Incision

h.

i.

Air evacuated

j.

Patch graft

Arterioplasty

Figure 2–9 Reconstruction of the vertebral artery.

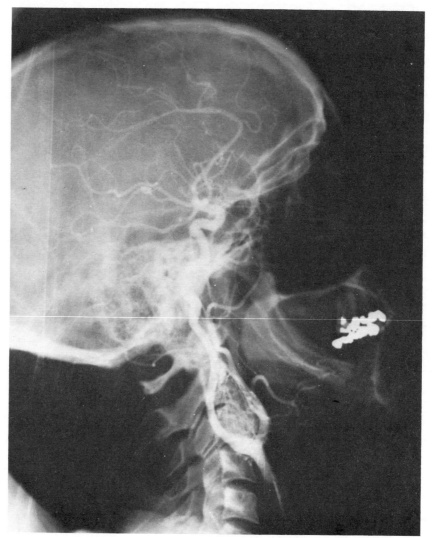

Figure 2–10 Right percutaneous lateral arteriogram in a 38-year-old woman, demonstrating characteristic features of carotid body tumor. Note vascularity of mass above carotid bifurcation symmetrically displacing internal and external carotid arteries outwardly. Tumor was satisfactorily resected subadventitially.

RESECTION OF CAROTID BODY TUMOR

The presence of a carotid body tumor is readily indicated by a pulsating mass over the carotid bifurcation, usually seen in young adults. Arteriography confirms the existence of a characteristic vascular tumor that is displacing the carotid bifurcation (Fig. 2–10).

Subadventitial resection usually results in complete removal of the tumor; the leg should be prepared for surgery and draped, however, in case resection and replacement of the common and internal carotid arteries with an autogenous saphenous vein becomes necessary. A roll is placed beneath the patient's shoulders, and the head is turned away from the side of the lesion. The skin incision is begun higher than in carotid endarterectomy, extending from just below the earlobe, parallel to the anterior border of the sternocleidomastoid muscle (Fig. 2–11, a and g). The major surgical hazard is damage to the hypoglossal nerve and, less frequently, to the vagus nerve. The surgeon should achieve orientation by initially exposing the common carotid artery proximal to the tumor (Fig. 2–11, a). The lateral aspect of the tumor is then dissected free of the sternocleidomastoid muscle and internal jugular

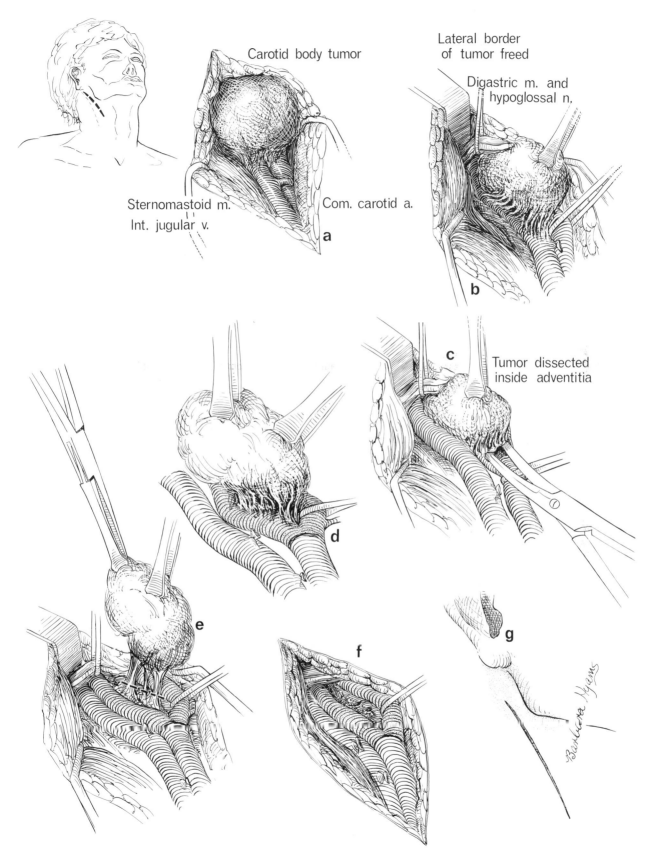

Carotid body tumor

Sternomastoid m.

Int. jugular v.

Com. carotid a.

a

Lateral border
of tumor freed

Digastric m. and
hypoglossal n.

b

c

Tumor dissected
inside adventitia

d

e

f

g

Figure 2–11 Resection of carotid body tumor.

vein (Fig. 2–11, *b*). Particular care is taken to dissect the hypoglossal nerve away from the tumor, thus avoiding injury to the nerve (Fig. 2–11, *b*).

By means of scissor dissection, a plane is created beneath the adventitial layer of the common carotid artery, and the tumor is dissected away from the artery in a cephalad direction (Fig. 2–11, *c* and *d*). *Emphasis is again placed on freeing the hypoglossal nerve from the cephalad aspect of the tumor before this step is initiated.* Subadventitial dissection of the tumor from the medial layer of the artery is facilitated by hypotensive anesthesia, which maintains the systolic blood pressure at approximately 70 mm Hg by means of nitrous oxide, oxygen, Fluothane, and a Nipride drip (50 mg sodium nitroprusside in 500 cc of 5% dextrose and water). The nerve to the carotid body, which is a well-defined structure, is then transected (Fig. 2–11, *e*). The residual carotid artery contains only the medial and endothelial layers and is extremely fragile (Fig. 2–11, *f*). Bleeding points resulting from dissection should be carefully sutured with 6–0 polypropylene suture. If the artery is damaged beyond repair by dissection that is too deep, resection and replacement of the involved common and internal carotid arteries with an autogenous saphenous vein graft may become necessary. In this event, the external carotid may be ligated without sequelae.

REFERENCES

1. Cooley, DA, DeBakey ME: Surgical considerations of intrathoracic aneurysms of the aorta and great vessels. Ann Surg 135:660, 1952.
2. DeBakey ME, Cooley DA: Successful resection of aneurysm of thoracic aorta and replacement by graft. JAMA 152:673, 1953.
3. Crawford ES, DeBakey ME, Garrett HE, Howell J: Surgical treatment of occlusive cerebrovascular disease. Surg Clin North Am 46:873, 1966.
4. Gowers WR: On a case of simultaneous embolism of central retinal and middle cerebral arteries. Lancet 2:794, 1875.
5. Hunt JR: The role of the carotid arteries in the causation of vascular lesions of the brain with remarks on certain special features of the symptomatology. Amer J Med Sci 147:704, 1914.
6. Moniz E: L'encephalographique arterielle; son importance dans la localization des tumeurs cérébrales. Rev Neurol 2:172, 1927.
7. Wells BA, Keats AS, Cooley DA: Induced tolerance to cerebral ischemia produced by general anesthesia during temporary carotid occlusion. Surgery 54:216, 1963.
8. Cossman D, Callow AD, Stein A, Matsumoto G: Early restenosis after carotid endarterectomy. Arch Surg 113:275, 1978.
9. Fields WS, Maslenikov V, Meyer JS, Hass WK, Remington RD, McDonald M: Joint study of extracranial arterial occlusion. V. Progress report of prognosis following surgery or nonsurgical treatment for transient cerebral ischemic attacks and cervical carotid artery lesion. JAMA 211:1993, 1970.
10. Hass WK, Fields WS, North RR, Kricheff II, Chase NE, Bauer RB: Joint study of extracranial arterial occlusion. II. Arteriography, techniques, sites, complications. JAMA 203:159, 1968.
11. Thompson J, Talkington C: Carotid endarterectomy. Ann Surg 184:1, 1976.
12. Beall AC, Crawford ES, Cooley DA, DeBakey ME: Extracranial aneurysms of the carotid artery. Report of seven cases. Postgrad Med 32:93, 1962.
13. Winslow N: Extracranial aneurysm of the internal carotid artery. Arch Surg 13:689, 1926.
14. Kaupp HA, Haid SP, Jurayj MN, Bergan JJ, Trippel OH: Aneurysms of the extracranial carotid artery. Surgery 72:946, 1972.
15. Rittenhouse EA, Radke HM, Sumner DS: Carotid artery aneurysm. Arch Surg 105:786, 1972.
16. Shipley AM, Winslow N, Walker WW: Aneurysm in the cervical portion of the internal carotid artery. An analytical study of the cases recorded in the literature between August 1, 1925 and July 31, 1936. Report of two new cases. Ann Surg 105:673, 1937.
17. Reivich M, Holling E, Roberts B, Toole JF: Reversal of blood flow through the vertebral artery and its effects on cerebral circulation. N Engl J Med 265:878, 1961.
18. Killen DA, Foster JH, Göbbel WG Jr, Stephenson SE Jr, Collins HA, Billings FT, Scott HW Jr: The subclavian steal syndrome. J Thorac Cardiovasc Surg 51:539, 1966.
19. Fred HL, Wukasch DC, Petrany Z: Transient compression of the left innominate vein. Circulation 29:758, 1964.

CHAPTER 3

Thoracic Outlet Syndrome and Lesions in Vessels of the Upper Extremity

THORACIC OUTLET COMPRESSION

INTRODUCTION

Like varicose veins and hemorrhoids, thoracic outlet compression is a price man has had to pay for assuming an upright position. In walking on all four extremities, the forward limbs extended anterior and cephalad to the trunk. In our present erect position, the arms hang caudad, posterior, and lateral to the shoulder girdle. This "abnormal" position results in stretching of the brachial plexus and axillary vessels, with compression by the first rib in some individuals. Trauma or occupational use of the upper extremities may also contribute to this condition.

The association of upper extremity symptoms with anatomic variations in the structures of the thoracic outlet has long been recognized.[1-3] However, only during the past decade has thoracic outlet syndrome (TOS) become accepted as a clinical entity with well-defined principles of treatment, to which Roos has made perhaps the most significant contribution.[4-6]

The optimum means of diagnosing and treating the TOS have remained controversial, and detailed discussion of the merits of the numerous proposed diagnostic tests are beyond the scope of this atlas. Roos[7] has described in a clear-cut manner the diagnostic concepts to which we adhere. The TOS is essentially compression of the brachial plexus by scissor-like action of the clavicle and first rib and/or congenitally anomalous fibromuscular bands. Roos emphasizes two points of particular importance:

"First, the symptoms are predominantly *neurologic* in nature, as a result of compression of the brachial plexus — *not vascular* as a result of compression of the subclavian artery in the thoracic outlet. Second, the examination of the *pulse* and its positional variations has little to do with the accurate diagnosis of TOS *in most cases*. . . . The idea of evaluating pulses in various neck and arm positions as a *sine qua non* of the diagnosis of TOS must be one of the most deeply entrenched fallacies in medical thought and practice."[7]

In ascertaining the diagnosis of TOS and excluding those conditions that must be considered in the differential diagnosis, the reader is referred to the excellent and complete chapter by David B. Roos in *Vascular Surgery*, edited by Robert B. Rutherford.[7] He lists the following differential diagnoses for thoracic outlet syndrome work-up: (1) cervical disc syndrome; (2) carpal tunnel syndrome; (3) orthopedic shoulder problems, such as shoulder sprain, rotator cuff injury, and tendinitis; (4) cervical spondylitis; (5) ulnar nerve compression at the elbow; (6) multiple sclerosis; (7) spinal cord tumor or disease; and (8) angina pectoris.[7]

It is significant in the diagnosis that symptoms usually involve aching discomfort, paresthesias that manifest as numbness with or without tingling, and headache. Vascular symptoms from arterial or venous compression are rare but may occur, including complications of arterial embolization[8] or subclavian aneurysms.[9] Various objective diagnostic tests, including nerve conduction velocity,[10] electromyography, and arteriography, have been proposed but have failed to provide the objective criteria desired to warrant their routine use.[11] Therefore, we no longer rely on these studies for the diagnosis of TOS, which we believe must be made on the basis of a careful and detailed history and physical examination. The most reliable diagnostic maneuver has been described by Roos as the "elevated arm stress test" (EAST).[7] This consists of having the patient place both arms in 90-degree abduction-external rotation with the shoulder and elbows stretched posteriorly. The hands are opened and closed for three minutes. This maneuver will reproduce the patient's usual symptoms in the presence of TOS.

ANATOMY

The thoracic outlet defines the area in which the brachial plexus passes posterior to the clavicle (retroclavicular fossa) and is joined by the subclavian artery and vein as they exit from the thoracic cavity by arching over the first rib (Fig. 3–1, *a*). The brachial plexus and subclavian artery pass through the interscalene triangle formed by the anterior and medius scalene muscles and the first rib. The subclavian

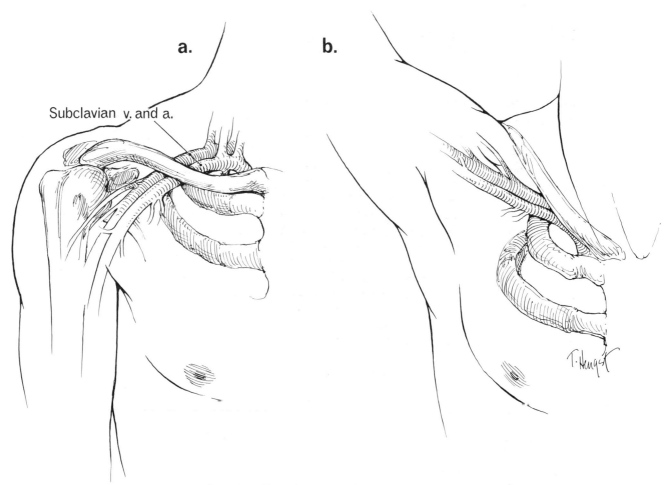

a.   **b.**

Subclavian v. and a.

Figure 3–1 Normal anatomy of the thoracic outlet.

vein passes anterior to the anterior scalene muscle (Fig. 3–2, b). Abduction of the arm associated with posterior and lateral displacement of the shoulder results in a scissor-like compression of the neurovascular structures between the clavicle and first rib (Fig. 3–1, b). Other anatomic variations and anomalies may contribute to and aggravate this costoclavicular scissor compression, including cervical ribs, abnormal transverse processes of the C–7 vertebra, exostosis of the first rib, abnormal variations of the anterior, medius, or minimus scalene muscles, or congenitally anomalous fibromuscular bands. Vascular complications are infrequent but may occur, including emboli to the upper extremities or vertebral arteries,[8] subclavian aneurysm,[9] and axillary vein thrombosis.[12]

TREATMENT

Many patients with mild symptoms will respond to conservative measures consisting of exercises to improve posture and strengthen shoulder girdle muscles.[13] Instructions are given to elevate and bring forward both shoulders; this maneuver opens the thoracic outlet. Elevation of the arms during work or sleep should be avoided Surgical treatment is indicated by failure of conservative measures to alleviate the symptoms of pain or paresthesias, development of loss of strength or function of the hand, or vascular symptoms.

OPERATIVE TECHNIQUE

Numerous operative approaches have been described and advocated. Resection of the clavicle[14] is only of historical interest. Scalenotomy[3] is obviously not acceptable in view of our current concept of the mechanism by which the TOS is produced.

Resection of the first rib has become accepted as the essential element in surgical relief of TOS. The first rib may be exposed by one of several approaches: anterior,[15] posterior,[16] or transthoracic. Although we have employed each of these approaches at various times, the transaxillary technique as first described by Roos[4] is, in our opinion, the preferable approach.

The patient is positioned laterally, with the arm suspended from the crossbar of an I.V. pole (Fig. 3–2, a). Care is taken not to stretch the arm unduly; when required for exposure, additional elevation of the shoulder may be achieved with the help of an assistant. A transverse incision 8 to 10 cm in length is made at the lower border of the axillary hairline between the posterior border of the pectoralis major muscle and the anterior aspect of the latissimus dorsi muscle (Fig. 3–2, a). Dissection is extended through the subcutaneous tissue and a plane is developed immediately anterior to the intercostal muscles (Fig. 3–2, c). The intercostobrachial nerve, which emerges from the second interspace, is preserved and retracted posteriorly when possible, but may be sacrificed with only a minimum of postoperative numbness and pain. The first rib is exposed by blunt dissection and is identified by palpation of its characteristic wide, flattened surface and smaller circumference. The attachments of the anterior and medius scalene muscles are dissected from the first rib, which is then exposed with a periosteal elevator (Fig. 3–2, d). Care is taken to avoid injury to the neurovascular bundle, which is gently retracted cephalad. The rib is transected with a large right-angle rib cutter (Fig. 3–2, e). Care is taken to stay anterior to the periosteum of the rib bed to avoid a pneumothorax.

The fascia surrounding the neurovascular bundle is incised for a length of 2 to 3 cm (Fig. 3–2, f). The rationale for this maneuver is that compression and chronic irritation by the first rib produces fibrosis and constriction of the fibrous sheath

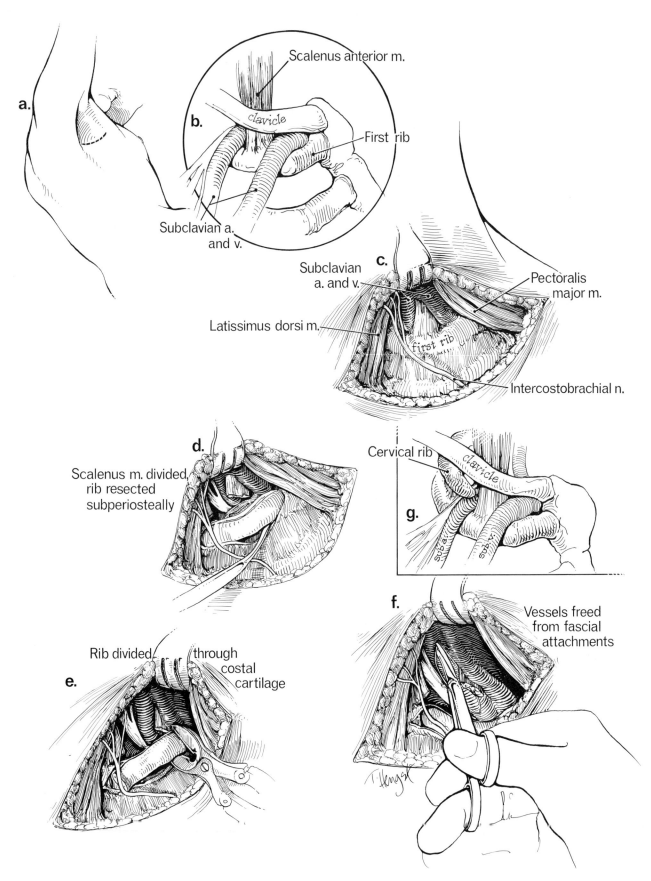

a.

b.
Scalenus anterior m.

clavicle

First rib

Subclavian a.
and v.

c.
Subclavian
a. and v.

Pectoralis
major m.

Latissimus dorsi m.

first rib

Intercostobrachial n.

d.
Scalenus m. divided,
rib resected
subperiosteally

Cervical rib

clavicle

g.

subcl.

a. subcl.

e.
Rib divided
through
costal
cartilage

f.
Vessels freed
from fascial
attachments

T. Hengst

Figure 3–2 Operative technique for relief of the thoracic outlet syndrome.

surrounding the neurovascular bundle, and if not released, such compression may continue to produce constriction. The wound is closed by approximating the subcutaneous layer and the skin with an absorbable subcuticular suture.

In the event that a pneumothorax occurs, a chest tube should be inserted in the fourth interspace. Although the lung may be expanded by the temporary placement of a small catheter through the pleural opening in the periosteal bed, which is removed following closure of the wound, this will sometimes result in a postoperative pleural effusion.

LESIONS IN VESSELS OF THE UPPER EXTREMITY

BYPASS OF OCCLUDED AXILLARY ARTERY

Axillary artery thrombosis may result from various forms of injury, ranging from mechanical trauma to irradiation for carcinoma of the breast. Baseball pitchers are particularly susceptible to thrombosis of the brachial artery because of repeated compression and intimal damage that occurs during the pitching maneuver.[17] The following technique was used to revascularize the thrombosed axillary artery of a major league baseball pitcher, who, following operation, pitched in a winning World Series.

The patient is placed in a supine position with a roll under the involved side, and the arm is abducted at 90°. The proximal axillary artery is exposed by an 8 cm subclavicular horizontal incision parallel to the inferior border of the clavicle (Fig. 3–3, a). The incision is extended through the pectoralis major muscle, the clavipectoral axillary fascia, and the subclavius muscle, thus exposing the proximal subclavian axillary artery (Fig. 3–3, b). The brachial artery is then exposed via a longitudinal incision along the medial aspect of the upper arm along the posterior border of the biceps muscle (Fig. 3–3, a and c). After administration of systemic heparin (2 mg/kg of body weight), an autogenous saphenous vein graft is anastomosed end-to-side to the proximal axillary artery with running 6–0 polypropylene suture (Fig. 3–3, b). A tunnel is made through the axillary space by *gentle finger dissection*. The vein graft is passed through the tunnel with a curved ring forceps and anastomosed end-to-side to the brachial artery in a similar fashion.

RESECTION OF ANEURYSM OF AXILLARY ARTERY

Although aneurysms of the axillary artery are rare (Fig. 3–4), they may be caused by either trauma or arteriosclerosis.[18, 19] Because these lesions tend to thrombose and produce embolization that results in ischemia of the upper extremities, excision with graft replacement is recommended.[20, 21]

The axillary artery is a continuation of the subclavian as it passes from the thoracic outlet over the first rib. Three segments are arbitrarily designated: proximal, middle, and distal, according to the corresponding relationship of the artery to the pectoralis minor muscle. The artery is in close proximity to the axillary vein, which lies medial to the artery and to the branches of the brachial plexus that encompass the artery. These structures course through the axillary space, which is bounded medially by the upper rib cage, anteriorly by the pectoralis major and minor muscles, and laterally by the humerus, coracobrachialis, and biceps muscles and medial shoulder joint.

Exposure of the axillary artery may be approached either through or lateral to

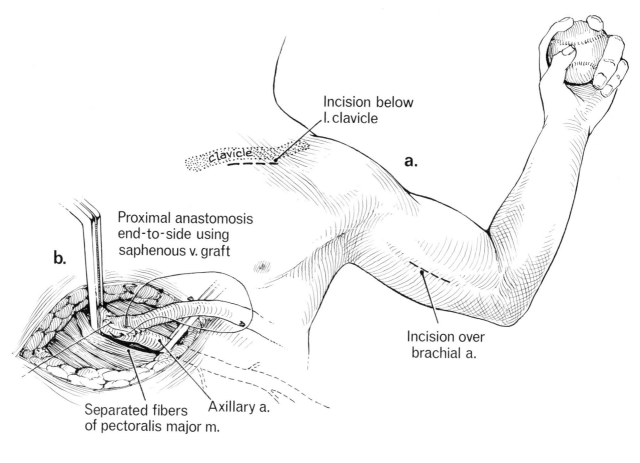

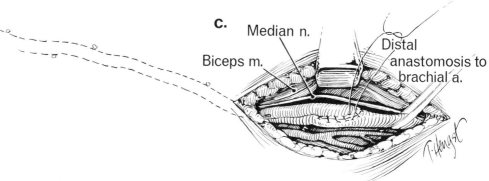

Figure 3–3 Technique for bypass of occluded axillary artery.

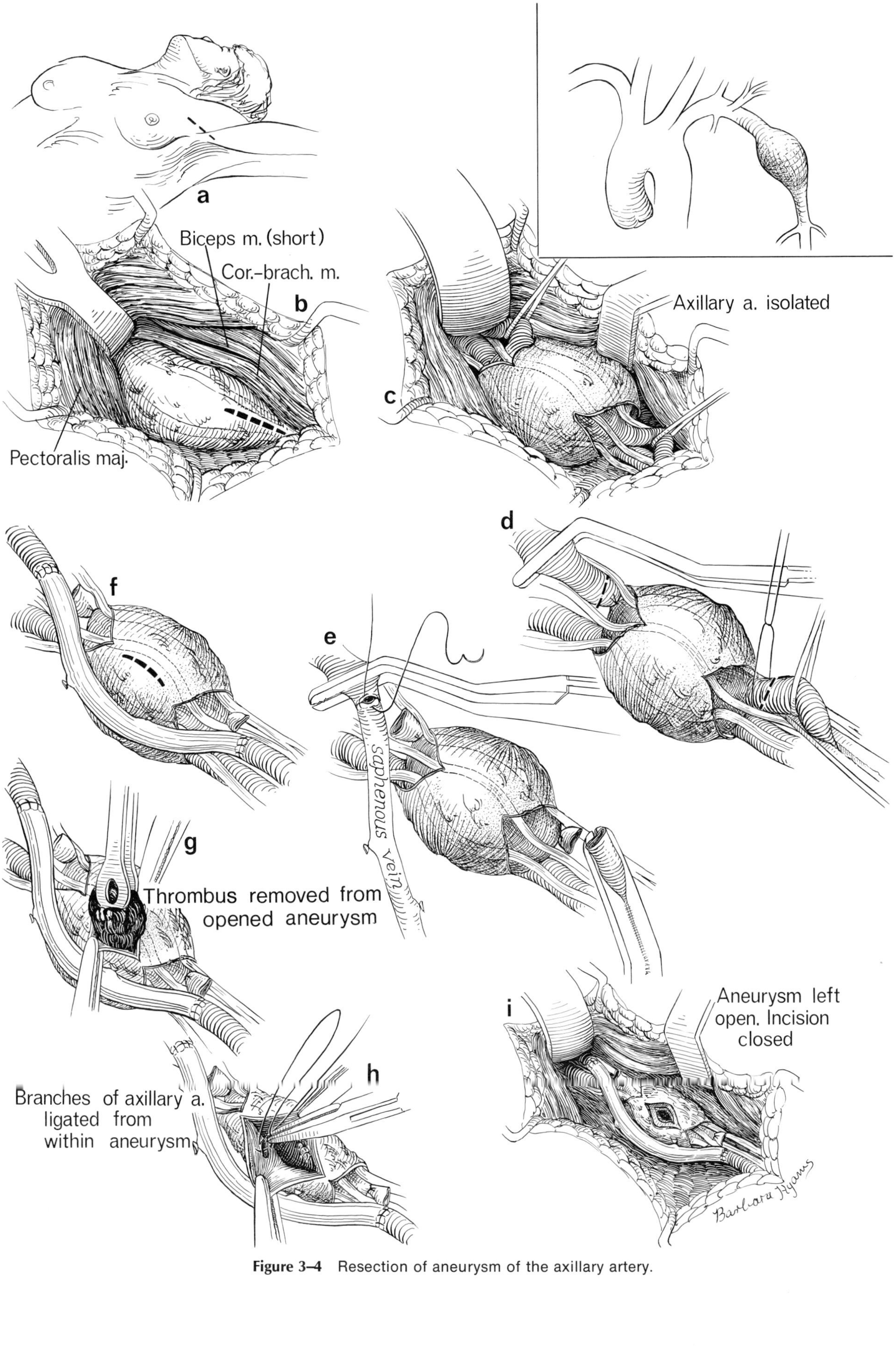
a
Biceps m. (short)
Cor.-brach. m.
b
Pectoralis maj.
Axillary a. isolated
c
d
f
e
saphenous vein
g
Thrombus removed from opened aneurysm
Aneurysm left open. Incision closed
i
h
Branches of axillary a. ligated from within aneurysm

Figure 3–4 Resection of aneurysm of the axillary artery.

the pectoralis major muscle. We prefer the lateral (subpectoral-axillary) approach, which provides adequate proximal and distal access to the axillary artery without transecting the pectoralis major muscle. The patient is positioned with a roll beneath the involved shoulder and the arm is abducted 90° (Fig. 3–4, *a*). A skin incision measuring approximately 10 cm is made parallel to the artery along the superior aspect of the axillary hairline (Figure 3–4, *a*). The pectoralis major muscle is retracted medially, and the coracobiceps and short biceps muscles are retraced laterally (Fig. 3–4, *b*). The axillary artery is then isolated proximally and distally to the aneurysm, and tapes are passed for control (Fig. 3–4, *c*). After systemic heparinization (2 mg/kg of body weight), the artery is ligated at both ends of the aneurysm with heavy Mersilene suture and transected proximally and distally (Fig. 3–4, *d*). An autogenous saphenous vein is anastomosed to both ends of the artery with running 6–0 polypropylene suture, and flow is restored to the arm (Fig. 3–4, *e* and *f*). The aneurysm is then incised and contained thrombus removed (Fig. 3–4, *g*). Branches of the axillary artery are ligated from within the aneurysm (Fig. 3–4, *h*), and the edges of the aneurysm wall are loosely reapproximated (Fig. 3–4, *i*).

SUBCLAVIAN ARTERY ANEURYSM

Aneurysms of the subclavian artery are uncommon,[20] and although, theoretically, they may result from arteriosclerosis, they are usually associated with thoracic outlet syndrome (TOS) and poststenotic dilatation of the artery.[2, 22] Although the natural history of these lesions has not been well defined, they do produce thrombosis of the subclavian artery and distal embolization to the vertebral circulation and upper extremity. Therefore, these lesions should be resected.

Most subclavian aneurysms are associated with TOS, and therefore operative treatment usually requires first rib resection (along with the cervical rib if present), as well as excision and replacement of the aneurysm. This is best accomplished by two separate incisions during the same period of anesthesia.

The patient is first placed in the lateral position, and resection of the first rib, cervical rib, and any congenital bands present is performed as described and shown in Figure 3–2. The transaxillary incision is closed and the patient is placed in the supine position with a roll beneath the shoulder. The subclavian aneurysm is approached through a supraclavicular incision as described in Chapter 2 (Fig. 2–4). Following systemic heparinization, the aneurysm is resected and replaced with a Dacron or saphenous vein graft as described in the preceding section on axillary artery aneurysm (Fig. 3–4); the only difference is in exposure — in this case it is obtained through a supraclavicular approach. This approach provides adequate exposure for resection of most subclavian aneurysms; however, in cases of large aneurysms, resection of the clavicle may be necessary.

SUBCLAVIAN–AXILLARY VEIN THROMBOSIS

Thrombosis of the subclavian and axillary veins and the resultant postphlebitic syndrome of the upper extremity present a difficult problem for which the optimum treatment has not yet been delineated. In cases of acute thrombosis of the subclavian axillary vein, the widely used treatment of heparinization and elevation results in a disabling postphlebitic syndrome in a majority of patients so treated.[12] Therefore, a more aggressive approach seems to be justified.

Although no one center, including our own, has accumulated sufficient experience to determine optimum treatment, the aggressive approach developed by Roos, combining urgent first rib resection and surgical thrombectomy of the subclavian vein via the transaxillary incision, appears to warrant continued evaluation.[4, 6, 7]

REFERENCES

1. Coote H: Pressure on the axillary vessels and nerve by an exostosis from a cervical rib: Interference with the circulation of the arm, removal of the rib and exostosis; recovery. Med Times Gaz 2:108, 1861.
2. Halsted WS: An experimental study of circumscribed dilation of an artery immediately distal to a partially occluding band, and its bearing on the dilation of the subclavian artery observed in certain cases of cervical rib. J Exp Med 24:271, 1916.
3. Oschner A, Gage M, DeBakey M: Scalenus anticus (Naffziger) syndrome. Am J Surg 28:669, 1935.
4. Roos DB: Transaxillary approach for the first rib resection to relieve thoracic outlet syndrome. Ann Surg 163:354, 1966.
5. Roos DB: Thoracic outlet syndrome. Rocky Mt Med J 64:49, 1967.
6. Roos DB: Experience with first rib resection for thoracic outlet syndrome. Ann Surg 173:429, 1971.
7. Roos DB: Thoracic outlet and carpal tunnel syndromes. In *Vascular Surgery* (edited by Rutherford RB). W.B. Saunders Company, Philadelphia, 1977, p 605.
8. Blank RH, Connar RG: Arterial complications associated with thoracic outlet compression syndrome. Ann Thorac Surg 17(4):315, 1974.
9. Mathes SJ, Salam AA: Subclavian artery aneurysm; sequela of thoracic outlet syndrome. Surgery 76(3):506, 1974.
10. Urschel HC Jr, Razzuk MA, Wood RE, Parekh M, Paulson DL: Objective diagnosis (ulnar nerve conduction velocity) and current therapy of the thoracic outlet syndrome. Ann Thorac Surg 12(6):608, 1971.
11. Daube JR: Nerve conduction studies in the thoracic outlet syndrome. Neurology 25:347, 1975.
12. Tilney NL, Griffiths HJG, Edwards EA: Natural history of major venous thrombosis of the upper extremity. Arch Surg 101:792, 1970.
13. Britt LP: Nonoperative treatment of the thoracic outlet syndrome symptoms. Clin Orthop 51:45, 1967.
14. Lord JW Jr: Surgical management of shoulder girdle syndromes. Arch Surg 66:69, 1953.
15. Nelson RM, Jenson CB: Anterior approach for excision of the first rib. Ann Thorac Surg 9:30, 1970.
16. Johnson CR: Treatment of thoracic outlet syndrome by removal of 1st rib and related entrapments through posterolateral approach: A 22-year experience. J Thorac Cardiovasc Surg 68:536, 1974.
17. Tullos HS, Erwin WD, Woods GW, Wukasch DC, Cooley DA, King JW: Unusual lesions of the pitching arm. Clin Orthop 88:169, 1972.
18. Stallworth JM, Bradham GB, Lee WH: Treatment of peripheral artery aneurysms. Am J Surg 27:785, 1961.
19. Inahara T: Arterial injuries of the upper extremity. Surgery 51:605, 1962.
20. Crawford ES, DeBakey ME, Cooley DA: Surgical considerations of peripheral arterial aneurysms. Arch Surg 78:226, 1959.
21. Crawford ES, Edwards WH, DeBakey ME, Cooley DA, Morris GC Jr: Peripheral arteriosclerotic aneurysm. J Am Geriatr Soc 9:1, 1961.
22. Holman E: The development of aneurysms. Surg Gynecol Obstet 100:599, 1955.

CHAPTER 4

Aneurysms of the Abdominal Aorta

In 1554, the French physician Fernel described an aneurysm as "a dilatation of an artery full of spiritous blood."[1] But resection of abdominal aortic aneurysms did not become generally accepted as the treatment of choice for this condition until first reported in Europe by DuBost and coworkers in 1952,[2] and in the United States at our medical center in 1953.[3, 4] After the first reported case of a successfully treated ruptured abdominal aortic aneurysm from our center in 1954,[5, 6] mortality associated with this condition decreased to approximately 20 percent as a result of improved surgical techniques.[7]

INDICATIONS AND PREOPERATIVE PREPARATION

The presence of an abdominal aortic aneurysm (AAA) is a universally acknowledged indication for resection unless associated with a terminal condition such as widespread malignancy. Numerous studies have shown that mortality in untreated patients with AAA is significantly higher than in those treated surgically, and the hospital mortality rate should not exceed 5 percent. The size of an aneurysm is not the only factor in deciding whether to operate, as small aneurysms rupture with almost the same frequency as large ones.[7]

The diagnosis of AAA may usually be made by palpation, along with lateral and anterior-posterior roentgenograms of the abdomen. Aortography is not necessary unless the patient is hypertensive or has evidence of distal arterial occlusive disease, in which case translumbar or retrograde aortography should be performed to rule out the presence of renal artery stenosis or significant aortoiliac occlusive disease. Associated renal artery lesions should be corrected at the time of resection of the AAA whether or not renal venous renin assays (RVRA) are abnormal.* Formerly, when the diagnosis of AAA was uncertain on the basis of palpation and plain roentgenograms of the abdomen, aortography was employed to confirm or exclude the diagnosis. However, recently developed computerized axial tomography (CAT) scans or echograms (sonograms) have provided satisfactory noninvasive methods of confirming or excluding the presence of an AAA.[8]

Preoperative evaluation should include careful assessment of carotid artery stenosis and coronary artery lesions, which frequently need surgical correction prior to resection of the AAA. Often, such associated lesions may be corrected concomi-

---

(See discussion in Chapter 6: Renal Artery Stenosis and Renovascular Hypertension.)

tantly with resection of the aneurysm. Adequate preoperative hydration is an important factor in preventing postoperative renal insufficiency.

SURGICAL TECHNIQUE OF NONRUPTURED ABDOMINAL AORTIC ANEURYSM

Following induction of general anesthesia, a Foley catheter is inserted into the bladder and a nasogastric tube is placed into the stomach. The groins should always be prepared for surgery in the event disease in the iliac arteries requires anastomosis of the distal limbs of the graft to the femoral arteries. However, most aneurysms can be replaced with a straight tube graft, even in the presence of extensive calcification of the common iliac arteries, if the patient has had no symptoms of intermittent claudication or physical signs of ischemia of the lower extremities.

The abdomen is entered through a midline incision, beginning at the xiphoid process of the sternum. Following exploration of the abdomen, the transverse colon and small bowel are reflected cephalad and laterally to the patient's right. The aneurysm is exposed by incising the peritoneum between the duodenum on the right and the inferior mesenteric vein on the left (Fig. 4–1, a to c). Mobilization of the left renal vein may be facilitated by ligating the left renal lumbar vein[7] and the testicular (or ovarian) and adrenal branches (see Fig. 6–1). This technique allows mobilization of the left renal vein 6 to 7 cm cephalad, precluding the necessity of transecting this vessel. When necessary, however, the left renal vein may be transected and reapproximated with running polypropylene sutures. Rarely, the left renal vein courses posterior to the aorta, and one must be cautious to avoid injury and hemorrhage, which may be difficult to control because of the posterior location.

The neck of the aneurysm is mobilized just below the renal arteries, but passing a tape around the aorta is not necessary and should be avoided because of the possibility of damaging a lumbar vein. When the aneurysm extends to the renal arteries, or when associated renal arterial lesions are present, it is necessary to clamp the aorta above the renal arteries following administration of heparin and, in some instances, 25 mg of mannitol intravenously. If dissection of the aorta above the renal arteries is not feasible because of adhesions from previous surgery or extension of the aneurysm above the renal arteries, the aorta may be clamped at the level of the diaphragm (the supraceliac bare area [SBA].[9] (See Fig. 9–2.)

The aortic clamp is applied to the aorta after administration of heparin (usually 1.0 mg per kg of body weight) (Fig. 4–1, d). To lessen the possibility of debris dislodgment into the distal circulation or renal arteries, the aorta should be cross-clamped *only once*. When the aneurysm extends proximal to the renal arteries, the aorta is first clamped above the renal arteries, the proximal anastomosis performed, and the renal arteries reanastomosed to the graft if necessary. A second clamp is then placed on the graft below the renal artery anastomosis, and the proximal clamp removed, allowing blood flow to the kidneys during performance of the distal anastomosis. However, if the total renal ischemic time is anticipated not to exceed one hour, leaving the proximal clamp in place during performance of the distal anastomosis may be preferred. This allows "internal flushing down" of the internal iliac artery instead of directing the flow and debris from the initial unclamping into the renal arteries. The period of "safe" renal ischemia can be prolonged by perfusing the renal arteries with cold Ringer's lactate solution at 0° C following aortic clamping.[10-12]

Following application of the proximal aortic clamp, the common iliac arteries are clamped (Fig. 4–1, d). There is no need to encircle the iliac arteries with tape, and injury to the underlying iliac veins is avoided. Should the aneurysm extend into the common iliac arteries, dissection and mobilization of these vessels is facilitated by

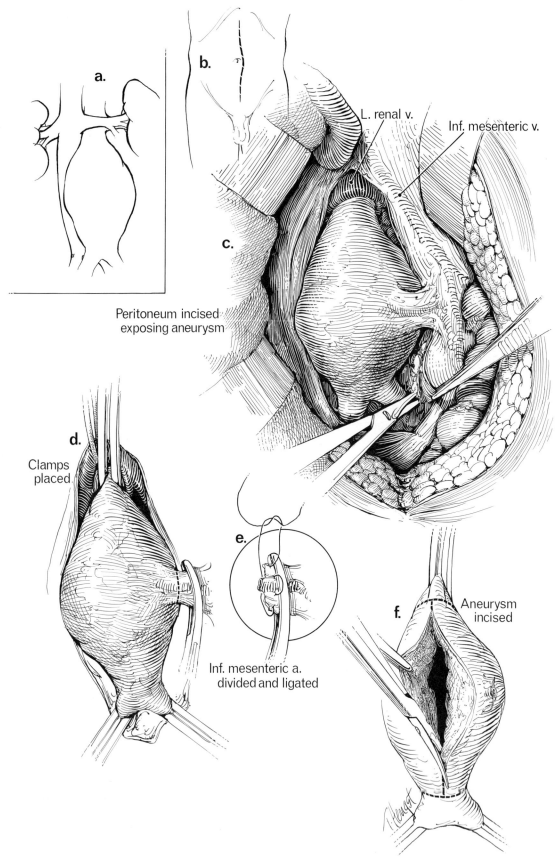

a.

b.

L. renal v.

Inf. mesenteric v.

c.

Peritoneum incised
exposing aneurysm

d.

Clamps
placed

e.

Inf. mesenteric a.
divided and ligated

f.

Aneurysm
incised

Figure 4–1   Technique of surgical repair of nonruptured abdominal aortic aneurysm.

Illustration continued on opposite page.

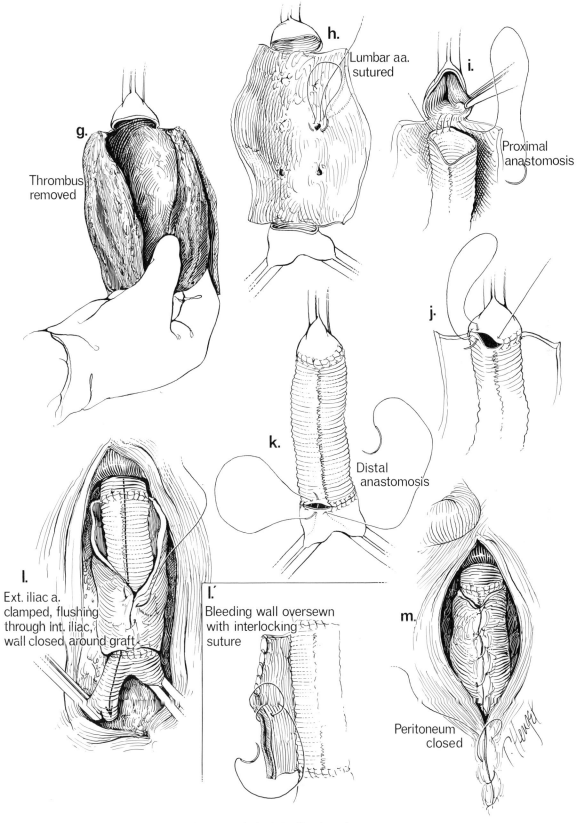

h. Lumbar aa. sutured

g. Thrombus removed

i. Proximal anastomosis

j.

k. Distal anastomosis

l. Ext. iliac a. clamped, flushing through int. iliac, wall closed around graft

l.' Bleeding wall oversewn with interlocking suture

m. Peritoneum closed

Figure 4–1 *Continued.*

first clamping the aorta to empty the distal vessels. Consideration is then given to choosing the type of distal anastomosis for the bifurcation graft. The three preferred alternatives are end-to-end to the common iliacs, end-to-end or end-to-side to the external iliacs, or end-to-side to the common femoral vessels. An effort should be made to preserve circulation to at least one internal iliac artery. Meticulous care is necessary to avoid injury to the ureters as they cross the external iliac arteries anteriorly; this is facilitated by clamping the proximal aorta, and thus decompressing the iliac arteries prior to their dissection. The inferior mesenteric artery is clamped, transected, and ligated with sutures (Fig. 4–1, e). A large inferior mesenteric artery, particularly a large marginal artery of Drummond, may be reanastomosed into the graft to preserve circulation to the sigmoid colon and rectum.

The aneurysm is incised (Fig. 4–1, f), and atheromatous and thrombotic material is evacuated (Fig. 4–1, g). The posterior wall of the aneurysm is left in place and the ostia of the lumbar arteries are ligated with sutures from within the aneurysm (Fig 4–1, h). An appropriately sized preclotted Dacron double velour graft is then tailored to approximate the diameter of the transected proximal aorta. If the question arises as to which of two sizes of grafts to use, the smaller should be chosen, because it is easier to enlarge the graft by tailoring it in an S-shaped fashion than to enlarge a friable aortic cuff. The proximal anastomosis is performed with a 3–0 braided polyester suture. The posterior wall of the aorta may be left in place and the posterior suture line accomplished first by sewing toward the surgeon (Fig. 4–1, i). The anterior suture line is then made in the same fashion (Fig. 4–1, j). A similar technique is used for the distal anastomosis (Fig. 4–1, k).

Prior to tying the final suture line, the common iliac arteries are flushed to evacuate debris. Internal flushing is accomplished by leaving the left common iliac clamp in place, moving the right iliac clamp down to the right external iliac artery, and, as the proximal aortic clamp is removed, flushing any loose debris from the proximal aorta into the right internal iliac artery (Fig. 4–1, l). Note that the aortic clamp has been applied and removed only once, thus lessening the dislodgment of debris and microemboli from the diseased aorta. Systemic heparinization is reversed at this point by intravenous protamine sulfate in a ratio of 1.5:1.0 to the heparin given prior to clamping the aorta. The edges of the aneurysm wall are oversewn with a continuous absorbable suture or are cauterized to prevent postoperative hemorrhage (Fig. 4–1, l), and the aneurysm wall and posterior peritoneum are reapproximated around the graft in separate layers (Fig. 4–1, m).

REPAIR OF LACERATION OF INFERIOR VENA CAVA OR ILIAC VEINS

Laceration of the inferior vena cava (IVC) or common iliac vein can be prevented by leaving the posterior wall of the aneurysm in place, by limiting the mobilization of the aorta, and by avoiding the passing of tapes around the aorta and common iliac artery. Should this complication occur, however, serious hemorrhage can result. If a laceration of the vein occurs, an important point to remember is *not* to attempt to suture the lacerated veins while they are distended, because an extension of the laceration can result. Decompression of the veins should be accomplished by proximal and distal compression, with the first assistant applying pressure with a folded "4-by-4" sponge held in ring forceps clamps (Fig. 4–2). In some instances the surgeon may control the hemorrhage with digital pressure while the assistant inserts the sutures. This simple maneuver provides a dry field and allows repair of the decompressed vein with carefully placed sutures. In some instances the hemorrhages may be controlled by applying a partial occlusion clamp to the vein and repairing the laceration with five monofilament sutures.

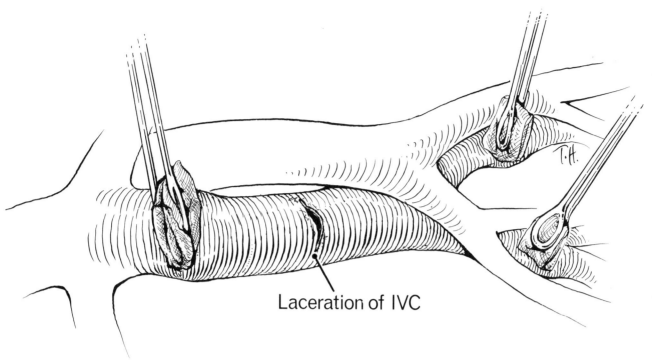

Figure 4–2 Repair of laceration of the inferior vena cava.

RESECTION OF ABDOMINAL AORTIC ANEURYSM IN THE PRESENCE OF HORSESHOE KIDNEY

This anomaly is reported to occur in one of every 600 persons. The resulting isthmus of the fused kidneys usually lies anterior to the aorta and inferior vena cava at the level of the fourth lumbar vertebra, but may lie posterior to these vessels. The ureters usually arise from the upper medial aspect of each kidney and course anterior to the renal isthmus.

The major technical problem in resection of an abdominal aortic aneurysm in the presence of horseshoe kidney is the frequently associated anomalous arterial supply. Thus the technique for resection of the aneurysm must be modified at the time of operation, depending upon the number and anatomic locations of the anomalous renal arteries that often arise from the aneurysm itself. The two most feasible techniques for handling these anomalous arteries are: (1) to reimplant the anomalous artery into the graft, or (2) to excise that portion of the horshoe kidney, usually the isthmus, that derives its blood supply from the anomalous arteries. The divided kidney may be reapproximated, or, alternatively, the transected renal surfaces may be repaired with the use of running absorbable sutures.

Resection of the aneurysm associated with a horseshoe kidney that has normal renal arteries is demonstrated in Figure 4–3. The standard dissection of the abdominal aorta is performed, and the arterial supply to the kidneys and the course of the ureters are delineated (Fig. 4–3, a). The isthmus of the horseshoe kidney is mobilized from the aneurysm and retracted in a caudad direction, and the proximal anastomosis is performed as in an uncomplicated aneurysm (Fig. 4–3, b). Following completion of the proximal anastomosis, the graft is passed posterior to the isthmus of the horseshoe kidney, which is retracted cephalad, and the distal anastomosis is performed as described in the previous section (Fig. 4–3, c). If anomalous renal arteries were transected, they are reanastomosed into the graft. But if because of their small

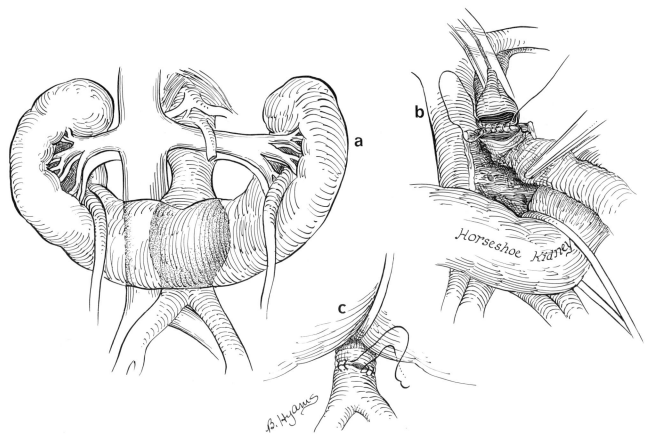

Figure 4–3 Resection of abdominal aortic aneurysm associated with a horseshoe kidney.

size this is not practical, to prevent subsequent renovascular hypertension, the ischemic isthmus of the horseshoe kidney is resected, thus assuring that infarcted renal tissue is not left in place.

RUPTURED ABDOMINAL AORTIC ANEURYSM

Rupture of an aneurysm of the abdominal aorta is the principal cause of death in patients with such lesions. According to Gliedman,[13] rupture occurs in 49 percent, and in a series described by Estes[14] the occurrence is 63 percent.

Since the first successful surgically treated ruptured abdominal aortic aneurysm (AAA) was reported from our center in 1954,[5] operative mortality has decreased from 60 percent in the initial series of five patients to 21 percent in our most recently reported series of 87 patients.[7]

Diagnosis of ruptured AAA can usually be made by clinical examination. Frequently, the patient has had a recently discovered AAA. Most patients experience typical symptoms, the most common of which in our series was sudden abdominal, flank, or back pain; this occurred in 80 percent.[7] Abdominal pain was reported in 77 percent, and back pain in 43 percent, radiating to the scrotum in 6 percent, the groin in 4 percent, and the legs in 3 percent. Thirty-five patients (40 percent) presented in shock, among whom nine (25.7 percent) died during the course of hospitalization. Among the 52 patients not in shock preoperatively, nine also died (17.3 percent).[7]

Following the diagnosis, which can usually be made upon the patient's admission to the emergency room, emergency celiotomy is performed. Routine preoperative preparation of the patient is usually unwarranted and may cause delay in controlling the hemorrhage. Blood transfusion and massive fluid infusions should not be done before operation. Every effort should be made to get the patient on the operating table and the proximal aorta cross-clamped as soon as possible after he or she enters the hospital. For patients in profound shock, induction of anesthesia is withheld until the abdomen is opened and hemorrhage controlled. A nasogastric tube is inserted to empty the stomach and prevent aspiration of gastric contents, and a Foley catheter is placed into the bladder to monitor urinary output. General anesthesia is induced, and the electrocardiogram and central venous pressure are monitored.

Upon entering the abdomen, the location of the retroperitoneal hematoma determines whether the aorta will be cross-clamped below the renal arteries or in the supraceliac "bare area" of the aorta at the level of the diaphragm (Fig. 4–4, a). The decision must be reached quickly. Heparin is administered before the aortic clamp is applied, since the hypovolemic patient with atherosclerosis has a strong tendency to develop intravascular thromboses during the period of circulatory arrest. The peritoneum overlying the hematoma and aneurysm is incised to the left of the duodenum (Fig. 4–4, b), the infrarenal aorta is isolated by blunt dissection with the left hand passing through the hematoma, the aorta is clamped below the renal arteries, and the upper clamp at the diaphragm is removed (Fig. 4–4, c). After clamps are placed at the common iliac arteries, the aneurysmal sac is incised. A woven Dacron graft of low porosity is anastomosed proximally and distally as described above in the section on nonruptured aneurysms (Fig. 4–4, d).

In some cases, the aneurysm extends to the level of the renal arteries, and thus precludes clamping of the aorta below the renal arteries (Fig. 4–4, e). In these instances, the clamp is left in place at the level of the diaphragm during creation of the proximal aortic anastomosis (Fig. 4–4, f). A second clamp is then placed across the graft and the proximal clamp at the diaphragm is removed during performance of the distal anastomoses (Fig. 4–4, g). Should the aneurysm involve the iliac arteries, these vessels are now dissected, inasmuch as they can be better exposed when decompressed. The iliac arteries are then clamped at a more distal level, and the distal limbs of the grafts are anastomosed to the common iliac, external iliac, or common femoral arteries, as appropriate (Fig. 4–4, g).

Among the 87 patients undergoing resection of ruptured AAA,[7] three died during operation and 15 during the early postoperative period. Total hospital mortality was 21 percent, providing a survival rate of 79 percent. Sudden cardiac arrest from arrhythmia, myocardial infarction or hypovolemia was the principal cause of death. Other early causes were renal failure (five patients), pulmonary edema (two patients), and intestinal obstruction (two patients). Thirty-two patients died after discharge. Among these, 15 died more than five years after operation, and 17 died during periods of equal distribution throughout the first five postoperative years. The most common causes of late mortality were myocardial infarction (ten patients), cerebrovascular accidents (five patients), and renal failure (two patients). Late death in seven patients was related to the operative procedure or to development of vascular disease in another area. In three patients undergoing surgery early in the series, pseudoaneurysms of the proximal suture line ruptured, and one of these patients died.[7]

FALSE ANEURYSMS

In false aneurysms (pseudoaneurysms), the aneurysmal sac is composed of only a fibrous capsule, whereas in true aneurysms, elements of the arterial wall are present. False aneurysms may be traumatic in origin, but are more often caused by disruption of the anastomotic suture line of a prosthetic graft. Numerous factors

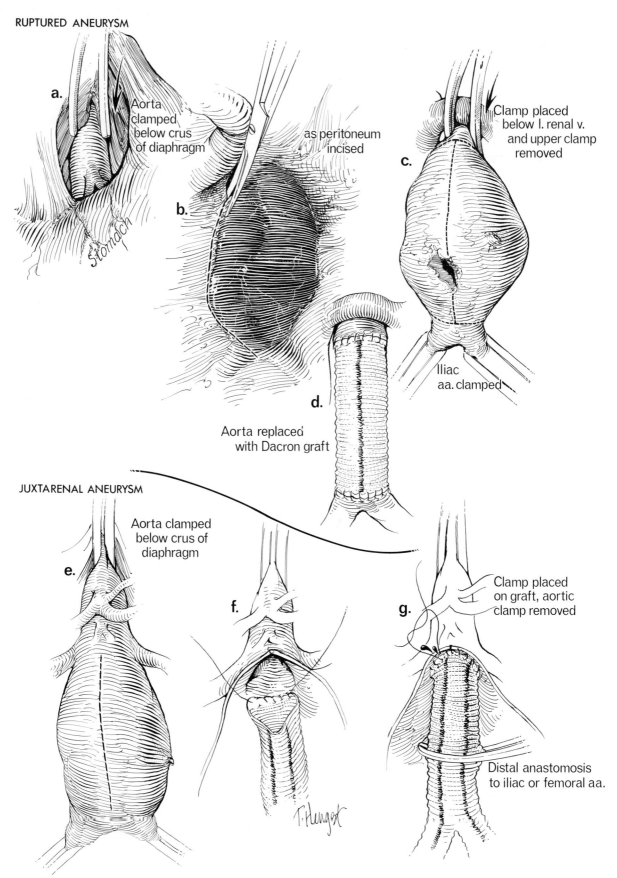

RUPTURED ANEURYSM

a. Aorta clamped below crus of diaphragm

Stomach

b. as peritoneum incised

c. Clamp placed below l. renal v. and upper clamp removed

Iliac aa. clamped

d. Aorta replaced with Dacron graft

JUXTARENAL ANEURYSM

e. Aorta clamped below crus of diaphragm

f.

g. Clamp placed on graft, aortic clamp removed

Distal anastomosis to iliac or femoral aa.

T. Hunggat

Figure 4–4   Repair of ruptured abdominal aortic aneurysm (*a* to *d*) and repair of a juxtarenal aneurysm (*e* to *g*).

have been blamed for predisposing false aneurysms; they include sepsis, type of graft material (i.e., woven), and stress on the suture line from limb motion. In our experience, however, the most frequent cause has been the type of suture used, i.e., late deterioration of silk, or breakage from "material fatigue" of monofilament nylon or polypropylene. Because a prosthetic graft anastomosis will never become permanently incorporated into an arterial wall, even after a number of years, the integrity of a prosthetic anastomosis depends upon the prolonged durability of the suture material used; therefore, we believe that braided polyester sutures should be used with prosthetic graft materials and that any monofilament suture, including the currently popular polypropylene, may be unreliable for suturing prosthetic grafts.

RESECTION OF AORTIC AND FEMORAL FALSE ANEURYSMS

Surgical resection and replacement of aortic and femoral false aneurysms is a relatively straightforward procedure and, in the absence of infection, should be associated with comparable risk and results as in resection of true aneurysms (Fig. 4–5, a). The presence of infection poses special problems, which will be discussed at the conclusion of this section.

Patients who have previously had aortic reconstruction with fabric grafts and who are suspected of having false aneurysms should undergo arteriography to visualize all anastomoses. A patient with a false aneurysm in any one of the three anastomoses of a previous aortofemoral graft will quite likely demonstrate false aneurysms in the other anastomoses. In addition to ascertaining the presence of other false aneurysms, arteriography is essential in delineating the status of the distal circulation, as it is frequently necessary to anastomose the new graft to a more distal site, i.e., the profunda femoris or superficial femoral arteries, or even the popliteal arteries. Translumbar aortography is the technique of choice for visualizing suspected false aneurysms of the abdominal aorta and iliac or femoral arteries. Retrograde transfemoral arteriography may cause dislodgment of thrombotic material into the distal circulation, thus producing microembolization ("trash foot"), or more major embolization and complete occlusion of a distal artery.

The abdominal and femoral areas are re-entered by excising the previous midline abdominal and femoral incisional scars (Fig. 4–5, b). The right and left femoral false aneurysms are exposed and the profunda femoris arteries mobilized distal to the false aneurysm (Fig. 4–5, c and d). When scar tissue is extensive, only proximal control of the arterial circulation is necessary before cross-clamping. Distal control may be obtained after the aneurysm is entered. Sometimes an intraluminal balloon catheter may be used for this purpose. When both superficial femoral arteries are chronically occluded, as in this illustration, these vessels can usually be sacrified as long as adequate circulation is restored to the profunda femoris arteries. If the superficial femoral vessels are patent, the distal limbs of the new graft may be anastomosed either into the common femoral vessels or, if not feasible, end-to-end to the profunda femoris artery, with a side graft to the superficial femoral or popliteal arteries. If the proximal common femoral vessel is patent, proximal control is more easily obtained by passing a No. 6 Fogarty catheter into this vessel after opening the false aneurysm.

The abdominal false aneurysm is then exposed, as described in previous sections, by dividing the peritoneum to the left of the duodenum. If feasible, the proximal aorta is isolated and clamped below the left renal vein following the preclotting of a Dacron double velour bifurcation graft and systemic administration of heparin (2 mg/kg of body weight) (Fig. 4–5, e). Frequently, proximal extension of the false aneurysm will make exposure and clamping of the aorta at this level impractical, and in such situations the "supraceliac" aorta should be clamped at the level of the aortic

Text continued on page 67.

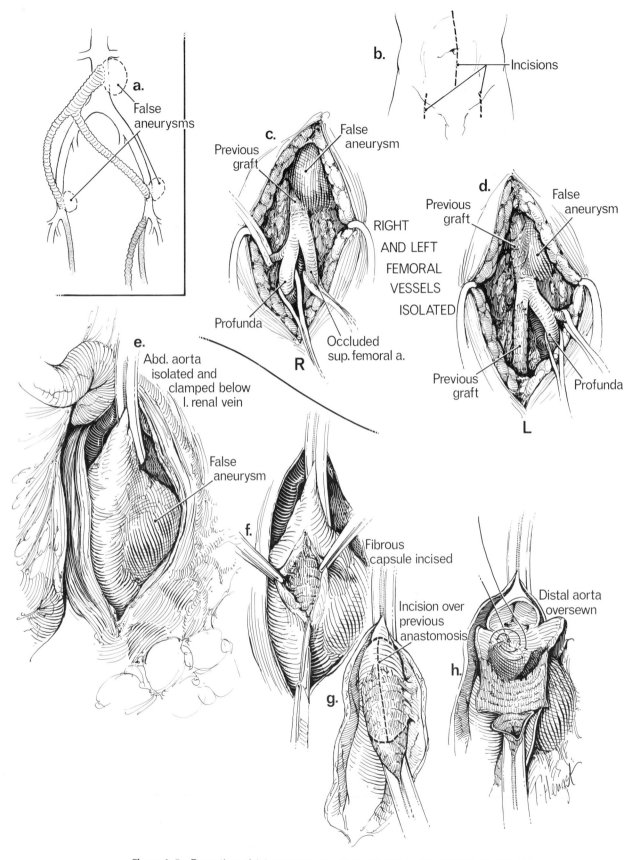

Figure 4–5 Resection of false aneurysms of abdominal aorta and femoral arteries.

Illustration continued on opposite page.

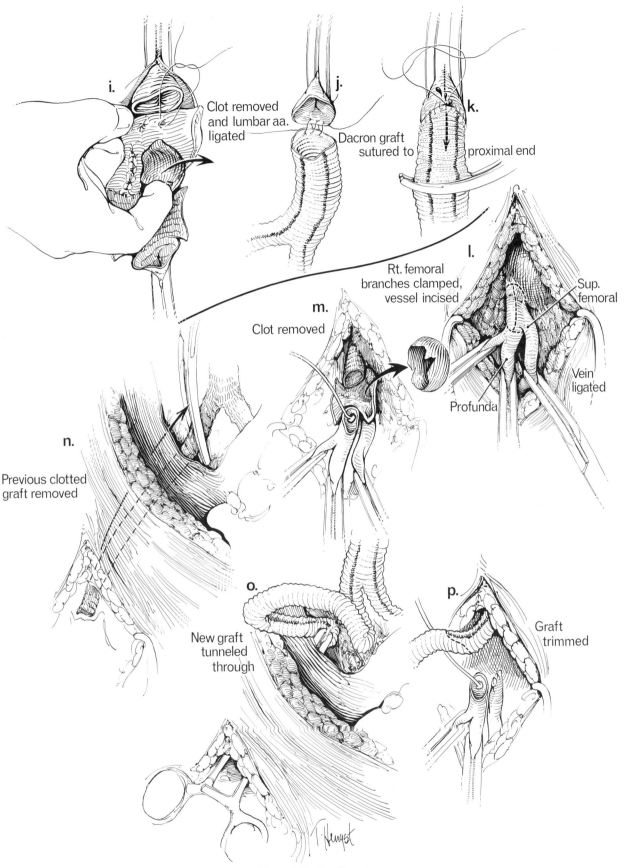

i. Clot removed and lumbar aa. ligated

j. Dacron graft sutured to proximal end

k.

l. Rt. femoral branches clamped, vessel incised

Sup. femoral

Vein ligated

Profunda

m. Clot removed

n. Previous clotted graft removed

o. New graft tunneled through

p. Graft trimmed

Figure 4–5 *Continued.*

Illustration continued on following page.

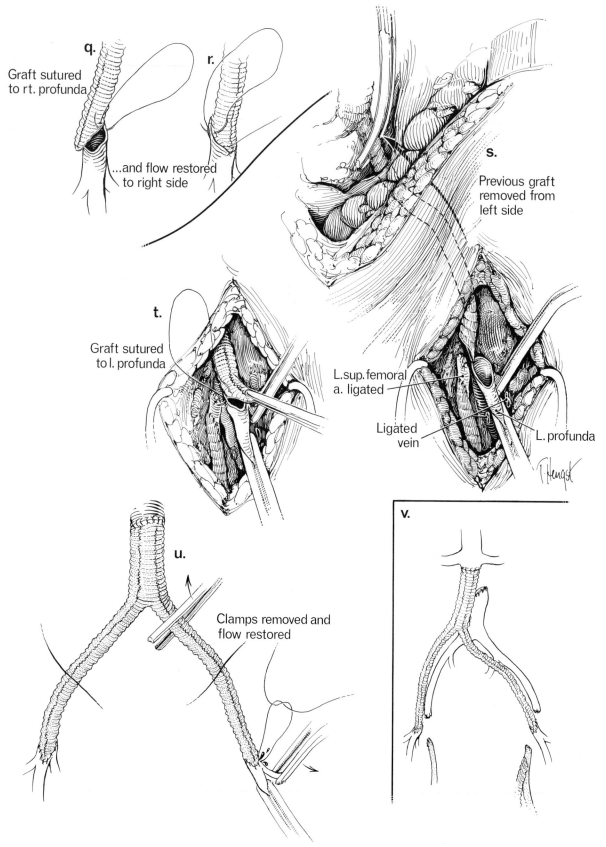

q. Graft sutured to rt. profunda

r. ...and flow restored to right side

s. Previous graft removed from left side

t. Graft sutured to l. profunda

L.sup.femoral a. ligated

Ligated vein

L. profunda

u. Clamps removed and flow restored

v.

Figure 4–5 *Continued.*

hiatus of the diaphragm. (See Fig. 9–2.) Exposure of the previous graft below the false aneurysm is obtained by incising the fibrous capsule surrounding the graft (Fig. 4–5, f). The graft is clamped distally and opened, and the incision extended cephalad over the previous anastomosis (Fig. 4–5, g). In cases where the previous anastomosis was placed end-to-end, the distal aorta will have been oversewn; however, if the previous proximal anastomosis was placed end-to-side to the aorta, the distal aorta will require oversewing at this point (Fig. 4–5, h). This may be facilitated by controlling back bleeding with a large Foley catheter inflated in the distal aorta, or by digital pressure applied by an assistant.

Thrombus within the false aneurysm is removed and any patent lumbar arteries are suture-ligated from within the aortic lumen (Fig. 4–5, i). A new Dacron graft is then anastomosed end-to-end to the transected proximal aorta (Fig. 4–5, j). Air is evacuated and the suture line tested by placing a second clamp on the graft and removing the proximal aortic clamp (Fig. 4–5, k).

The branches of the right profunda femoris artery (and superficial femoral artery if patent) are then clamped and the right femoral false aneurysm incised (Fig. 4–5, l). Thrombus within the false aneurysm is removed and the profunda femoris artery tailored for end-to-end anastomosis (Fig. 4–5, m). If significant backflow is present from the proximal common femoral artery, an attempt is made to preserve retrograde flow into the proximal common femoral and iliac artery system on at least one side to maintain flow into the pelvis. Removal of the old graft is accomplished by withdrawing it retrograde through the tunnel (Fig. 4–5, n), with the right limb of the new graft passed retroperitoneally beneath the inguinal ligament (Fig. 4–5, o). It is not advisable to reuse the old tunnel, which is almost always contracted with dense scar tissue. A new tunnel should be made by gentle blunt finger dissection from above and below; when completed, the surgeon's two index fingers should meet in the middle without constriction from surrounding tissues. Enlargement of the old tunnel, or creation of a new tunnel, should *never* be attempted with a firm instrument, such as a ring forceps, because of possible injury to the ureter, bladder, or even the sigmoid colon on the left.

The right distal limb of the graft is then trimmed in an S-shaped fashion (Fig. 4–5, p), and anastomosed end-to-end to the profunda femoris artery (Fig. 4–5, q). The left limb of the graft is clamped and flow is restored to the right lower extremity by gradually removing the proximal clamp (Fig. 4–5, r). The left femoral aneurysm is excised and circulation restored in a similar fashion (Fig. 4–5, s to v).

The presence of infection in a false aneurysm presents a much more complicated situation, with a grave prognosis. Many plans of management have been suggested and utilized in our institution, including complete removal of the graft and entirely bypassing the area of infection by axillo-femoral or obturator foramen grafts. Unsatisfactory results from all these procedures have led us to take a more conservative approach in recent years, which has resulted in lowered mortality. Since radical treatment of an infected graft is usually fatal, we believe that treatment should not be based upon drastic measures but upon palliative therapy. Application of this approach will be described as related to the two most common situations: first, the infected bifurcation (or aortic tube) graft with generalized sepsis and an infected proximal false aneurysm (with or without aortoduodenal fistula), and second, an infected false aneurysm of the distal anastomosis without generalized sepsis — with the possibility that the infection is confined to the femoral area and not the entire graft.

In the instance of a proximal false aneurysm, there is danger of rupture with exsanguinating hemorrhage into the adjacent duodenum, and therefore urgent removal of the false aneurysm and repair of the aortoduodenal fistula is imperative. Because of the unsatisfactory hemodynamic results and the high reinfection rate of axillo-femoral grafts, we have virtually abandoned this procedure. Instead, following resection of the false aneurysm, removal of the infected graft, and repair of the duodenal fistula if present, a new graft is inserted as indicated by the anatomic condition of the proximal aorta. This procedure is coupled with local debridement of necrotic tissue, local irrigation with an antibiotic solution, and prolonged massive appropriate intravenous antibiotic therapy.

If the quality of the aortic cuff below the renal arteries is suitable, the new graft is reanastomosed at this level; but if the aortic cuff is insufficient or extremely friable at this level, the proximal aorta is oversewn just below the renal arteries, and the proximal anastomosis of the new graft is made end-to-side to the "supraceliac bare area" (SBA) of the aorta at the level of the diaphragm. Although patients treated by this approach have experienced approximately a 40 percent reinfection rate with recurrent complications, 60 percent of a small number of patients thus treated have survived one to three years without evidence of reinfection or recurrent complications.[15]

The results of this conservative approach in patients with infected pseudoaneurysms of one or both femoral anastomoses have been gratifying. In such patients, following exclusion of a false aneurysm of the proximal anastomosis by aortography, our approach has been to treat only the complications of the infected femoral false aneurysm, i.e., femoral abscess formation or hemorrhage from the distal anastomosis through the fistulous sinus tract. In such cases, if only a femoral abscess develops, it is incised and drained, with subsequent inspection of the suture line for leakage. A chronic, draining fistulous sinus is more desirable than radical removal of the entire graft, which results in an extremely high mortality rate. If hemorrhage occurs from the infected distal anastomosis, the anastomosis is either reinforced with sutures or a short segment of distal graft is replaced and the wound is drained to promote a chronic draining sinus.

Comment

One such case involved a 63-year-old male who underwent a bilateral aortofemoral bypass for aortoiliac occlusive disease in 1955. The left femoral anastomosis became infected during the early postoperative period and was managed as described above. For 16 years thereafter, the patient experienced several complications from graft infection but remained physically active and continued his practice as a judge until he died at the age of 80 of a myocardial infarction.

(See Chapter 20 for a complete history of this patient.)

REFERENCES

1. Fernel J.: *Medicine*, published by Andreas Wechel, Paris, 1554.
2. Dubost C, Allary M, Oeconomos N: Resection of an aneurysm of the abdominal aorta; reestablishment of continuity by preserved human arterial graft, with result after 5 months. Arch Surg 64:405, 1952.
3. DeBakey ME, Cooley DA: Surgical treatment of aneurysm of abdominal aorta by resection and restoration of continuity with homograft. Surg Gynecol Obstet 97:257, 1953.
4. DeBakey ME, Cooley DA: Successful resection of aneurysm of thoracic aorta and replacement by graft. JAMA 152:673, 1953.
5. DeBakey ME, Cooley DA, Creech O Jr: Surgical treatment of aneurysms and occlusive disease of the aorta. Postgrad Med 15:120, 1954.
6. Cooley DA, DeBakey ME: Ruptured aneurysm of abdominal aorta. Excision and homograft replacement. Postgrad Med 16:334, 1954.
7. Chiariello L, Reul GJ Jr, Wukasch DC, Sandiford FM, Hallman GL, Cooley DA: Ruptured abdominal aortic aneurysm: Treatment and review of 87 patients. Am J Surg 128:735, 1974.
8. Gerson LP: Computerized axial tomography: A brief survey. Cardiovascular Diseases, Bulletin of the Texas Heart Institute 4(#3):237, 1977.
9. Wukasch DC, Leigh IG, Iverson MD, Rubio PA: The left renal lumbar vein: Importance in exposure of the renal arteries. Cardiovascular Diseases, Bulletin of the Texas Heart Institute 3(#2):233, 1975.

10. Gontijo B, Pereira de Sousa R, Grace RR: Renal autotransplantation for renovascular hypertension. Cardiovascular Diseases, Bulletin of the Texas Heart Institute 4(#2):161, 1977.

11. Stanley JC, Ernest CB, Fry WJ: Fate of 100 aortorenal bypass grafts: Characteristics of late graft expansion, aneurysmal dilation and stenosis. Surgery 74:931, 1973.

12. Hoffman RM, Stilper KW, Johnson RWG, Belzer FO: Renal ischemic tolerance. Arch Surg 109:550, 1974.

13. Gliedman ML, Ayers WB, Vestel BL: Aneurysms of the abdominal aorta and its branches. A study of untreated patients. Ann Surg 146:207, 1957.

14. Estes JE Jr: Abdominal aortic aneurysm: Study of 102 cases. Circulation 2:258, 1950.

15. Statistical information from the Texas Heart Institute, 1978.

CHAPTER 5

Thoracic Aneurysms

Excisional therapy of aortic aneurysms has almost completely replaced techniques previously employed to reinforce the weakened aortic wall. Except in small localized sacciform lesions where tangential excision and lateral aortorrhaphy is possible, circumferential excision with graft replacement is the technique of choice.[1-4] Excision and graft replacement require that aortic circulation be interrupted for various periods of time. The consequences of circulatory cessation, therefore, must be considered when selecting the optimal method of surgical treatment.[5, 6]

In temporary aortic occlusion of the thoracic aorta, the major concerns are with myocardial strain due to hypertension, adequate coronary circulation, and circulation to the brain and spinal cord. Of somewhat secondary importance is hepatic, renal, and intestinal circulation, but these organs usually have sufficient tolerance to ischemia to permit enough time for aortic excision and graft replacement. Thus, the method of aortic resection varies according to the anatomic location of the aneurysm.[7, 8]

ANEURYSMS OF THE ASCENDING AORTA WITH AORTIC VALVE INSUFFICIENCY

Fusiform aneurysms of the ascending aorta are not rare and are often associated with aortic regurgitation. Cystic medial necrosis of the elastic fibers of the aortic wall is the most common histologic finding, but some luetic and arteriosclerotic aneurysms are also encountered. Intramural dissection of the ascending aorta may be present as the primary cause or as the result of the degenerative aortic disease.

The operation is performed through a median sternotomy. In the presence of large aneurysms care should be taken to prevent injury to the aneurysm with the sternal saw while opening the sternum. Full cardiopulmonary bypass with cannulation of the right atrium or of both venae cavae is used for these lesions (Fig. 5–1, a). The ascending aorta may be cannulated more distally than usual, with the cannula placed in the transverse rather than the anterior ascending portion of the aortic arch. In some instances, particularly with dissecting aneurysms, the catheter for arterial return should be placed in the common femoral artery. The caval clamps are applied and the aorta is cross-clamped. A cold solution containing potassium, magnesium, and calcium ions at 10° C is injected into the ascending aorta until cardiac arrest occurs. Cold saline solution at 5° C is applied topically to the heart for several minutes and then removed. We have used this method of cold ischemic arrest for periods in excess of 120 minutes without myocardial complication. Usually, resection of the ascending aorta with replacement of the aortic valve and the ascending aorta can be accomplished in less than half this period. We believe that coronary perfusion is unnecessary; the potential risks to the coronary circulation and myocardium outweigh the possible advantages.

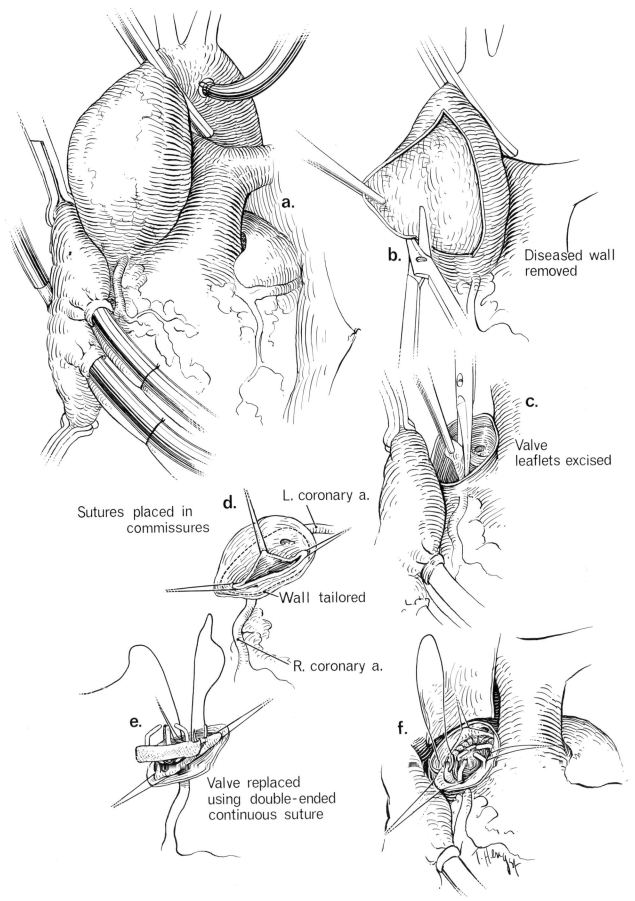

a.

b. Diseased wall removed

c. Valve leaflets excised

Sutures placed in commissures

d. L. coronary a.

Wall tailored

R. coronary a.

e. Valve replaced using double-ended continuous suture

f.

Figure 5–1 Technique for repair of aneurysm of the ascending aorta with aortic valve insufficiency.

Illustration continued on following page.

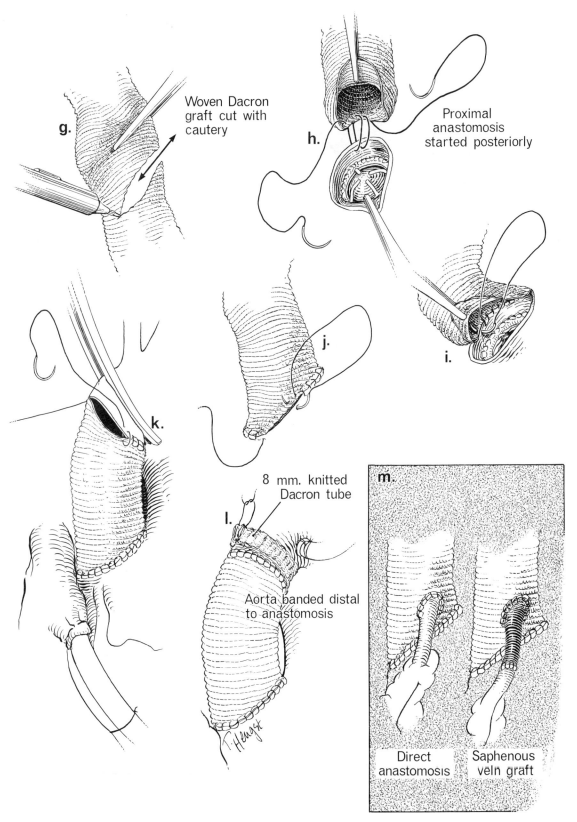

g. Woven Dacron graft cut with cautery

h. Proximal anastomosis started posteriorly

i.

j.

k.

l. 8 mm. knitted Dacron tube

Aorta banded distal to anastomosis

m. Direct anastomosis

Saphenous vein graft

Figure 5–1 *Continued.*

After the aorta is cross-clamped proximal to the origin of the innominate artery and the blood is aspirated from the left side of the heart through the left atrial sump, the ascending aorta is opened (Fig. 5–1, b). Although the aortic leaflets may appear normal, valvuloplasty will infrequently restore complete competence to the valve. The deformity of the commissural suspensions caused by the annular dilatation remains and, therefore, the aortic valve must be replaced (Fig. 5–1, c). The remainder of the aortic wall cephalad to the coronary ostia is resected, thus avoiding injury to the ostia (Fig. 5–1, d). While in the past we used a continuous suture technique for implantation of the valve prosthesis, we now prefer an interrupted technique that utilizes 2–0 braided polyester sutures. Sutures of alternating blue or green with white facilitate identification of the ends and tying of the sutures (Fig. 5–1, e and f).

A preclotted, tightly woven Dacron graft is used to restore continuity. The proximal end of the graft is tailored and cut obliquely to accommodate the enlarged aortic annulus (Fig. 5–1, g). To prevent fraying of the edges, a disposable hot cautery may be used to prepare the edges of the graft. The graft is sutured with a double-armed 3–0 or 4–0 braided polyester suture. The smaller-sized thread and needles preclude large needle holes in the thin and sometimes friable proximal aorta (Fig. 5–1, h). Suturing is done carefully to avoid tearing the aortic wall as the anastomosis is completed (Fig. 5–1, i and j).

After the proximal anastomosis is finished, the graft is tailored for the distal anastomosis by making the end oblique so that the long side will fit the convex surface of the aortic arch (Fig. 5–1, k). The distal anastomosis is completed with a 4–0 suture. Additional interrupted sutures are placed in both anastomoses to control bleeding. The distal anastomosis may be reinforced with a collar graft of 8- to 10-mm woven Dacron tubing or a strip of felt material (Fig. 5–1, l). When the right or left coronary artery originates high in the aorta, the excision and proximal anastomosis may be performed below the coronary ostium. After the anastomosis to the Dacron graft, the coronary vessel may be reimplanted into the graft, either directly or by interposing a short segment of autologous saphenous vein graft (Fig. 5–1, m).

DISSECTING ANEURYSM OF THE ASCENDING AORTA

When the aneurysm is produced by an acute or chronic aortic dissection, the technique of repair varies only slightly from that used for a fusiform aneurysm of the ascending aorta. The cavae are occluded over the cannulae with caval clamps as total perfusion is started (Fig. 5–2, a). After the clamp is placed across the distal portion of the ascending aorta, the outer false lumen is opened and blood and thrombi are removed (Fig. 5–2, b). The point of intimal tear is usually identified just above the aortic valve and coronary ostia, located proximally. Often the dissecting process has extended proximally and separated the aortic commissures from their mural attachments, a condition which causes the leaflets to prolapse downward and produce aortic regurgitation. While repair of such valves may be occasionally successful, our experience indicates that the valve should almost always be replaced with a prosthesis (Fig. 5–2, c).

After the proximal portion of the dissecting aneurysm is resected down to the annulus, the distal end is repaired. Usually the dissection has extended beyond the level of the aortic clamp. An attempt is made to obliterate the false lumen by suturing the inner and outer coats together (Fig. 5–2, d). This may not be totally effective in obliterating the distal process, but application of an encircling band of graft to reinforce the anastomosis discourages extension of the dissecting process. Long-term results have been acceptable, and recurrence of the aneurysm in the transverse aortic arch rarely causes complications.

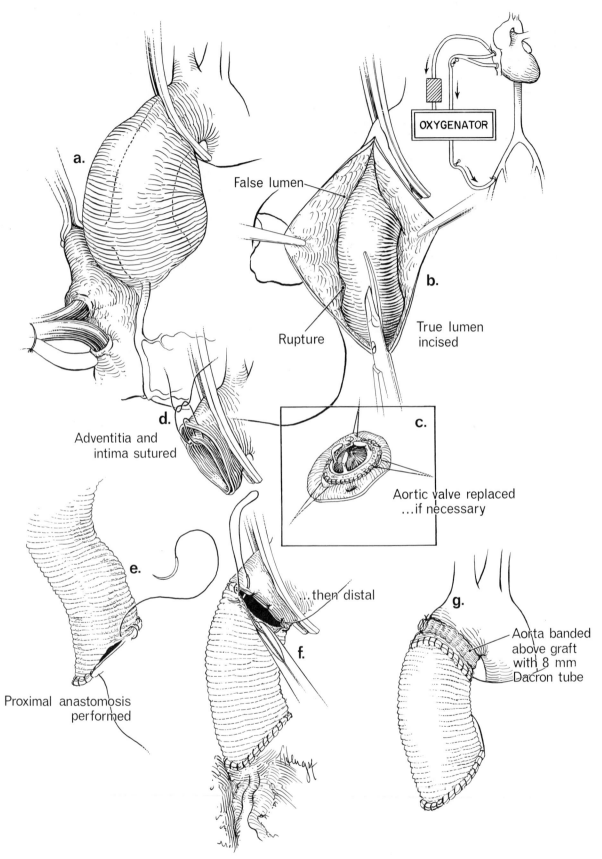

a.

False lumen

Rupture

True lumen
incised

b.

d.

Adventitia and
intima sutured

c.

Aortic valve replaced
...if necessary

OXYGENATOR

e.

Proximal anastomosis
performed

...then distal

f.

g.

Aorta banded
above graft
with 8 mm
Dacron tube

Figure 5–2 Repair of dissecting aneurysm of the ascending aorta.

After the proximal end of the graft is beveled to fit the shape and diameter of the proximal aorta, the anastomosis is effected with a continuous running suture of 3–0 or 4–0 polyester (Fig. 5–2, e). Distally, the anastomosis is performed in a similar fashion. After the air has been evacuated from the left ventricle and ascending aortic graft, the caval and aortic clamps are released (Fig. 5–2, f). To prevent disruption of the distal anastomosis or aneurysm formation at or beyond the suture line, the important final step is to apply a Dacron tube as a reinforcing collar (Fig. 5–2, g).

ANEURYSMS OF THE ASCENDING AORTA AND TRANSVERSE AORTIC ARCH

These lesions present a major technical problem for successful surgical treatment because resection requires that the cerebral circulation through the carotid and vertebral arteries be temporarily interrupted.[9] Preservation of cerebral viability in our experience has been difficult to accomplish with acceptable consistency when techniques of individual perfusion of arch tributaries have been employed (Fig. 5–3, a to e). Recently, we have induced so-called "deep" total body hypothermia to protect the brain during the period of circulatory arrest, and results have improved substantially (Fig. 5–3, f and g). Other techniques involving temporary bypass grafts have been discontinued (Fig. 5–3, h to l).

ARCH ANEURYSM — RESECTION UNDER DEEP HYPOTHERMIA WITH CIRCULATORY ARREST

Usually a median sternotomy incision is employed for arch resection. Under hypothermia with circulatory arrest, cannulation of each of the venae cavae for venous outflow is preferred, but when the aneurysm is large, a single catheter in the right atrium may be adequate. In extremely large lesions a venous catheter may be inserted first by way of a common femoral vein into the inferior vena cava, even before making the thoracotomy incision. Cannulation for return of oxygenated blood from the pump oxygenator should be through the common femoral artery. To ensure a more even distribution of cooling throughout the body, particularly the brain, a separate cannulation of the ascending aorta is desirable if it can be accomplished without disturbing the aneurysm or producing embolization from a laminated thrombus or from atherosclerotic debris.

Cooling proceeds at a gradual rate. When the body temperature falls below 25° C, ventricular fibrillation often occurs, and, if the aortic valve is incompetent, the left ventricle should be protected against overdistention by occasional manual cardiac compression. The cooling process should continue slowly for approximately 30 minutes to assure uniform distribution of the hypothermic state.

During the period of cooling, the arteries on the aortic arch (innominate, left common carotid, and left subclavian) are dissected in the superior mediastinum. In the actual case depicted (Fig. 5–4, a to g), the patient had severe aortic incompetence. Therefore, while the hypothermic state was being produced slowly, the aortic valve was excised and replaced with an aortic valve prosthesis (Cooley-Cutter low profile valve). After cooling was completed, these vessels (which now contained cold blood) were cross-clamped before arterial perfusion was discontinued.

At 12 to 14° C the pump to the arterial line was stopped and the arterial line was clamped to prevent air from backing up into it (Fig. 5–4, b). The venous outlet cannulae were permitted to drain into the reservoir in the extracorporeal line until no

Text continued on page 80.

TOTAL PERFUSION:

PROXIMAL ARCH

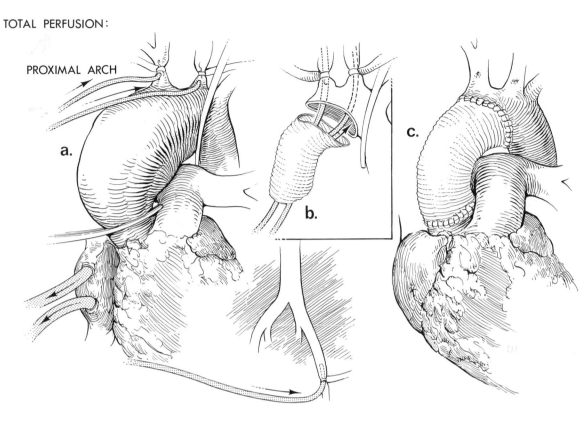

ENTIRE ARCH

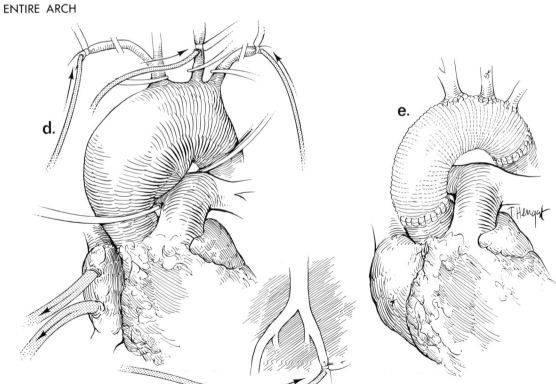

Figure 5–3 *a* to *g* Techniques of perfusion during arch resection that have been used successfully in previous years. Continuous perfusion of carotid and vertebral arteries may be utilized by individual cannulation of these vessels, using a connector to the arterial line from the pump oxygenator.

Illustration continued on opposite page.

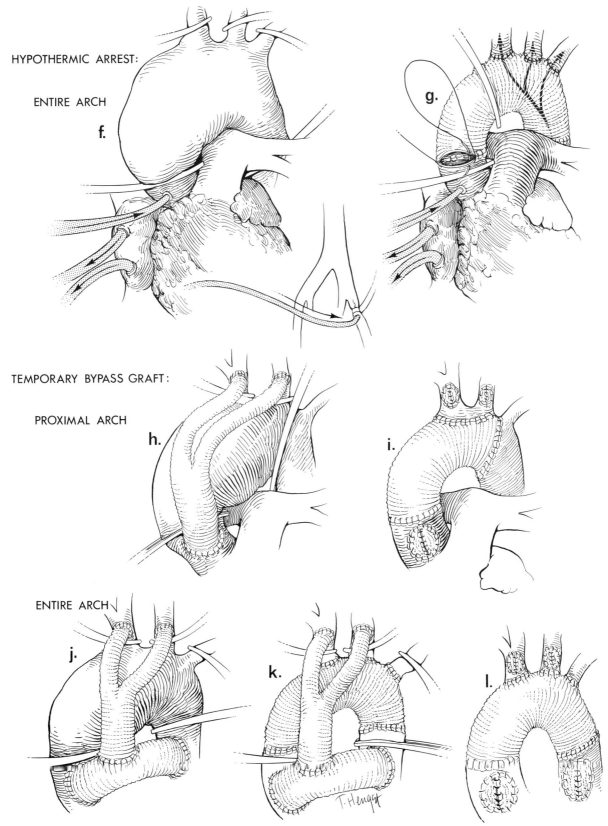

HYPOTHERMIC ARREST:

ENTIRE ARCH

f.

g.

TEMPORARY BYPASS GRAFT:

PROXIMAL ARCH

h.

i.

ENTIRE ARCH

j.

k.

l.

T. Henage

Figure 5–3 *Continued.*   *h* to *i*   When anatomic conditions are favorable, and when facilities for cardio-pulmonary bypass are not available, carotid perfusion may be obtained by implantation of a temporary Dacron bifurcation graft from the proximal ascending aorta to the common carotid arteries. If the aneurysm is confined to the aortic arch proximal to the subclavian artery, the excised segment may be replaced by a Dacron fabric graft (*h, i*). After this is accomplished, the temporary graft may be removed. For more extensive arch aneurysms, the techniques shown in *j, k,* and *l* may be employed.

These techniques were used in previous years and, while still useful under special circumstances, they have been generally replaced by more direct methods, using pump oxygenators.

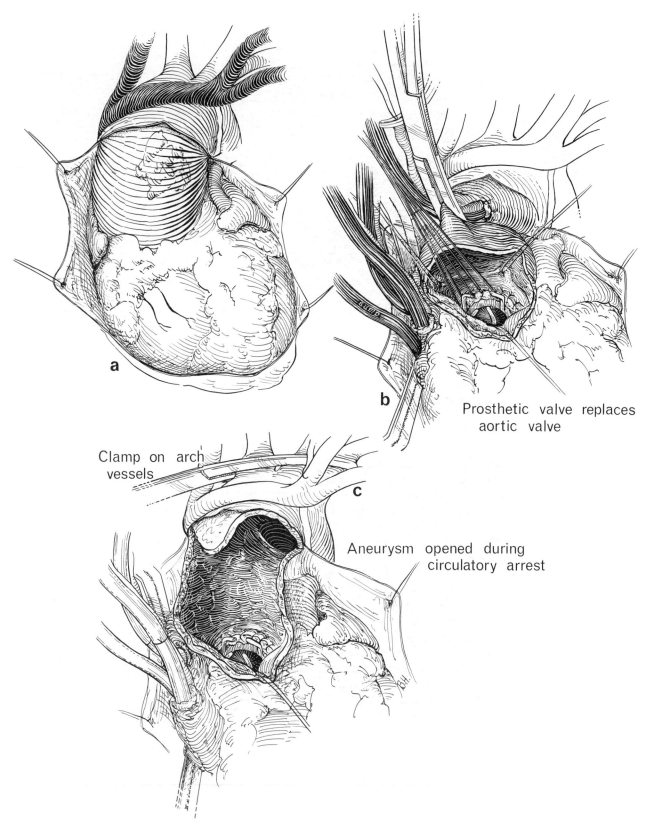

a

b

Prosthetic valve replaces
aortic valve

Clamp on arch
vessels

c

Aneurysm opened during
circulatory arrest

Figure 5–4 Resection of arch aneurysm under deep hypothermia with circulatory arrest.

Illustration continued on opposite page.

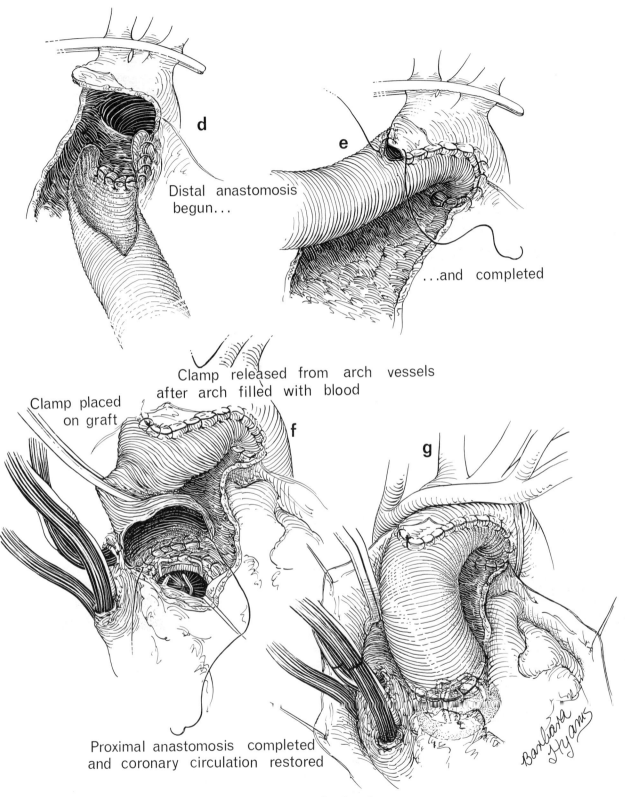

d Distal anastomosis begun...

e ...and completed

Clamp released from arch vessels after arch filled with blood

Clamp placed on graft

f

g

Proximal anastomosis completed and coronary circulation restored

Barbara Hyams

Figure 5–4 *Continued.*

more blood would drain. With the arch vessels cross-clamped and with cold oxygenated blood entrapped, cerebral air embolism could not occur.

After total circulatory arrest had been obtained, the ascending aorta and aneurysm were incised widely (Fig. 5–4, c). The outer curvature of the transverse arch was preserved intact and sutured into the Dacron graft as a unit without performing individual anastomoses (Fig. 5–4, d). A tightly woven low-porosity Dacron graft was then tapered and tailored to conform to the defect in the arch. Excision of the entire aneurysmal wall was not indicated and the distal anastomosis was accomplished expeditiously by suturing inside the evacuated aneurysm (Fig. 5–4, d and e). The distal anastomosis was performed with a 48-inch double-armed braided 3–0 polyester suture. The distal dissection and anastomosis were accomplished without injury to the left recurrent laryngeal nerve encircling the aorta distal to the ligamentum arteriosum.

When the distal anastomosis was completed and the arch vessels were properly implanted into the graft, the arterial pump was restarted, infusing blood into the femoral arterial cannula, and the aorta was refilled with cold oxygenated blood (Fig. 5–4, f). When all the air was driven out of the aorta and graft, the graft was clamped proximal to the innominate artery. The clamp was then removed from the arch vessels and the anastomosis was carefully inspected for leaks, which were repaired with individual sutures (Fig. 5–4, g).

Rewarming of the patient was commenced and gradually continued over the ensuing 45 minutes. During the rewarming period, the proximal aortic anastomosis was performed. The graft was cut and tapered to conform to the aortic root. *(The tendency in our experience has been to make the new ascending limb too short, and this may place tension on the proximal suture line.)* The proximal anastomosis was completed with a 3–0 braided polyester suture. *(A monofilament polyester or polyethylene suture is never used. It is our opinion that whenever an aortic or arterial anastomosis is performed to a fabric graft a braided suture should be used. The rigid textile graft places excessive stress on monofilament sutures and subsequently may cause them to fracture.)*

When the patient's body temperature rose to 36° C and cardiac output was restored by defibrillation and electrical countershock, the cardiopulmonary bypass was discontinued.

Most patients recover consciousness within four to six hours, as did this patient.

ANEURYSM OF A CERVICAL AORTIC ARCH

Rarely, aneurysms of the aortic arch are found with congenital anomalies. Cervical aortic arch is an anomaly which results when embryologic vascular arches fail to fuse and resorb in the normal manner, so that continuity between the ascending and descending aorta is established through a circuitous route, with the arch rising high in the cervical region.

A young adult patient presented at our institution with a pulsation on the right side of his neck that was progressively increasing in size. The lesion was demonstrated angiographically to be an aneurysm of a right cervical aortic arch (Fig. 5–5). Repair of the anomaly was achieved without using extracorporeal circulation and by creating a new intrathoracic arch.

The steps in the correlation are illustrated in Figure 5–6, a to l. A midline sternotomy incision was made with extension into the right supraclavicular space (Fig. 5–6, b). The patient had a ventricular septal defect, which was repaired in the standard manner by using temporary cardiopulmonary bypass (Fig. 5–6, c). The septal defect was closed with interrupted sutures and the ventriculotomy incision was repaired. Cannulae were removed from the venae cavae and the vascular repair was accomplished. Dissection of the cervical arch and arch vessels revealed that the

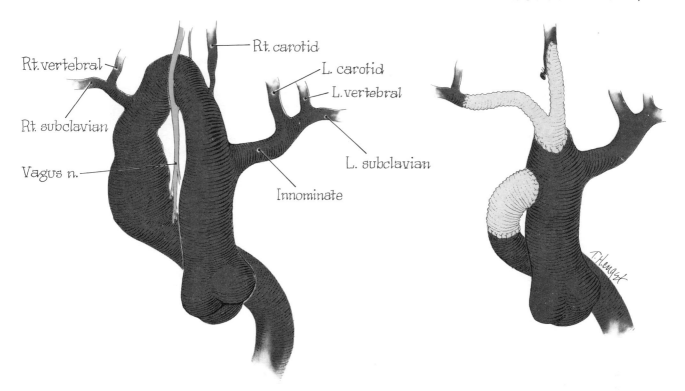

Figure 5–5 Right cervical arch with aneurysm.

right common carotid artery was stenotic at its orifice, and pulsation in the artery was almost absent.

The first step in the operation was to bypass the anomalous aneurysmal arch. The descending limb of the arch was cross-clamped and the aorta was divided (Fig. 5–6, *d*). A 16 mm woven Dacron graft was sutured to the distal descending thoracic aorta with braided polyester suture (Fig. 5–6, *e*). A curved vascular clamp was then applied tangentially to the side of the ascending aorta and the graft was anastomosed to the aorta (Fig. 5–6, *f*). Interruption of circulation to the lower body did not exceed 30 minutes, and there were no neurologic sequelae from the temporary spinal cord ischemia. The proximal portion and remainder of the anomalous arch were then excised. A woven Dacron bifurcation graft 12 × 6 mm was utilized to restore continuity (Fig. 5–6, *h* to *l*).

The final three anastomoses were done in the following sequence: an end-to-side carotid anastomosis (Fig. 5–6, *g* to j), an end-to-end aortic anastomosis (Fig. 5–6, *k*), and finally an end-to-end subclavian anastomosis (Fig. 5–6, *l*). A total of five anastomoses were performed. The patient recovered fully from the repair of this complex anomaly without neurologic sequelae.

This case serves to illustrate the technique of repairing complex anomalies with the use of vascular prostheses and an assortment of vascular clamps with different shapes and configurations. Other similar techniques for vascular reconstruction of congenital anomalies of the aortic arch are found in the chapter dealing with vascular ring and retroesophageal subclavian artery (Chapter 12, Congenital Arterial Anomalies).

FUSIFORM AND SACCIFORM ANEURYSMS OF THE DESCENDING THORACIC AORTA

Resection of aneurysms of the descending thoracic aorta is complicated by the need for protection of the spinal cord from ischemic damage during the period of

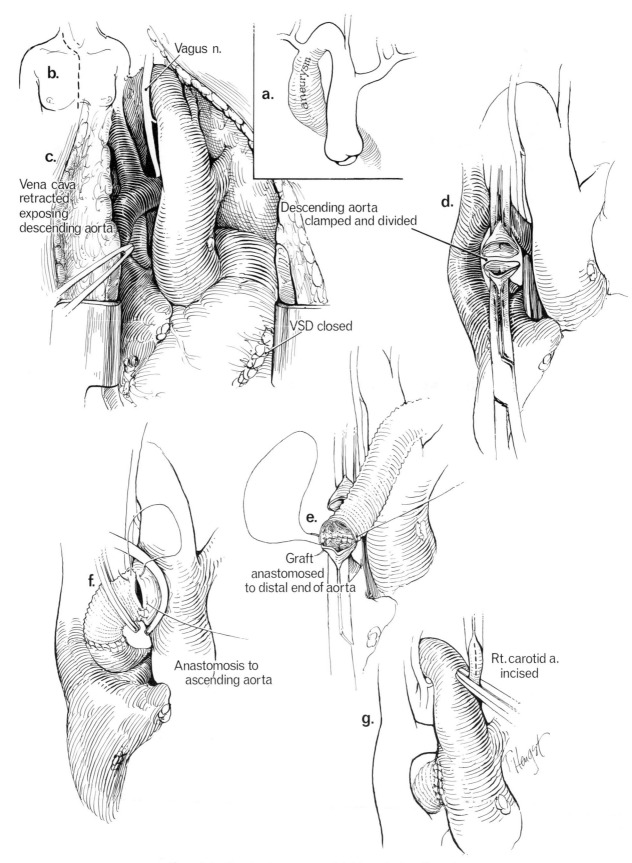

Vagus n.

a.

b.

c.

Vena cava
retracted
exposing
descending aorta

Descending aorta
clamped and divided

d.

VSD closed

e.

Graft
anastomosed
to distal end of aorta

f.

Anastomosis to
ascending aorta

g.

Rt. carotid a.
incised

Figure 5–6 Repair of aneurysm of right cervical aortic arch.

Illustration continued on opposite page.

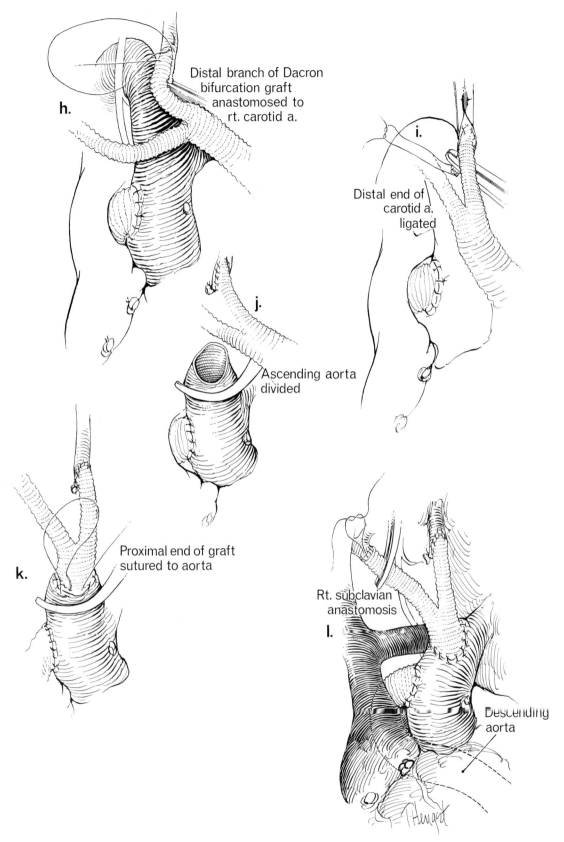

h. Distal branch of Dacron bifurcation graft anastomosed to rt. carotid a.

i. Distal end of carotid a. ligated

j. Ascending aorta divided

k. Proximal end of graft sutured to aorta

l. Rt. subclavian anastomosis

Descending aorta

Figure 5–6 *Continued.*

temporary interruption of aortic circulation.[10] Our first experience with such operations involved the use of extracorporeal circuits to provide for perfusion of the lower half of the body during this period. In the majority of patients so managed, neurologic sequelae did not occur, and renal and hepatic functions were not impaired. We attributed this success to the extracorporeal circulatory support system. Another technique, in which a pump oxygenator was used for bypass by femoral vein to femoral artery, was employed for several years; results were moderately satisfactory. Recently, however, we discontinued the use of such temporary circulatory conduits and results were equally good.

By eliminating the bypass technique, certain complications that occasionally resulted from left atrial or vascular cannulations were avoided. Also, in those patients in whom a pump oxygenator was placed in the circuit for perfusion by femoral vein or inferior vena cava to femoral artery, full heparinization of the patient was necessary. This, plus the use of a bubble oxygenator, seemed to increase the amount of postoperative bleeding.

At present, we believe that all aneurysms of the descending thoracic aorta may be resected without the use of extracorporeal circuits. The surgeon should proceed with a carefully planned strategy to minimize the period of aortic occlusion. In most instances this period is less than 30 minutes. We believe that partial systemic heparinization protects the spinal cord, abdominal viscera, and lower body from thromboses, particularly microthromboses. Before cross-clamping the aorta, we administer heparin, 2.0 mg/kg of body weight, intravenously.

For aneurysm of the proximal descending aorta, the patient is placed in the right true lateral position with the left arm extended forward. An arterial line is placed in the right radial artery for continuous monitoring of blood pressure. If the pressure exceeds 180 mm Hg the anesthesiologist may cautiously increase the depth of anesthesia or administer vasodilator drugs. A standard posterolateral incision is made by entering the fourth intercostal space. The incision usually extends forward, below, and medial to the nipple. The fifth rib may be divided posteriorly to give adequate exposure. The proximal aorta is dissected first, usually dividing the ligamentum arteriosum (Fig. 5–7, a). An attempt should always be made to preserve the recurrent laryngeal nerve. The aorta proximal and distal to the aneurysm is then cross-clamped and the aneurysm incised longitudinally (Fig. 5–7, b). Segmental intercostal, bronchial, and mediastinal vessels that appear in the aorta are oversewn.

The proximal and distal ends of the aorta are prepared for anastomosis. It is not necessary to divide the aorta completely since the anastomosis can be made to an open orifice with the aorta still attached to the aneurysm posteriorly. A woven low-porosity Dacron graft is selected that conforms to the aortic diameter (usually 26 to 30 mm). Both anastomoses are performed with double needle, 3–0 polyester braided suture, 48 inches in length (Fig. 5–7, c to f). When the aneurysm extends far distally, it may be easier to begin with the distal anastomosis, but usually the proximal one is done first.

After both anastomoses are completed, the distal aortic clamp is released (Fig. 5–7, h). A 19-gauge needle is inserted into the graft to evacuate air. The proximal clamp is released gradually, and the blood pressure is constantly observed to prevent atrial hypotension. A proper valvular clamp facilitates this step. If the aneurysm extends proximal to the origin of the left subclavian artery, a 10 mm woven Dacron graft may be used to restore continuity of that vessel. The subclavian artery should never be simply ligated because in adult patients ischemic damage to the left forearm and hand will almost always result. Bleeding points in the anastomoses are controlled with individual sutures. Each anastomosis should have a Dacron velour graft collar wrap applied for hemostasis and reinforcement. Heparin is reversed by injection of protamine sulfate.

The final step consists in removing the remaining thrombus from the aneurysm and closing the residual aneurysm walls on the graft. One should avoid the impulse

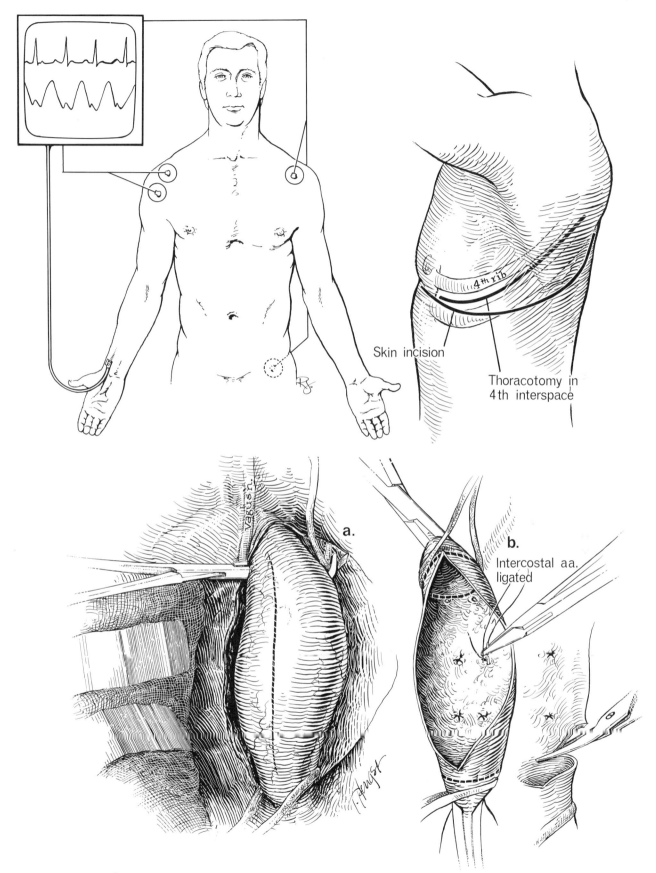

Skin incision

Thoracotomy in
4th interspace

Figure 5–7   Repair of fusiform and sacciform aneurysms of the descending thoracic aorta.

Illustration continued on following page.

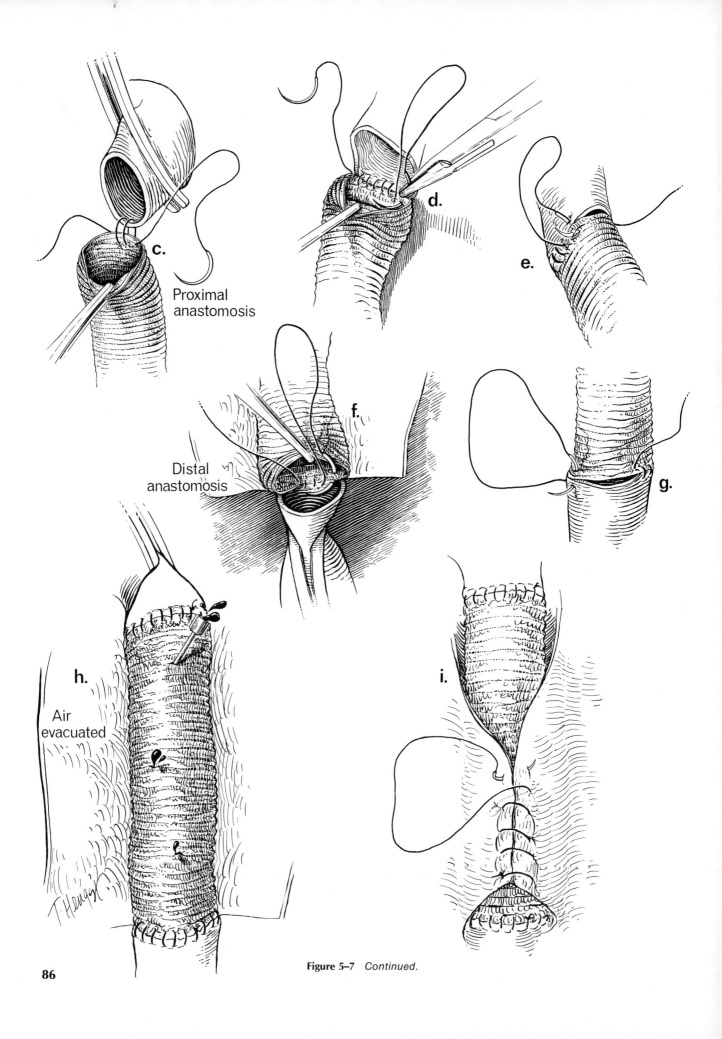

c.

Proximal
anastomosis

d.

e.

Distal
anastomosis

f.

g.

h.

Air
evacuated

i.

T. Henry

86

Figure 5–7 *Continued.*

to resect the aneurysm completely because extensive dissection of the lesion may lead to pulmonary trauma and troublesome hemorrhage from surrounding structures. If the aneurysm is extensive, a double thoracotomy through the posterolateral skin incision may enhance the performance of proximal and distal anastomoses. Thus an upper fourth intercostal opening may be used for exposing the proximal suture line, and an additional second incision may be made lower, in the eighth interspace, to expose the distal anastomosis.

DISSECTING ANEURYSM OF THE DESCENDING THORACIC AORTA

Surgical treatment of this lesion differs only slightly from the methods outlined for fusiform aneurysm of the descending aorta. The site of origin for the dissecting process is often the region just distal to the ligamentum arteriosum and the origin of the left subclavian artery from the aortic arch. The dissecting process may be confined to the thoracic aorta distally but often extends below the diaphragm and into the abdominal aorta and branches.[11]

The lesion is approached through a left posterolateral thoracotomy, entering the fourth intercostal space (Fig. 5–8, a). The fifth rib may be divided posteriorly for additional exposure. The aorta proximal to the aneurysm is mobilized and encircled with an umbilical tape. Usually the tape should be passed proximal to the origin of the left subclavian artery and distal to the common carotid. An effort should be made to spare the vagus and recurrent laryngeal nerves in the surgical dissection, but this is not always possible if extensive fibrosis is present. Distally, the aorta below the aneurysm is encircled with a tape.

Preparations are then made for circulatory bypass by using cannulation of the femoral vein and artery. Heparin, 2.0 mg/kg of body weight, is administered. The aorta proximal and distal to the aneurysm is cross-clamped and the aneurysm is opened. Back bleeding from intercostal and bronchial vessels is controlled with multiple sutures (Fig. 5–8, b). A tightly woven preclotted Dacron tube graft of appropriate size is used to restore aortic continuity.

Either anastomosis may be done first. When the distal anastomosis must be made deep in the cardiophrenic recess just proximal to the origin of the celiac axis in the abdominal aorta, we find it technically easier to do the distal anastomosis first, so that the free end of the graft may be manipulated for better exposure. In the drawing, the proximal anastomosis is performed first by using a continuous running suture of 3–0 braided polyester suture (Fig. 5–8, c). When this anastomosis is completed, the suture line is tested by partially releasing the proximal clamp to identify gaps in the anastomosis. These are closed with interrupted sutures and the proximal clamp is reapplied.

The distal anastomosis is then completed in a similar manner by suturing both walls of the aneurysm to the graft (Fig. 5–8, d). Several sutures, or even a continuous suture, may be used to approximate the two walls before the anastomosis is performed. The distal clamp is partially released and again gaps in the anastomosis are closed with interrupted sutures. When bleeding from the anastomosis has been controlled, the proximal clamp is released. Protamine sulfate, 3.5 mg/kg of body weight, is administered. As coagulability is restored, bleeding from the graft and anastomotic sites ceases. The proximal and distal anastomoses are then reinforced with collars by using tubes of woven Dacron. If necessary, several such reinforcements may be applied distally to prevent dilatation of the lower segment (Fig. 5–8, e).

Finally, the residual portion of the aneurysm wall is sutured over the graft and the mediastinal pleura is closed. The chest is closed with underwater sealed drainage.

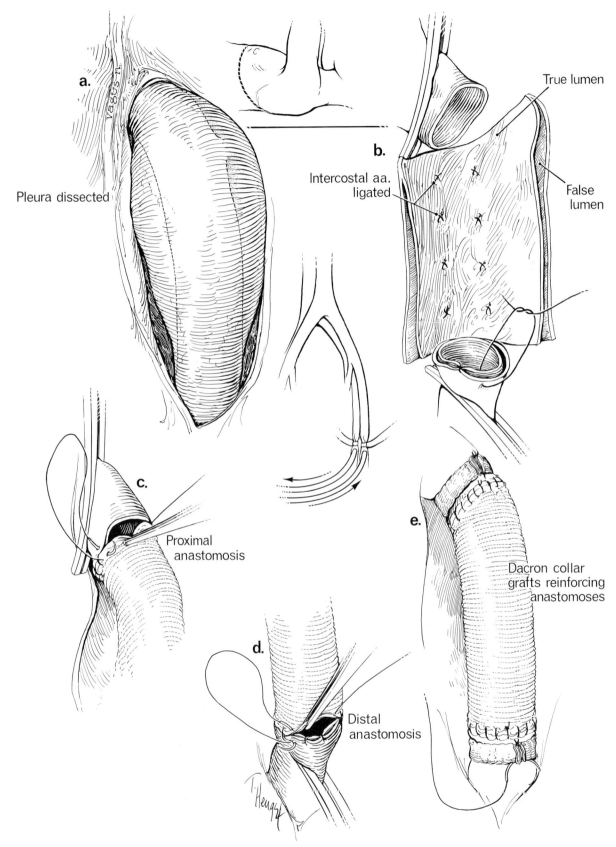

a.

Pleura dissected

Vagus n.

b.

True lumen

Intercostal aa.
ligated

False
lumen

c.

Proximal
anastomosis

e.

Dacron collar
grafts reinforcing
anastomoses

d.

Distal
anastomosis

T. Henry

Figure 5–8   Repair of dissecting aneurysm of the descending thoracic aorta.

LARGE DISSECTING ANEURYSM OF THE DESCENDING AORTA EXTENDING INTO THE ABDOMINAL AORTA

When a dissecting aneurysm reaches an enormous size and the diameter is large at the aortic hiatus in the diaphragm, the distal anastomosis may be impossible to achieve through the thoracotomy incision (Fig. 5–9, a). In these situations the distal anastomosis may be performed through a separate incision into the left upper abdomen (Fig. 5–9, b).

The patient is placed in a semilateral or lateral position on the operating table and the fourth or fifth intercostal space is opened in standard fashion. After it is determined that the distal aortic anastomosis would be difficult or impossible to complete through the thoracotomy, an incision may be made through the ninth intercostal space to enter the abdomen. The abdominal aorta is exposed extraperitoneally. After heparin, 2.0 mg/kg of body weight, is administered intravenously, the aorta is cross-clamped below the renal arteries but proximal to the aortic bifurcation (Fig. 5–9, c). A longitudinal incision is made in the aorta and a 20 to 24 mm Dacron graft is sutured by an end-to-side technique with the use of 3–0 braided polyester suture. A clamp is placed on the graft and the aortic clamps are released. Bleeding points on the anastomosis are repaired with individual sutures.

Attention is directed to the proximal anastomosis. The aorta proximal to the origin of the left subclavian artery and ligamentum arteriosum is cross-clamped. The left subclavian artery is clamped separately (Fig. 5–9, d). A distal clamp is applied at the diaphragmatic hiatus and the aneurysm is incised longitudinally; thrombus is removed from the false lumen and the true lumen is identified and opened widely. Segmental vessels, which may be found in both the true and false lumens, are then oversewn inside the aneurysm. An incision is made through the diaphragm and the graft is drawn up to the level of the proximal aorta. The origin of the dissecting process can usually be found just distal to the ligamentum and the left subclavian artery at the aortic isthmus. The proximal anastomosis is completed end-to-end. The clamp on the distal end of the graft is released first and air is evacuated from the graft with a 19-gauge needle. The clamp is then released on the left subclavian artery and bleeding points on the proximal anastomosis are repaired. Finally, the clamp on the proximal aortic arch is removed gradually, permitting redistribution of blood supply between the upper and lower halves of the body. Protamine sulfate is administered to reverse the heparin.

The final step in the operation consists of oversewing and ligating the distal stump of the thoracic aorta (Fig. 5–9, f and g). This must be done carefully and securely because both early and late hemorrhage may occur from the aortic stump. The aneurysmal wall is then sutured over the graft in the usual manner (Fig. 5–9, g and h). The completed surgical technique is shown in Figure 5–9, i.

There are several advantages in the use of this technique. Since the distal anastomosis is performed below the anatomic zone of the aorta from which blood supply to the spinal cord and vital abdominal viscera is minimized, the period of circulatory interruption for those organs is spared, and confined only to the period during the proximal anastomosis — a time interval that may be less than 15 or 20 minutes. Another advantage of this abdominal bypass procedure is that the distal anastomosis is performed to a more normal aorta than if the anastomosis were made at the aortic hiatus in the diaphragm.

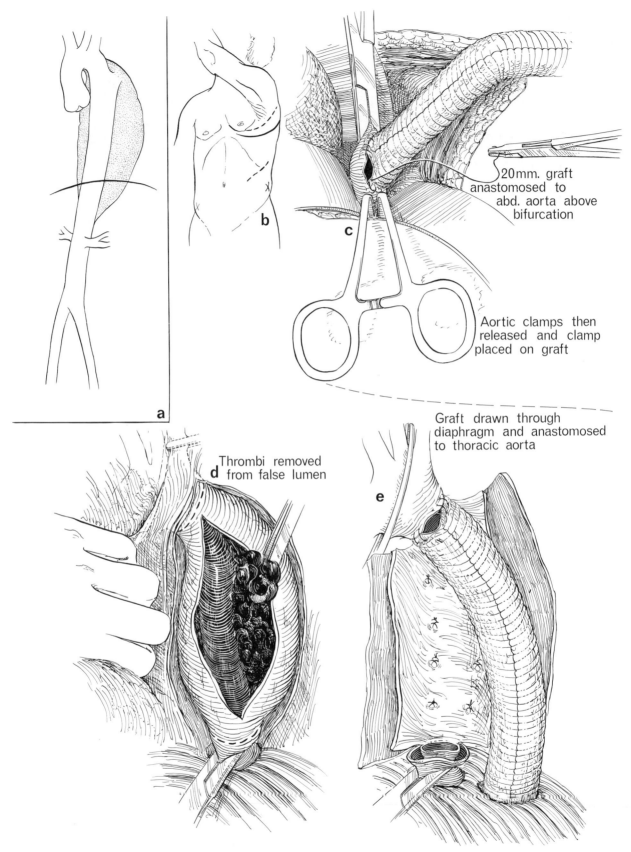

20mm. graft
anastomosed to
abd. aorta above
bifurcation

Aortic clamps then
released and clamp
placed on graft

Graft drawn through
diaphragm and anastomosed
to thoracic aorta

d Thrombi removed
from false lumen

Figure 5–9   Repair of large dissecting aneurysm of the descending aorta extending into the abdominal aorta.

Illustration continued on opposite page.

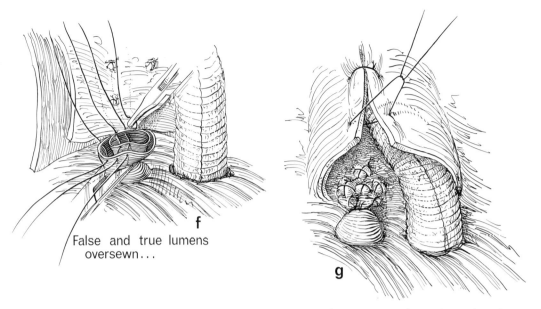

False and true lumens
oversewn...

and aneurysmal aorta sutured
around graft

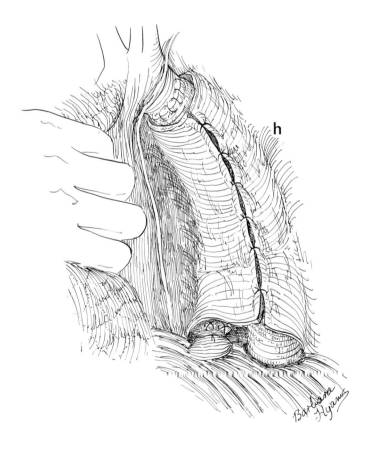

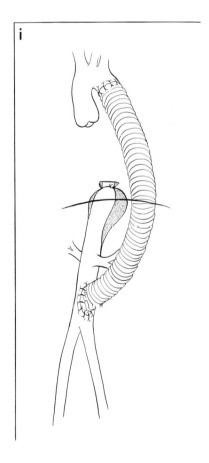

Figure 5–9 *Continued.*

FUSIFORM ANEURYSMS INVOLVING THE THORACIC AND ABDOMINAL AORTA (THORACIC ABDOMINAL ANEURYSMS)

These lesions provide a major technical challenge to the vascular surgeon and usually require exceptional surgical technique to achieve a successful result without disastrous complications. We do not believe the safety of the operation is enhanced by temporary extracorporeal circulation. The indications for operation should be carefully assessed and the risks explained to the patient. In the past, complicated and tedious techniques of restoring circulation to the abdominal viscera were utilized, and operations sometimes required eight to ten hours and use of multiple blood transfusions. We presently employ a simpler, more direct approach with emphasis on expeditious surgery, which limits the length of time that circulation to the abdominal viscera is interrupted. The accompanying drawings were made from a patient with an extensive aneurysm that involved the critical segment of aorta which provided circulation to the spinal cord, entire gastrointestinal tract, and kidneys (Fig. 5–10, *a*). The patient had no complications after operation and recovered completely.

Exposure of the aneurysm was obtained with a thoracoabdominal incision through the seventh intercostal space and by dividing the diaphragm (Fig. 5–10, *c*). Retroperitoneal dissection was used by reflecting the abdominal viscera toward the right. In some instances, removal of the spleen may be necessary. The left kidney was left in its natural position (Fig. 5–10, *d*). *We believe that leaving the kidney in the normal anatomic bed allows renal function to be preserved during and after operation.* After heparin, 3.0 mg/kg of body weight, was administered, the aorta proximally and the common iliac arteries distally were cross-clamped (Fig. 5–10, *e*). The left renal vein was then divided between vascular clamps, with the intention of restoring continuity later.

Vascular clamps were applied to the various visceral vessels as they were identified (Fig. 5–10, *f*). The aneurysm was opened widely and the orifices exposed inside the aneurysm. *This technique avoids the tedious dissection of the individual vessels before occluding the aorta.* The smaller intercostal and segmental vessels were oversewn, but one large pair of arteries was subsequently anastomosed to the graft. Proximal and distal anastomoses were performed first and aortic flow was re-established (Fig. 5–10, *h*).

Most of the remaining anastomoses were performed by using a strong partial occlusion clamp on the side of the Dacron graft. The anastomoses were performed in sequence as follows: right renal artery, celiac artery, superior mesenteric artery, and left renal artery (Fig. 5–10, *j* to *l*). The final arterial anastomosis was between the large intercostal vessels that presumably supplied the spinal cord. The left renal vein was anastomosed end-to-end. In some instances it may be possible to anastomose the celiac and superior mesenteric arteries as a single unit into the side of the graft (Fig. 5–10, *j* and *k*). The final result provided restoration of blood supply to all major arteries (Fig. 5–10, *m*).

REINFORCEMENT OF THORACIC ANEURYSMS

Resection of aneurysms of the thoracic aorta has been established as the procedure of choice whenever (1) circumstances warrant definitive surgery, (2) the anatomic factors permit resection with acceptable risk, and (3) the threat of rupture is imminent. Most of the indirect methods for control of aneurysms that were applied several decades ago have been discarded. In those days, attempts at reinforcement

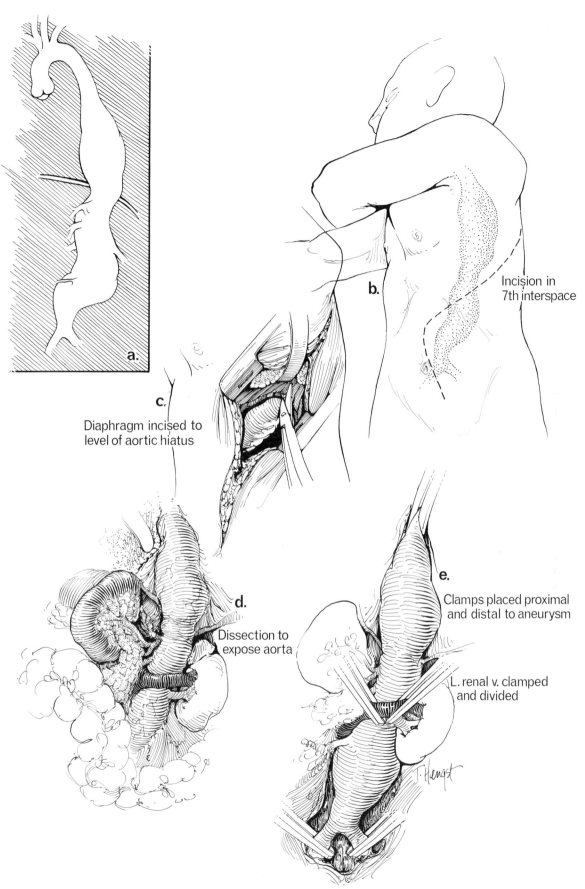

a.

b.

Incision in
7th interspace

c.

Diaphragm incised to
level of aortic hiatus

d.

Dissection to
expose aorta

e.

Clamps placed proximal
and distal to aneurysm

L. renal v. clamped
and divided

Figure 5–10 Repair of fusiform aneurysms involving the thoracic and abdominal aorta (thoraco-abdominal aneurysms).

Illustration continued on the following page.

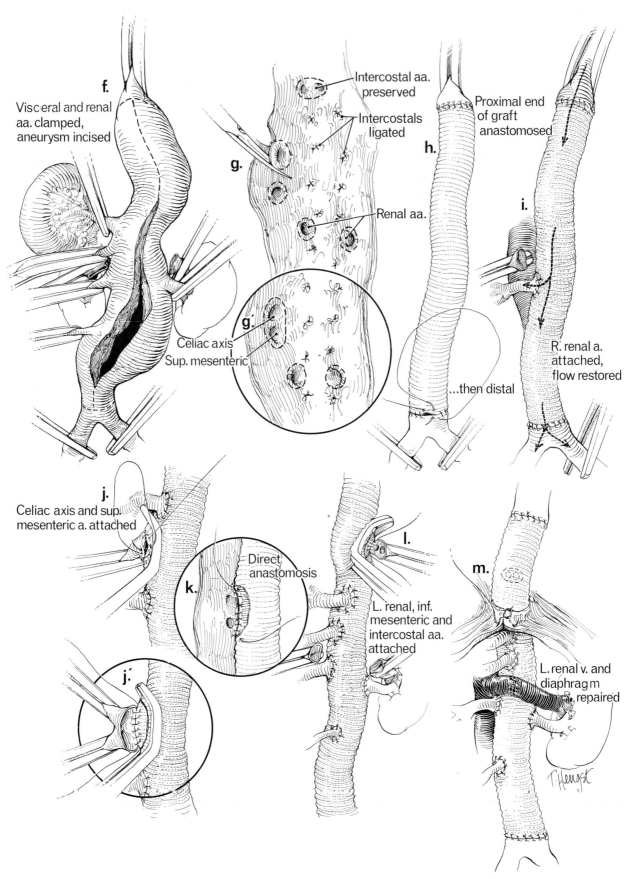

f. Visceral and renal aa. clamped, aneurysm incised

g. Intercostal aa. preserved

Intercostals ligated

Renal aa.

g. Celiac axis
Sup. mesenteric

h. Proximal end of graft anastomosed

...then distal

i. R. renal a. attached, flow restored

j. Celiac axis and sup. mesenteric a. attached

k. Direct anastomosis

j.

l. L. renal, inf. mesenteric and intercostal aa. attached

m. L. renal v. and diaphragm repaired

Figure 5–10 *Continued.*

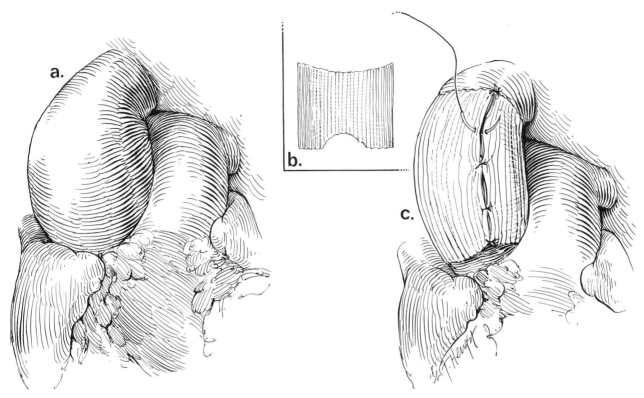

Figure 5–11 In some instances, a fusiform aneurysm of the thoracic aorta may be controlled by the use of a woven Dacron "wrap around" as shown.

were confined to the stimulation of thrombosis inside the sac, or to the promotion of fibrous thickening of the aneurysmal wall, which added strength, retarded expansion, and prevented possible rupture. Owing to lack of success, such methods of treatment were largely discarded.

Recently, however, these concepts of surgical treatment have been revived in a modified form. For example, we advocate the use of a woven Dacron tube to be used as a reinforcing collar on the aorta adjacent to aortic anastomoses to Dacron grafts. In some operations on the thoracic aorta, as many as six such tubes have been wrapped around a weak position of the vessel. This has helped in the repair and control of bleeding from the aortotomy site in those patients with severe poststenotic dilatation of the ascending aorta caused by long-standing aortic valve stenosis.[6]

In some instances a fusiform aneurysm of the thoracic aorta may be controlled by wrapping it with Dacron fabric. In the case shown in the illustration, a fusiform aneurysm of the ascending aorta is present (Fig. 5–11, a). Such lesions may be caused by either primary cystic medial necrosis or poststenotic dilatation.

Standard resection of an asymptomatic aneurysm by the use of temporary cardiopulmonary bypass could subject the patient to risk from serious complications, such as bleeding and embolism. If the intimal surface is known to be free from thrombus and atherosclerotic debris, satisfactory control may be achieved by using a woven Dacron "wrap-around" (Fig. 5–11, b and c). This method has proved to be satisfactory for many problems involving repair of the ascending aorta. The wrap technique and the collar-graft technique are also applicable to fusiform aneurysms involving the transverse aortic arch which have not become large enough to be densely adherent to the trachea or left mainstem bronchus. In the descending thoracic aorta, smaller fusiform aneurysms may be wrapped with Dacron fabric without interrupting aortic circulation. Therefore, external reinforcement of a weakened aortic wall may still have a place in aortic surgery.

REFERENCES

1. DeBakey ME, Cooley DA, Crawford ES, Morris GC Jr: Aneurysms of the thoracic aorta: Analysis of 179 patients treated by resection. J Thorac Cardiovasc Surg 36:393, 1958.
2. DeBakey ME, Beall AC Jr, Morris GC Jr, Garrett HE: Resection and graft replacement of aneurysms involving the transverse arch of the aorta. Surg Clin North Am 46:1057, 1966.
3. Wheat MW Jr: Treatment of dissecting aneurysms of the aorta: Current status. Prog Cardiovasc Dis 16:87, 1973.
4. Gore I, Hirst AE Jr: Dissecting aneurysm of the aorta. Prog Cardiovasc Dis 16:103, 1973.
5. Seybold-Epting W, Meyer J, Hallman GL, Cooley DA: Surgical treatment of acute dissecting aneurysm of ascending aorta. J Thorac Surg 18:43, 1977.
6. Buxton B, Harlan BJ, Cooley DA: Techniques of reinforcing the ascending thoracic aorta. Aust NZ J Surg 47:99, 1977.
7. Cooley DA, Mullins CE, Gooch JB: Aneurysm of right-sided cervical arch: Surgical removal and graft replacement. J Thorac Cardiovasc Surg 72:106, 1976.
8. Kidd JN, Reul GJ Jr, Cooley DA, Sandiford FM, Kyger ER III, Wukasch DC: Surgical treatment of aneurysms of the ascending aorta. Circulation 54 (Suppl 3):118, 1976.
9. Ventemiglia R, Oglietti J, Wukasch DC, Hallman GL, Cooley DA: Interruption of the aortic arch: Surgical considerations. J Thorac Cardiovasc Surg 72:235, 1976.
10. Buxton B, Harlan BJ, Cooley DA: Surgical treatment of fusiform thoracic aortic aneurysms by external reinforcement. Cardiovascular Diseases, Bulletin of the Texas Heart Institute, 3(#1):35, 1976.
11. Reul GJ Jr, Cooley DA, Hallman GL, Reddy SB, Kyger ER II, Wukasch DC: Dissecting aneurysm of the descending aorta: Improved surgical results in 91 patients. Arch Surg 110:632, 1975.

CHAPTER **6**

Renal Artery Stenosis and Renovascular Hypertension

INTRODUCTION

The role of hypertension as a contributing factor in mortality from cardiovascular disease has focused attention upon its diagnosis and treatment. Although hypertension is best controlled by medical therapy in the vast majority of patients, in many, surgical treatment may provide a more definitive result. Obstructive lesions of the renal arteries can produce so-called renovascular hypertension (RVH), primarily diastolic, and surgical correction of these lesions can produce complete relief.[1-3]

DEVELOPMENT OF SURGICAL TREATMENT FOR RENOVASCULAR HYPERTENSION

The relationship between blood pressure elevation and kidney function was first described in 1836 by Bright,[4] whose name is still associated with this syndrome. It was not until almost 100 years later, however, in 1926, that Callahan et al.[5] first performed direct renal artery surgery, ligating an aneurysm of a renal artery. Shortly thereafter, in 1934, Goldblatt[6] reported his classic experiment demonstrating that constriction of a renal artery produces atrophy of the involved kidney, resulting in hypertension. In a case of hypertension due to pyelonephritis, remission by nephrectomy was reported in 1937 by Butler.[7] The initial, significant description of fibromuscular dysplasia of a renal artery was reported in 1938 by Leadbetter et al.[8]

The mechanics of experimental renal hypertension were first explained in 1940 and 1941 by Page and associates,[9, 10] who investigated renin, the pressor substance in the kidney, and found that it required another substance, *renin activator,* working with it to produce pressor action.

In 1948, Mathé[11] first successfully resected an aneurysm of the renal artery, preserving the involved kidney. Thromboendarterectomy of both renal arteries for relief of hypertension was first reported in 1954 by Freeman et al.[12] During the years from 1957 to 1964, the interest stimulated by these initial successes led to rapid refinements in surgical techniques, which were described by Poutasse and Dustan,[1] DeCamp and Birchall,[2] and surgeons from our own center.[3]

Although these reports demonstrated that renovascular hypertension could be relieved in some cases, criteria for proper selection of patients awaited the development of more specific diagnostic tests. By means of intravenous pyelography (IVP), renal scans and renograms, attempts were made to determine which patients would benefit from surgical treatment.[13] Conclusive indications for patient selection awaited the significant development of split renal function studies by Stamey et al. in

1961[14] and Howard in 1962,[15] and for the description of a positive renal venous renin assay (RVRA) by Michelakis, Foster, et al. in 1967.[16] The role of renin in the production of RVH has been described previously by Irving Page[9] in his 1941 Janeway lecture at Mt. Sinai Hospital.

In recent years, major developments in the surgical treatment of RVH have included technical contributions such as the use of autogenous saphenous vein grafts by Wylie,[17] the development of a technique for dilatation of the renal arteries in fibromuscular dysplasia by Fry,[18] and a description from our institution of the "left renal lumbar vein" and its importance in facilitating exposure of the renal arteries.[19] Subsequent to the evolvement of effective surgical techniques, the major contribution to the surgical treatment of RVH has been the establishment of valid criteria for the diagnosis of RVH by Dean and Foster,[20] with indications for surgical treatment.

INCIDENCE OF RENOVASCULAR LESIONS

During our early experience with the management of RVH, the incidence of renovascular lesions was believed to approach 20 percent.[3] Subsequent experience, however, suggests that this figure was an overestimate resulting from the preselection of patients in our center. Although the exact incidence of RVH is unknown, we now concur with Foster[21] that approximately 5 to 10 percent of persons with predominant elevation of diastolic blood pressure will also have RVH.

PATHOPHYSIOLOGY

Page's theory, proposed in 1940,[9, 10] is still considered the best explanation of RVH production. This concept is that an obstructive lesion in a renal artery results in reduced renal artery perfusion or pulse pressure or both, triggering the release of renin by the juxtaglomerular apparatus of the kidney. Renin passes into the systemic circulation by way of the inferior vena cava and is converted into angiotensin, which produces hypertension. Although this mechanism forms the basis for one of the most reliable diagnostic tests for RVH, recent experimental evidence reported by Louis et al.[22] has questioned its validity.

CAUSES OF RENOVASCULAR HYPERTENSION

Arteriosclerotic occlusive lesions are the most common cause of RVH, occurring in approximately 73 percent of cases in our experience. The occlusive process originates in the proximal segment of the renal artery in 71 percent of patients. Such arteriosclerotic lesions most frequently involve the left renal artery, occur in an older age group, and are twice as common in men as in women.[13, 34]

Fibromuscular dysplasia, the second most common cause of RVH, was the contributing factor in approximately 12 percent of the patients in our series. This condition, for which the etiology is unknown, most often involves the right renal artery. The obstruction usually presents as diffuse involvement of the middle or distal renal artery, occurring more frequently in women by a ratio of nine to one, and in a younger age group with a mean age of 40 years.[13] This condition in the renal arteries is often associated with concomitant symptomatic fibromuscular dysplasia of the internal carotid arteries.[34] Dissection of the renal artery affected by fibromuscular dysplasia can occur spontaneously, producing partial or complete obstruction of the artery.[34] Revascularization of advanced fibromuscular dysplasia of the renal arteries in cases where it extends to the branch arteries may present a difficult technical problem. The technique of dilatation described by Fry[18, 23] appears to offer the best solution; however, the method of in vitro renal vascular reconstruction utilizing extracorporeal hypothermic continuous perfusion with transplantation of the kidney, as first described by Ota, Mori, and associates,[24] and modified by Blezer et al.,[25, 26] offers the best possibility of corrective surgery for otherwise inoperable lesions.

Renal artery aneurysms, the third most common kind of lesions that produce RVH, were seen in approximately 4 percent of our patients.[34] Controversery exists as to whether excision is indicated in the absence of definite evidence that the aneurysm is producing hypertension. If hypertension exists, lateralizing renal venous renin assays (RVRA) and split renal function studies (SRFS) should be performed to determine suitability for operation. Fry and associates[27] advise excision in all cases of ruptured renal artery aneurysms. The preferred method of excision in the distal renal artery includes transection of the renal artery and vein, extracorporeal hypothermic continuous perfusion, resection of the aneurysm and reconstruction of the renal artery with the use of microsurgical techniques, and autotransplantation of the kidney into the iliac fossa.[24, 25, 28]

Emboli to the renal arteries are usually manifest by acute renal insufficiency. When renal emboli are suspected, selective renal arteriography should be done and a Fogarty catheter embolectomy performed on an emergency basis.

Multiple renal arteries with or without stenotic lesions may be associated with hypertension.[34] Until recently, this syndrome was usually considered inoperable, but new microsurgical techniques with the use of extracorporeal hypothermic continuous perfusion may be applicable in these situations.[24, 25, 28, 29]

The crossing of two ipsilateral renal arteries can result in impingement, stenosis, and poststenotic dilatation, leading to RVH.[34] Thoracoabdominal aneurysms often produce renal artery occlusion by dissection of one or both renal arteries. Surgical treatment involves resection and replacement of the descending thoracic segment of the dissected thoracic aorta, restoring blood flow through the true lumen of the abdominal aorta, and thereby into the true lumen of the renal arteries.[30] Iatrogenic dissection of a normal renal artery (usually as a complication of aortography) can also produce renal artery obstruction and subsequent RVH.

DIAGNOSTIC TECHNIQUES AND INDICATIONS FOR OPERATION

After a history and physical examination, along with routine laboratory studies, the hypertensive patient is screened by means of rapid sequence intravenous pyelography (IVP). In our experience, IVP has disclosed an abnormality in only 70 percent of documented cases of RVH.[13] False negative IVP in patients with RVH has been reported at 31 percent by Foster et al.,[21] one-half of such instances occurring in patients with bilateral renal artery stenosis.

Because of the proven inadequacy of IVP as a screening technique, renal arteriography is also performed in all hypertensive patients to be evaluated for RVH. Translumbar aortography provides simplicity of performance as a screening procedure. Because of the posterior origin of the left renal artery and the posterior course of the renal arteries, both selective and oblique views may be necessary for visualizing lesions in the origin or distal third of these arteries. To demonstrate renal arterial anatomy, retrograde aortography will yield more precise information than will translumbar aortography. Retrograde or even antegrade selective renal arteriography may not be technically feasible, however, and actually may be contraindicated in the presence of diffuse arteriosclerotic disease; therefore, we believe that translumbar aortography continues to be the technique of choice in RVH evaluation of most patients who have diffuse aortoiliac occlusive disease.

The usefulness of split renal function tests (SRFT) and renal venous renin assays (RVRA) in predicting response to renal artery revascularization has been described by Dean and Foster,[20] and Buda et al.[31] The following considerations should be borne in mind: (1) Not all patients with renal artery lesions and hypertension have RVH; therefore, not all will respond to surgical therapy. (2) The hypertensive patient with unilateral renal artery stenosis and grossly elevated venous renin activity from the affected kidney will usually respond to surgical therapy. However, these two well-documented concepts concerning patient management raise problems involving the evaluation of patients with bilateral renal artery lesions, the interpretation of false positive or false negative SRFS and RVRA, and those situations in which deferring treatment to await RVRA results is not practical for optimum patient care. Our experience indicates a high correlation between operative pressure gradients and favorable surgical results.

Although the usefulness of SRFS and RVRA is duly recognized, these studies are not always practical, and operation is often recommended in the absence of conclusive test results. The presence of an arteriosclerotic obstructive lesion of a renal artery in a hypertensive patient is a valid indication for surgical treatment; otherwise, progression of the lesion to complete occlusion may result in ultimate loss of the kidney. This approach is particularly relevant if the patient is to undergo another intraabdominal vascular surgical procedure for abdominal aortic aneurysm or occlusive disease of the aorta and iliac or visceral arteries.

SURGICAL TECHNIQUES

Various surgical techniques of renal artery revascularization have been developed and described for individual renal artery lesions. Adequate exposure of the renal arteries is the key to obtaining optimum technical results.

EXPOSURE

A midline abdominal incision extending from the xiphoid to a point below the umbilicus provides maximum exposure and allows access for any concomitant procedures. The peritoneum overlying the aorta is incised, mobilizing the inferior mesenteric vein to the left and the duodenum to the right. The left renal vein overlying the left renal artery is transfixed by three major branches which limit its mobilization (Fig. 6–1, a). The most important of these branches is the left renal lumbar vein, which is present in 95 percent of patients in our experience.[19] When this large left renal lumbar vein and the testicular and adrenal tributaries are ligated, the left renal vein may be mobilized 6 to 7 cm in a cephalad direction (Fig. 6–1, b). By increasing the mobility of the left renal vein and the inferior cava, this maneuver provides excellent exposure of both renal arteries and precludes the necessity of transecting the left renal vein.[19]

LEFT RENAL ARTERY BYPASS

After mobilization and cephalad retraction of the left renal vein as described above, the left renal artery is occluded with vascular clamps and a 1 to 2 cm longitudinal arteriotomy is made in the artery (Fig. 6–2, a to c). An autogenous saphenous vein graft (Fig. 6–2, d) or a 7 mm double velour knitted Dacron graft*[32] is

---

*Meadox-Cooley Double Velous Graft, Meadox Medicals, 6 Raritan Road, Oakland, New Jersey 07436.

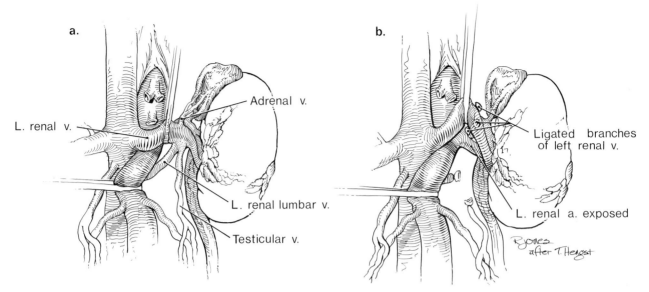

Figure 6–1 *a*, Drawing of branches of left renal vein demonstrating posterior location of left renal lumbar vein. *b*, Transected branches of left renal vein demonstrating mobility of left renal vein obtained by maneuver. (From Cooley DA, Wukasch DC: Surgical treatment of renovascular hypertension. Conn Med 42(7):423, 1978.)

tailored to match the arteriotomy (Fig. 6–2, *d*). An end-to-side anastomosis is performed using continuous polypropylene suture if a vein graft is used, or multifilament polyester suture if a Dacron graft is used (Fig. 6–2, *e* and *f*). The anastomosis is made by applying a partial occluding clamp to the abdominal aorta, and anastomosing the proximal end of the graft end-to-side to the aorta (Fig. 6–2, *g*).

RIGHT RENAL ARTERY LATERAL TO INFERIOR VENA CAVA

Lesions in the middle or distal third of the right renal artery require exposure of the artery lateral to the inferior vena cava (IVC), which is facilitated by first ligating the left renal lumbar vein, as described above, to obtain maximum cephalad mobilization of the left renal vein. The origin of the right renal artery is identified and the artery dissected posterior to the IVC. The IVC is mobilized and retracted to the left. The artery is dissected and the distal anastomosis is made as described above (Fig. 6–2, *h*). The graft is passed anterior to the IVC and anastomosed end-to-side to the abdominal aorta (Fig. 6–2, *i*).

RIGHT RENAL ARTERY BYPASS MEDIAL TO THE INFERIOR VENA CAVA

A proximal right renal artery lesion (Fig. 6–3, *a*) may be bypassed medial to the inferior vena cava (IVC). In such cases, the IVC is mobilized and retracted to the right (Fig. 6–3, *b*). This maneuver is facilitated by mobilizing the left renal vein after ligation of its three major tributaries, the most important being the left renal lumbar vein.[19] The distal and proximal anastomoses are made as described above.

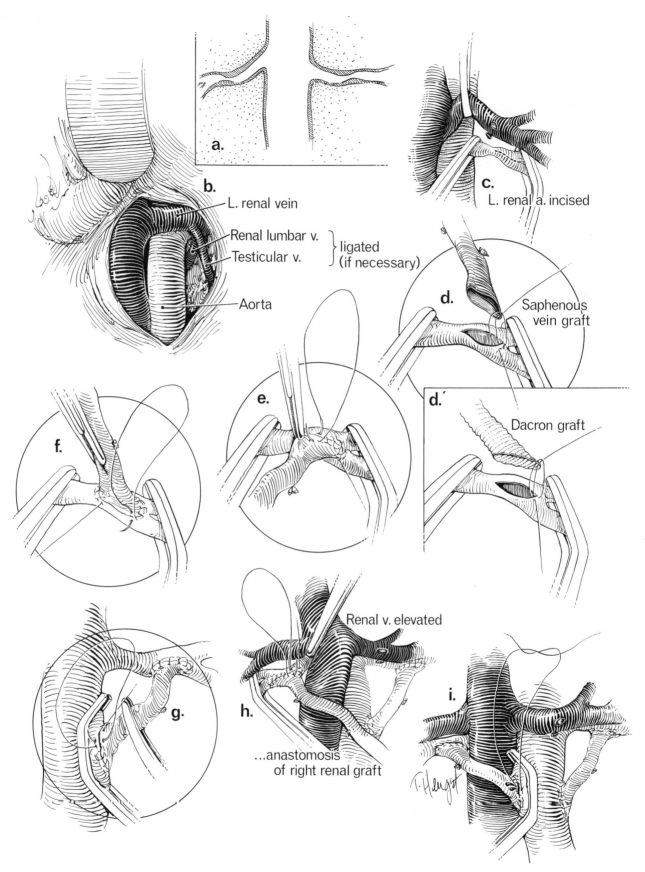

a.

b.

L. renal vein

Renal lumbar v.
Testicular v. } ligated
(if necessary)

Aorta

c.
L. renal a. incised

d.
Saphenous
vein graft

d.´
Dacron graft

e.

f.

g.

h.
...anastomosis
of right renal graft

Renal v. elevated

i.

Figure 6–2 Various surgical techniques of renal artery bypass. (From Cooley DA, Wukasch DC: Surgical treatment of renovascular hypertension. Conn Med 42(7):423, 1978.)

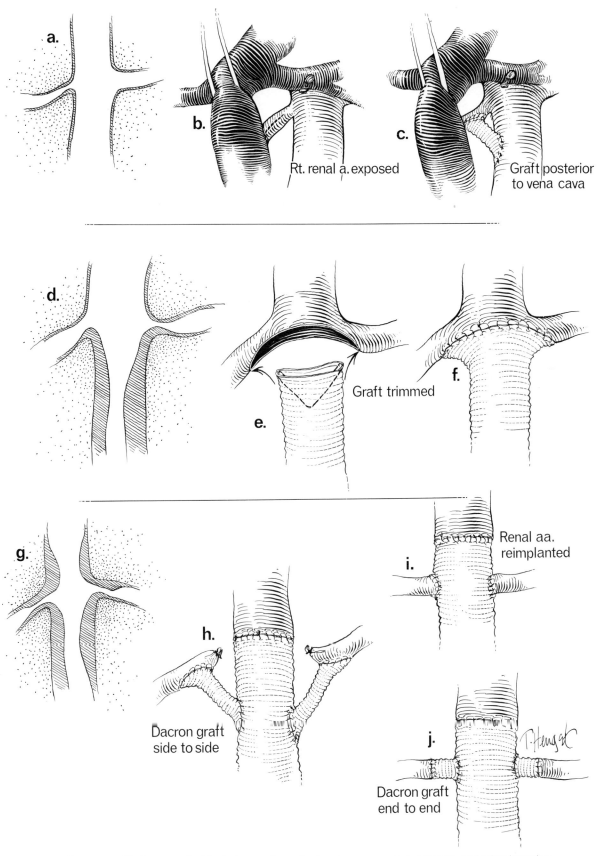

Figure 6–3 Various surgical techniques of renal artery bypass, endarterectomy, and reimplantation. (From Cooley DA, Wukasch DC: Surgical treatment of renovascular hypertension. Conn Med 42(7):423, 1978.)

ENDARTERECTOMY AND ARTERIOPLASTY

Patients having renal artery stenosis associated with aneurysms of the abdominal aorta (AAA) or aortoiliac occlusive disease (AIOD) and requiring concomitant aortic graft replacement are often best treated by this technique (Fig. 6–3, d). The proximal aorta is clamped above the renal arteries following intravenous administration of heparin and mannitol. The aorta is transected at the level of the renal arteries and an endarterectomy is performed under direct vision (Fig. 6–3, e). A double velour knitted Dacron graft[32] is tailored so that it forms "dog ears" to extend out each renal artery (see hyphenated line of Fig. 6–3, e). The graft is then anastomosed end-to-end to the proximal aorta and renal arteries (Fig. 6–3, f). The graft is clamped just distal to the anastomosis and the proximal aortic clamp is released to provide renal perfusion during performance of the distal graft anastomosis.

REIMPLANTATION OF RENAL ARTERIES

Patients with aneurysm of the abdominal aorta or with aortoiliac occlusive disease extending above the renal arteries require detachment of the renal arteries and reimplantation, with or without extension of these arteries by side grafts (Fig. 6–3, g). Adequate exposure of the aorta proximal to the renal arteries is facilitated by clamping the proximal aorta at the level of the diaphragm at the supraceliac bare area.[33] The renal arteries are then transected and reanastomosed into the aortic graft by one of the techniques shown in Figure 6–3, h to j.[34]

In all procedures described above, heparin (2 mg/kg body weight) is administered prior to occlusion of the renal arteries or aorta and reversed with protamine sulfate (ratio 1.5 mg protamine to 1.0 mg heparin) following restoration of flow.

RENAL ARTERY ANEURYSM

Aneurysms of the renal arteries may be of four types: (1) saccular, (2) fusiform distal to a stenotic lesion, (3) intrarenal, or (4) dissecting.[35, 36] When an aneurysm is associated with renal hypertension, as shown by lateralizing renal venous renin assays (RVRA), operative treatment is indicated. Another absolute indication for surgical intervention is in patients with acute dissection of a renal artery aneurysm. Because the natural history and incidence of rupture of renal artery aneurysms has not been clearly delineated, the rationale for operation to prevent rupture remains controversial.[27, 37, 38] The evidence available indicates that the factors associated with the propensity of renal artery aneurysms to rupture are noncalcification[37, 38] and large size.[36] In asymptomatic, normotensive patients without dissection, our policy is to recommend operation only when the aneurysm is noncalcified and greater than 2 cm in diameter.

Surgical technique necessarily varies according to the anatomy of the lesion. Proximal or midrenal artery aneurysms may be resected and the renal artery reconstructed, as described above for stenotic lesions (Fig. 6–3). Distal aneurysms in the main renal artery or its branches are best managed by renal autotransplantation, using microsurgical techniques.[24, 28] The renal artery and vein are divided, leaving the ureter intact. The kidney is brought out to the abdominal wall, cooled, and irrigated with Ringer's lactate at 5° C. The renal artery is reconstructed with an autogenous saphenous vein graft anastomosed to the iliac artery, the renal vein implanted into the iliac vein, and the kidney autotransplanted into the iliac fossa. The technique of renal autotransplantation[24, 28] offers the possibility of salvaging many kidneys which previously were sacrificed by nephrectomy.[39]

REFERENCES

1. Poutasse EF, Dustan HP: Arteriosclerosis and renal hypertension: Indications for aortography in hypertensive patients and results of surgical treatment of obstructive lesions of renal artery. JAMA 165:1521, 1957.
2. DeCamp PT, Birchall R: Recognition and treatment of renal arterial stenosis associated with hypertension. Surgery 43:134, 1958.
3. DeBakey ME, Morris GC Jr, Morgen RO, Crawford ES, Cooley DA: Lesions of the renal artery: Surgical technique and results. Am J Surg 107:84, 1964.
4. Bright R: Cases and observations illustrative of renal disease accompanied with the secretion of albuminous urine. Guy's Hosp Rep 1:338, 1836.
5. Callahan WP, Schlitz FH: Aneurysm of the renal artery. Surg Gynecol Obstet 43:724, 1926.
6. Goldblatt H: Studies on experimental hypertension. J Exp Med 59:347, 1934.
7. Butler AM: Chronic pyelonephritis and arterial hypertension. J Clin Invest 16:889, 1973.
8. Leadbetter WF, Burkland CE: Hypertension in unilateral renal disease. J Urol 39:611, 1938.
9. Page IH: Nature of clinical and experimental arterial hypertension (Janeway lecture). J Mt Sinai Hosp 8:3, 1941.
10. Page IH, Helmer OM: Crystalline pressor substance (angiotonin) resulting from interaction between renin and renin activator. J Exper Med 71:29, 1940.
11. Mathé CP: Aneurysm of the renal artery: Report of five cases, one treated by resection of aneurysm without sacrificing the kidney. J Urol 60:543, 1948.
12. Freeman NE, Leeds FH, Elliott WG, Roland SI: Thromboendarterectomy for hypertension due to renal artery occlusion. JAMA 156:1077, 1954.
13. Morris CG Jr, DeBakey ME, Crawford ES, Cooley DA, Zanger LCC: Late results of surgical treatment for renovascular hypertension. Surg Gynecol Obstet 122:1255, 1966.
14. Stamey TA, Nudelman IJ, Good PH, Schwentker FN, Hendricks F: Functional characteristics of renovascular hypertension. Medicine 40:347, 1961.
15. Howard JE, Connor TB: Hypertension produced by unilateral renal disease. Arch Intern Med 109:8, 1962.
16. Michelakis AM, Foster JH, Liddle GW, Rhamy RK, Kuchel O, Gordon RD: Measurement of renin in both renal veins: Its use in the diagnosis of renovascular hypertension. Arch Intern Med 120:444, 1967.
17. Wylie EJ, Perloff DL, Stoney RJ: Autogenous tissue revascularization techniques in surgery for renovascular hypertension. Ann Surg 170:416, 1969.
18. Fry WJ, Brink BW, Thompson NW: New techniques in the treatment of extensive fibromuscular disease involving the renal arteries. Surgery 68:959, 1970.
19. Wukasch DC, Iverson LIG, Rubio PA: The left renal lumbar vein: Importance in exposure of the renal arteries. Cardiovascular Diseases, Bulletin of the Texas Heart Institute 3(2): 233, 1976.
20. Dean RH, Foster JH: Criteria for the diagnosis of renovascular hypertension. Surgery 74:926, 1973.
21. Foster JH, Dean RH, Pinkerton JA, Rhamy RK: Ten years experience with the surgical management of renovascular hypertension. Ann Surg 177:755, 1973.
22. Louis WJ, Renzini V, MacDonald GJ, Boyd GW, Peart WS: Renal-clip hypertension in rabbits immunised against angiotensin II. Lancet 1:333, 1970.
23. Lamis PA, Stanton PE, Wilson JP, Letton AH: Fibromuscular disease of the segmental renal arteries. Arch Surg 106:109, 1973.
24. Ota K, Mori S, Awane Y, Ueno A: Ex situ repair of renal artery for renovascular hypertension. Arch Surg 94:370, 1967.
25. Belzer FO, Keaveny, TV, Reed TW, Pryor JP: New method of renal artery reconstruction. Surgery 68:619, 1970.
26. Belzer FO, Salvatierra O, Perloff D, Grausz H: Surgical correction of advanced fibromuscular dysplasia of the renal arteries. Surgery 75:31, 1974.
27. Cerny JC, Chang CY, Fry WJ: Renal artery aneurysms. Arch Surg 96:653, 1968.
28. Lim RC, Eastman AB, Blaisdell FW: Renal auto-transplantation: Adjunct to repair of renal vascular lesions. Arch Surg 105:847, 1972.
29. Lawson RK, Hodges CV, Pitre TM: Nephrectomy, microvascular repair and autotransplantation. Surg Forum 23:539, 1972.
30. Cooley DA, Norman JC: Repair of dissecting aneurysms of the descending aorta. In *Techniques in Cardiac Surgery,* Houston, Texas Medical Press, 1975, p 191.
31. Buda JA, Baer L, Parra-Carrillo JZ, Kashef MM, McAllister FF, Voorhees AB Jr, Priani CL: Predictability of surgical response in renovascular hypertension. Arch Surg 111:1243, 1976.
32. Cooley DA, Wukasch DC, Bennett JG, Trono R, Barton BB: Double velour knitted Dacron grafts for aortoiliac vascular replacements. In *Vascular Grafts — Current Status and Future Trends* (Philip N. Sawyer and Martin J. Kaplitt, editors). New York City, Appleton-Century-Crofts, 1978, pp 197–208.
33. Wukasch DC, Cooley DA, Sandiford FM, Nappi G, Reul GJ Jr: Ascending aorta-abdominal aorta bypass: Indications, technique, and report of 12 patients. Ann Thorac Surg 23:442, 1977.
34. Cooley DA, Wukasch DC: Surgical treatment of renovascular hypertension. Conn Med 42(7):423, 1978.
35. Poutasse EF: Renal artery aneurysms: Their natural history and surgery. J Urol 95:297, 1966.
36. Poutasse EF: Renal artery aneurysms. J Urol 443:113, 1975.
37. Harrow BR, Sloane JA: Aneurysm of renal artery: Report of five cases. J Urol 81:35, 1959.
38. McCarron JP Jr, Marshall VF, Whitsell JC II: Indications for surgery on renal artery aneurysms. J Urol 114:117, 1975.
39. Guerriero WG, Scott R Jr, Joyce L: Development of extracorporeal renal perfusion as an adjunct to bench surgery. J Urol 107:4, 1972.

CHAPTER 7

Dialysis Shunts

INTRODUCTION AND GENERAL PRINCIPLES

Acute renal failure is a complication that will inevitably occur in any vascular center, particularly after aortic aneurysm resection and renal artery revascularization.[1] Therefore, the vascular surgeon must be prepared to perform external arteriovenous (AV) shunting and to create internal arteriovenous fistulae for the treatment of acute and chronic renal failure. An experienced nephrology and renal dialysis group is an integral part of the team in any hospital where vascular surgery is performed. To support such a renal dialysis unit with a full-time nephrologist, a chronic renal dialysis program is advantageous. This in turn requires the availability of a kidney transplant team.

Renal dialysis may be performed by peritoneal dialysis or hemodialysis. If treatment of acute renal insufficiency requires more than one or two episodes of peritoneal dialysis, hemodialysis — which is significantly more effective and associated with fewer complications — will usually become necessary.

Access for hemodialysis may be obtained by either temporary external shunting, as described by Scribner,[2] or by the creation of an internal arteriovenous fistula.[3] External arteriovenous shunts with Teflon-Silastic catheters, using the Scribner technique, will remain patent for four weeks or longer. If renal function fails to return during this period, an internal fistula should be considered.

Because the patient who requires renal hemodialysis has usually undergone a period of intensive treatment requiring prolonged intravenous therapy, the availability of suitable veins is almost always a major problem. Therefore, the selection of the site and type of shunt or fistula to be performed is equally as important as the technique of performing the operation. Several general principles are applicable:

(1) A temporary external shunt rather than an internal fistula is indicated in patients whose recovery of renal function is possible.

(2) Other conditions being equal, use of the patient's nondominant upper extremity is preferred. In a right-handed patient, the left forearm should be used before the right. When a combined temporary shunt and an internal fistula are performed in a right-handed patient, the logical approach is to place the permanent internal fistula into the left forearm and the temporary Scribner shunt into either ankle or the right forearm.

(3) Whether using temporary or permanent shunts, the initial site selected should be the most distal on the extremity, so that subsequent fistulae, should they become necessary, can be "moved up." Using this approach, as many as two or three shunts can be applied to a single extremity if required.

(4) When creating permanent internal fistulae, the patient's autogenous vessels should be utilized when possible. The radial artery and cephalic vein or other wrist veins are the vessels of first choice. Should use of these vessels in both upper extremities be unsatisfactory, the shunt may be "moved up" the forearm, utilizing

106

either the radial or ulnar arteries. When all satisfactory sites in the forearm have been exploited, various graft materials may be used in different locations.

(5) Graft materials in order of our preference are: (a) autogenous saphenous veins, (b) Dardik umbilical vein homografts,* and (c) bovine heterografts.

(6) A reasonable sequence of sites and types of permanent AV fistulae could include: (a) Radial-cephalic AV fistula at the wrist; (b) radial or ulnar-brachio-cephalic AV fistula in the upper forearm or arm; (c) graft AV fistula in the forearm; (d) autogenous saphenous vein mobilized to the knee and anastomosed to the femoral artery; (e) axillary artery to axillary vein prosthetic graft; and (f) graft from the femoral artery to the femoral vein.

Other general considerations include the desirability of local rather than general anesthesia because of the poor general condition of most patients who require dialysis. Although it is possible to insert a Scribner shunt at the bedside, we prefer to perform all such procedures in the operating room. A double tourniquet, "sitting stools," optic magnification, and illumination for the surgeon and his assistant facilitate the procedure.

The recent application of plasmaphoresis in the treatment of various collagen diseases[4] has provided a new demand for arteriovenous fistulae. The procedure is particularly challenging in severely debilitated patients with dermatomyositis, lupus erythematosus, and rheumatoid arthritis or a combination of two or more of these (mixed collagen) diseases. Patients with dermatomyositis are perhaps the most difficult group in which to obtain long-term patency of the fistula because of the "rock hard" consistency of the tissues that compress the vessels.

SCRIBNER EXTERNAL SHUNT TECHNIQUE

The upper extremity is prepped and draped completely and placed on an arm board at 90° to the patient's body. After injection of local anesthesia (1% Xylocaine), vertical incisions 3 to 5 cm in length are made over the radial artery and cephalic veins just above the wrist. The use of vertical rather than transverse incisions allows proximal extension and dissection of the vessel in the event that the artery or vein is unsatisfactory at the site initially selected. Should the cephalic vein be thrombosed, as is frequently the case following prolonged intravenous therapy, the basilic or any of the other venous collaterals distributed throughout the volar aspect of the forearm may be used (Fig. 7–1, a). A helpful maneuver for locating a satisfactory vein is to place around the forearm a rubber tourniquet that occludes venous return but not arterial flow. Infiltration of the artery and vein to be used with several cc's of papaverine will prevent spasm and facilitate insertion of the cannulae. The vessels are ligated distally, and a single 2–0 silk suture is passed around the vessel prox-imally. Following insertion of the largest caliber Teflon vessel tip possible, a single silk suture is tied to hold the Teflon tip in place (Fig. 7–1, b). Use of only a single suture to fix the tip will allow its removal by simply withdrawing it without having to reopen the incision. Silastic tubings that were connected to the Teflon vessel tip prior to their insertion into the vessels are then brought out through separate skin incisions, and the wounds are closed with interrupted absorbable suture in both the subcutaneous layers (Fig. 7–1, c).

Properly managed external shunts can often be kept functioning for several months. The most important aspect of shunt care is regular, around-the-clock irriga-tion of the cannulae with a dilute heparin solution. When external shunts do throm-bose acutely, the thrombus can sometimes be extracted with a small Fogarty cath-eter inserted through the external tubing.

Alternate sites for placement of Scribner external shunts, using the posterior

*Meadox Medicals, P.O. Box 530, Oakland, New Jersey 07436.

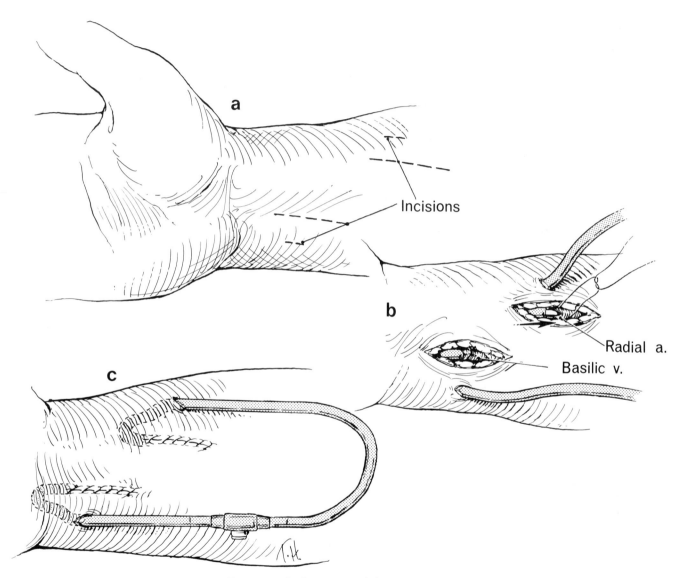

a

Incisions

b

Radial a.

Basilic v.

c

Figure 7–1 Scribner external shunt technique.

tibial artery and greater saphenous vein, are the mid- or proximal forearm and the lower leg just above the ankle. When these sites are unsatisfactory, as in children, whose vessels may be too small for satisfactory cannulation at any of the above sites, the shunts can be placed in the groin via a branch of the profunda femoris artery and greater saphenous vein.[5]

PERMANENT INTERNAL ARTERIOVENOUS FISTULAE

The description of surgical creation of an autogenous internal arteriovenous fistula by Brescia et al. in 1966[3] has provided the means for repeated hemodialysis for chronic renal failure. Application of such internal fistulae for plasmaphoresis by Brewer[4] has opened the door to a new means of treating mixed collagen diseases.

The radial artery and basilic vein are exposed above the wrist or higher in the forearm, as described for performing an external shunt (Fig. 7-1). Systemic heparinization is instituted, using 2 mg/kg of body weight, and vascular clamps are applied. The cephalic (or basilic or median antecubital) vein is then anastomosed end-to-side to the radial (or ulnar) artery, using running 6-0 polypropylene suture. The anastomosis is identical to that described in aortocoronary bypass.[6, 7] It should be approximately 5 mm in length. In most cases, approximately 10 to 14 days is required for the fistula to "mature"; that is, to become sufficiently dilated to facilitate easy puncture for dialysis. Thus, when immediate dialysis is required, it is desirable to place an external shunt in the ankle concomitantly.

CREATION OF ARTERIOVENOUS FISTULAE WITH GRAFTS

When the vessels in the wrist, forearm, or ankle are no longer satisfactory for creation of an autogenous end-to-side or side-to-side anastomosis, use of a graft between any small artery and vein can provide adequate access for dialysis or plasmaphoresis. As mentioned above, the order of our preference for graft materials is: autogenous saphenous vein, Dardik umbilical vein homograft,[8] and bovine heterograft.[9]

An example of utilizing a bovine heterograft for creating an internal fistula between the radial artery and median antecubital vein in the left forearm is shown in Figure 7-2. Because of the multiple incisions and extensive dissection required, general anesthesia is preferred. Multiple incisions are made over the artery, the vein, and in a distribution to create a subcutaneous tunnel in the shape of a gentle loop. The radial artery is dissected distal to the bifurcation of the brachial artery (Fig. 7-2, b). Following systemic heparinization (2 mg/kg of body weight), the artery is clamped and the graft anastomosed end-to-side with 6-0 polypropylene running suture (Fig. 7-2, c). Performing the arterial anastomosis first allows distention of the graft, with the arterial flow passing through the tunnel in such a manner as to prevent kinking (Fig. 7-2, d). The graft is then anastomosed end-to-side to the median or other appropriate vein.[10]

AXILLARY ARTERY TO AXILLARY VEIN GRAFT

When the above described attempts have failed or do not appear feasible, a shunt created between the axillary artery and axillary vein is a useful technique.[11] Under general anesthesia, the patient is placed in a supine position with both arms extended and a roll beneath the shoulder blades (Fig. 7-3, a). The axillary artery and

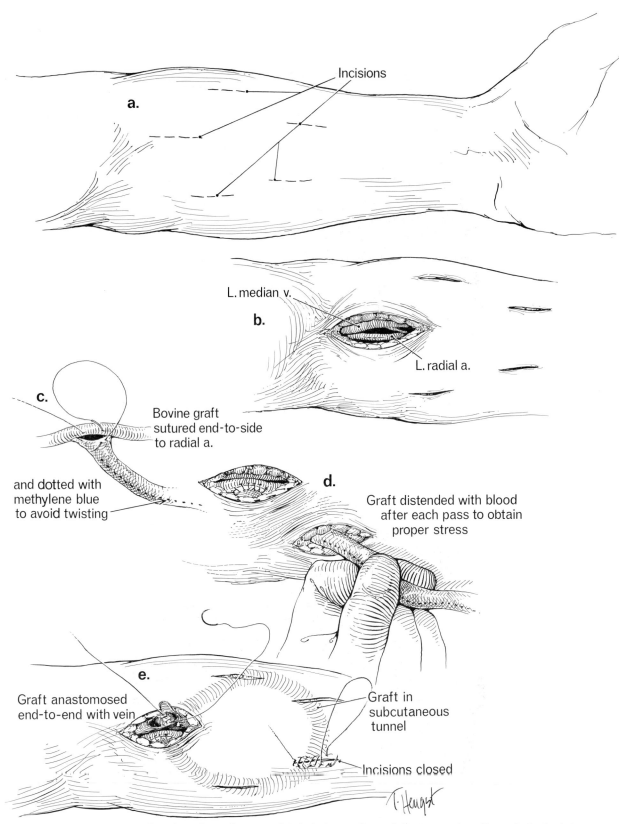

a.

Incisions

b.

L. median v.

L. radial a.

c.

Bovine graft
sutured end-to-side
to radial a.

and dotted with
methylene blue
to avoid twisting

d.

Graft distended with blood
after each pass to obtain
proper stress

e.

Graft anastomosed
end-to-end with vein

Graft in
subcutaneous
tunnel

Incisions closed

Figure 7-2 Creation of arteriovenous fistula between the radial artery and median vein in the left forearm, with bovine heterograft.

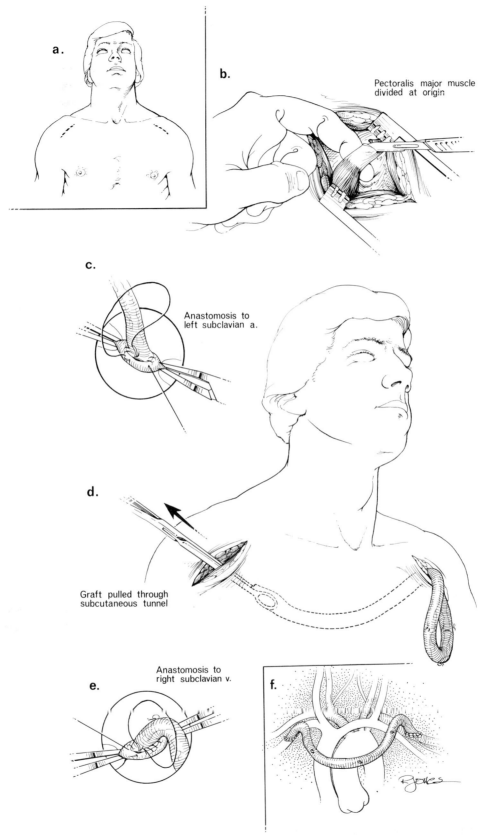

a.

b.

Pectoralis major muscle
divided at origin

c.

Anastomosis to
left subclavian a.

d.

Graft pulled through
subcutaneous tunnel

Anastomosis to
right subclavian v.

e.

f.

Figure 7–3   Axillary artery to axillary vein graft.

vein are exposed on opposite sides via a deltopectoral approach between the deltoid muscle and pectoralis major muscle. To allow for proper angulation of the graft, a transpectoral approach is used by dividing the fibers of the pectoralis major muscle to gain exposure of the axillary artery (Fig. 7–3, b). A Dardik umbilical vein homograft or bovine heterograft is used to create an internal shunt between the axillary artery and the opposite axillary vein. The graft is tunneled through the fibers of the pectoralis major muscle into a subcutaneous tunnel across the anterior chest, with a single transverse incision being made over the midsternum at approximately the second space (Fig. 7–3, c to f).

REFERENCES

1. Cooley DA, Wukasch DC: Surgical treatment of renovascular hypertension. Conn Med 42(7):423, 1978.
2. Quinton WE, Dillard DH, Scribner BH: Cannulation of blood vessels for prolonged hemodialysis. Trans Am Soc Artif Intern Organs 6:104, 1960.
3. Brescia MJ, Cimino JE, Appel K, Hurwich BI: Chronic hemodialysis using venipuncture and surgically created arteriovenous fistula. N Engl J Med 275:1089, 1966.
4. Brewer EJ: *Juvenile Rheumatoid Arthritis, 2nd ed.* WB Saunders Company, Philadelphia (in press).
5. Belzer FO, Kountz SL: Arteriovenous Quinton-Scribner shunt with the profunda femoris artery and saphenous vein. Surgery 70:443, 1971.
6. Wukasch DC, Cooley DA, Sandiford FM, Nappi G, Reul GJ Jr: Ascending aorta–abdominal aorta bypass: Indications, techniques and report of 12 patients. Ann Thorac Surg 23:442, 1977.
7. Cooley DA, Norman JC: *Techniques in Cardiac Surgery,* Texas Medical Press, 1975, pp 24–29.
8. Dardik I, Ibrahim I, Dardik H: Femoral popliteal bypass employing modified human umbilical cord vein: An assessment of early clinical results. Cardiovascular Diseases, Bulletin of the Texas Heart Institute 3(3):314, 1976.
9. Kaplitt MJ, Frantz SL, Vagnini FJ, Gulotta SJ, Vellore T, Padmanabhan VT, Oka N: Clinical evaluation of a new negatively charged 4-mm bovine heterograft (Bio-Surgi graft). In Sawyer PN, Kaplitt MJ (eds): *Vascular Grafts,* New York, Appleton-Century-Crofts, 1978, pp 393–397.
10. Lefrak EA, Noon GP: Surgical technique for creation of an arteriovenous fistula using a looped bovine graft. Ann Surg 182:782, 1975.
11. Garcia-Rinaldi R, Von Koch L: The axillary artery to axillary vein bovine graft for circulatory access: Surgical considerations. Am J Surg 135:265, 1978.

CHAPTER 8

Lesions of the Visceral Arteries

With increasing emphasis upon a direct surgical approach to vascular lesions involving the extremities and carotid circulation, considerable interest has been focused upon the abdominal visceral circulation. Various syndromes have been identified and related to specific occlusive lesions, and the symptoms and physical findings have been correlated with diagnostic angiography. Aneurysmal lesions have been less well defined clinically, since symptoms of pain tend to occur late, or only after frank rupture. Some order has been developed even with visceral aneurysms, however, and the surgeon should now be able to recognize the need for operation in most cases. He should be well enough acquainted with the techniques to correct the basic defect, whether it is an occlusive or aneurysmal lesion.

ACUTE OCCLUSIVE LESIONS

Visceral ischemia caused by superior mesenteric artery obstruction with acute onset is usually an urgent surgical problem, although the results of surgery may be disappointing, depending upon the specific pathologic condition involved. Three major types of acute occlusion occur, and the delineation of each may be difficult.[1, 2]

ACUTE EMBOLIC OCCLUSION

This type of lesion most often occurs in cardiac patients with mitral stenosis, intracardiac myxoma, atrial fibrillation or ischemic heart disease and intracardiac thromboses.[3, 4] The onset of symptoms is usually sudden, with cramping and upper abdominal pain that becomes generalized. Almost explosive evacuation of the bowel may occur as the intensive spasm occurs. Such a dramatic onset is relatively characteristic, and in addition to the usual laboratory and radiographic studies, diagnosis should be confirmed by immediate selective arteriography if possible. The characteristic angiographic appearance is of a sharply defined occlusion of the superior mesenteric artery, beginning distal to the first few jejunal branches. At laparotomy, the small intestine may be ischemic or frankly infarcted, but the proximal jejunum and most of the transverse colon are usually spared, making possible surgical correction by embolectomy or intestinal resection. In all such patients, we advocate a "second-look concept," which may make the difference as to their survival or nonsurvival. With this approach, the surgeon deliberately plans to re-explore the abdomen 24 to 36 hours after the initial procedure to establish the viability of the bowel. The success of surgery usually depends upon the elapsed time from onset of the embolism, the size and location of the embolus, the extent of bowel necrosis, and the general condition of the patient. In some instances, even when the ischemic bowel has been revascularized successfully, death may result from bacteremia or some other toxic factor caused by revascularizing the marginally viable bowel.

ACUTE THROMBOTIC OCCLUSION

Spontaneous thrombosis of the superior mesenteric artery caused by an atherosclerotic lesion or coagulopathy usually has a more insidious onset, with continuous and progressively severe abdominal pain, punctuated by colicky episodes. This condition progresses gradually until the abdomen is distended, the bowel sounds are absent, and the patient becomes severely obtunded. A history of abdominal discomfort preceding the acute attack may assist in the differential diagnosis from acute embolism. Oliguria proceeds to anuria, and leukocytosis of 20,000 to 40,000 occurs. Bloody diarrhea signals the onset of bowel infarction and mucosal necrosis. Diagnosis is usually difficult in the early period of the illness, but it can be based on clinical findings and a blood count after 24 hours. An abdominal x-ray film reveals generalized bowel distention, including distention of the colon. Selective mesenteric arteriography shows an occlusion which is located more proximally in the artery than is seen with embolic occlusion. Moreover, the shape of the occlusion at its proximal end may appear to be more tapered than expected with an acute embolus.

Operation often reveals an extensive bowel infarction involving the fourth portion of the duodenum, the proximal jejunum, and the transverse colon. If the inferior mesenteric artery and gastric arteries are also thrombosed, the entire gastrointestinal tract may be infarcted. An attempt to revascularize the mesenteric artery after spontaneous thrombosis is seldom successful. Thrombectomy is usually futile, particularly for that portion of the thrombus located in the proximal 2 or 3 cm of the vessel. In some instances, a saphenous vein graft between the side of the infrarenal abdominal aorta and the side of the superior mesenteric artery may be successful if the distal arterial bed still has some patency as shown by retrograde distal flow into the arteriotomy. Usually, the only procedure possible is an extensive bowel resection, removing the entire jejunum, ileum, and transverse colon.[5] Few patients survive this form of therapy. A "second look" may be advisable 24 to 48 hours later if the patient is still alive. Breakdown of the suture line is common in these cases, and the rare patient who survives becomes an "intestinal cripple." The prognosis is worse for spontaneous thrombosis than for embolic occlusion.

PRIMARY MESENTERIC INFARCTION (PERIPHERAL SPASM)

The onset of symptoms may vary, simulating either of the above types of acute mesenteric syndromes.[6-8] Often the condition results from some distant trauma such as a crushing body injury or a severe thermal burn. Exploratory laparotomy may reveal a hemorrhagic appearance of the mesentery adjacent to the bowel, with segmental infarctions of the small and large intestines. The pathologic process begins peripherally in the intestinal arterioles or venules and involves the capillary bed, which thromboses. Thus, pulsations are characteristically palpable in the proximal mesentery and distally into the intestinal arcade. Surgical treatment in these cases may be confined to intestinal resection of several segments of bowel, or, in advanced cases, to more extensive resections. The "second-look procedure" may be extremely important to these patients, since the process may extend into other areas. Unfortunately, long-term survival is not common. After operation, treatment of all patients with acute mesenteric occlusion should include continuous dextran infusion and the cautious use of heparin to combat the thrombotic tendency.[9-13]

CHRONIC OCCLUSIVE LESIONS

The knowledge that ischemia of the bowel and abdominal viscera could cause symptoms, notably gradual weight loss, is a relatively recent acquisition in medical practice.[14] While other symptoms may be produced by ischemia, unexplained weight loss must always arouse the physician's suspicion of either celiac or superior mesenteric artery stenosis, or of complete occlusion. Malabsorption from the intestinal tract as evidenced by the presence of undigested fat or carbohydrates may be the cause of the weight loss.[15, 16] Much more common, however, is a so-called "food fear" or "small meal syndrome" in patients who have learned that ingestion of larger quantities of food causes abdominal pain or cramps (abdominal angina).[17, 18] Increased peristalsis from food ingestion leads to intestinal claudication in much the same manner as rapid walking causes calf pain in patients with occlusion of the iliac or femoral circulation. The pain usually begins in midabdomen, progressing to the epigastrium, and is related directly to the quantity of food ingested. Usually the pain is relieved spontaneously in less than one hour. Sometimes the onset and progress of symptoms, along with weight loss, are rather subtle, and the patient may be unaware of their cause-and-effect relationship. Patients gradually develop a state of cachexia, and are often suspected of having carcinomatosis. Other symptoms, such as diarrhea, are relatively inconstant and, instead, patients may be constipated because of the small amounts of food eaten. A history of chronic weight loss should cause the physician to suspect the true cause[19]; auscultation and the presence of an upper abdominal bruit are contributory to a diagnosis, although bruits are relatively common in many patients in the primary atherosclerotic age group.

Aortography is the *sine qua non* of diagnosis in the visceral ischemia syndrome. In the anteroposterior projection, the aortogram may reveal no abnormality. Collateralization of the chronic occlusions of the superior mesenteric and celiac arteries from the inferior mesenteric artery through Riolan's arch may reveal the striking dilation of a marginal artery in the colonic mesentery — the wandering artery of Drummond. The precise diagnosis and definition of the exact location and extent of the occlusion depend upon a lateral projection of the aortogram. The occlusion may involve the celiac artery (most common), the superior mesenteric, or the inferior mesenteric. Complete occlusion of both of the major arteries to the abdominal viscera is not uncommon, and in some patients all three vessels may be severely stenotic or even completely occluded. Thus, in chronic occlusion, collateral circulation may derive from proximal or distal vessels which normally have no significant connections with the visceral vessels. This tendency for the body to compensate for circulatory deficiency explains the known clinical features of insidiousness and chronicity.[20]

SURGICAL TREATMENT OF CHRONIC VISCERAL OCCLUSION

A midline abdominal incision will provide adequate exposure for surgical treatment of all types of chronic visceral occlusion. The technique to re-establish normal pulsatile flow depends upon the location of the obstruction. The surgeon may have a choice of doing a thromboendarterectomy with or without patch graft angioplasty or of using a synthetic or autologous saphenous vein graft to bypass the obstruction. Exposure of the abdominal aorta for the bypass is necessary, and both the supraceliac and infrarenal segments may be used for the proximal anastomosis.[21]

Exposure of the supraceliac aorta is accomplished by gently retracting the liver upward with a curved retractor, and the stomach in a caudad direction (Fig. 8–1, *a*, and *b*).[22] The posterior peritoneum is incised above the upper margin of the pancreas. The overlying muscular crus of the diaphragm is incised, providing an exposure

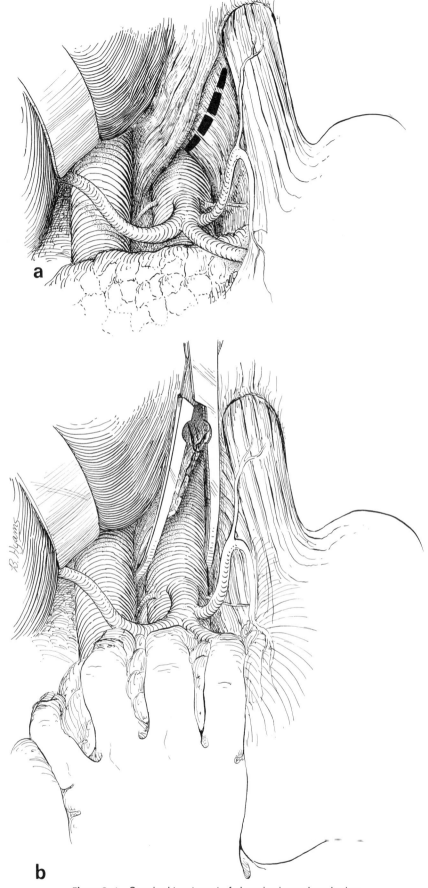

Figure 8–1 Surgical treatment of chronic visceral occlusion.

of 4 to 6 cm of a "bare area" of the abdominal aorta. This segment of the aorta may then be cross-clamped or partially occluded tangentially during the attachment of grafts.

The infrarenal abdominal aorta is exposed by a more routine approach, such as is used in cases of aortoiliac occlusive disease or infrarenal abdominal aortic aneurysm.

Celiac Artery Revascularization

Revascularization of the celiac artery may be done in several ways, including endarterectomy with or without patch graft, bypass, or division and reimplantation of the artery. Shown in Figure 8–2 is a technique employed in an elderly patient with a celiac band syndrome, in which the fibrous edge of the diaphragmatic crus produced a chronic impingement on the celiac artery, thus causing severe weight loss, abdominal discomfort, and cachexia (Fig. 8–2, a). The diagnosis was established by lateral aortography, and the lesion was approached by an upper midline abdominal incision (Fig. 8–2, b). Dissection and division of the offending fibromuscular band eliminated the extrinsic compression of the artery. Although the artery was freed of the compression, the proximal lumen did not enlarge sufficiently to provide normal distal pulsation, indicating a probable congenital underdevelopment of the artery (Fig. 8–2, c); therefore, the proximal narrow segment of artery was ligated and excised (Fig. 8–2, d, and e). A partial occlusion clamp was placed on the aorta, and a new opening was made distal to the normal site of origin of the celiac artery (Fig. 8–2, f). The celiac artery was reconnected to the aorta using a 4.0 polypropylene suture and a continuous suture technique (Fig. 8–2, g and h). Normal flow was then directed into the celiac artery (Fig. 8–2, i), and the patient made a strikingly prompt recovery.

Superior Mesenteric Artery Revascularization

Revascularization of the superior mesenteric artery may be accomplished by either thromboendarterectomy or by using the bypass technique. Exposure of the proximal origin of the artery from the aorta is somewhat tedious, and may be difficult because of the extensiveness of sympathetic nerve fibers in the vicinity. Moreover, the abdominal aorta may be sclerotic at that point, making endarterectomy and patch grafting unsatisfactory. Usually we prefer to use the bypass technique as depicted in Figure 8–3.

When the lesion is confined to the superior mesenteric artery (Fig. 8–3, a), an upper midline abdominal incision extending slightly below the umbilical level provides adequate exposure (Fig. 8–3, b). The transverse colon is retracted cephalad and the small bowel is eviscerated from the peritoneal cavity and retracted to the right (Fig. 8–3, c). The posterior peritoneum is incised along the left lateral margin of the distal duodenum dividing the ligament of Treitz. The inferior mesenteric vein is an important landmark, and the peritoneal incision should be made between the duodenum and the vein to avoid an unnecessary and sometimes messy dissection into the mesocolon. The superior mesenteric artery is dissected out of the root of the mesentery and freed from the extensive surrounding network of autonomic nerves (Fig. 8–3, d). While soft pulsations may be palpable in the vessel of the partially or totally obstructed artery, the proximal stenosis still must be corrected. The infrarenal aorta is cleared on the ventral surface adjacent to the superior mesenteric artery. In the case depicted, a 7.0 mm double velour knitted Dacron graft was used. Some surgeons may prefer a segment of autologous vein for the interposition graft. Satisfactory long-term results have been obtained with both types of substitutes, and a few late failures have also been encountered with both.

Text continued on page 121.

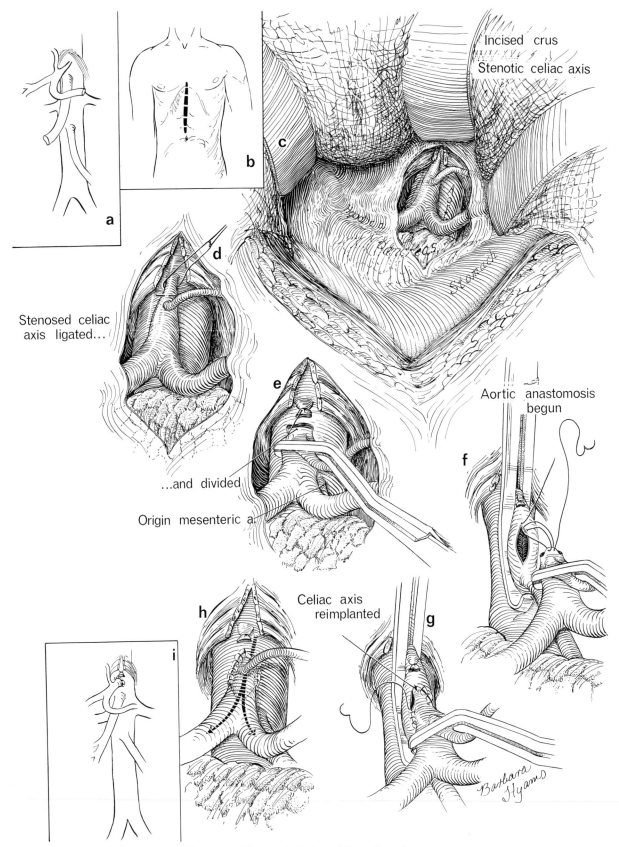

Incised crus

Stenotic celiac axis

Stenosed celiac axis ligated...

...and divided

Origin mesenteric a.

Aortic anastomosis begun

Celiac axis reimplanted

Figure 8–2 Revascularization of the celiac artery.

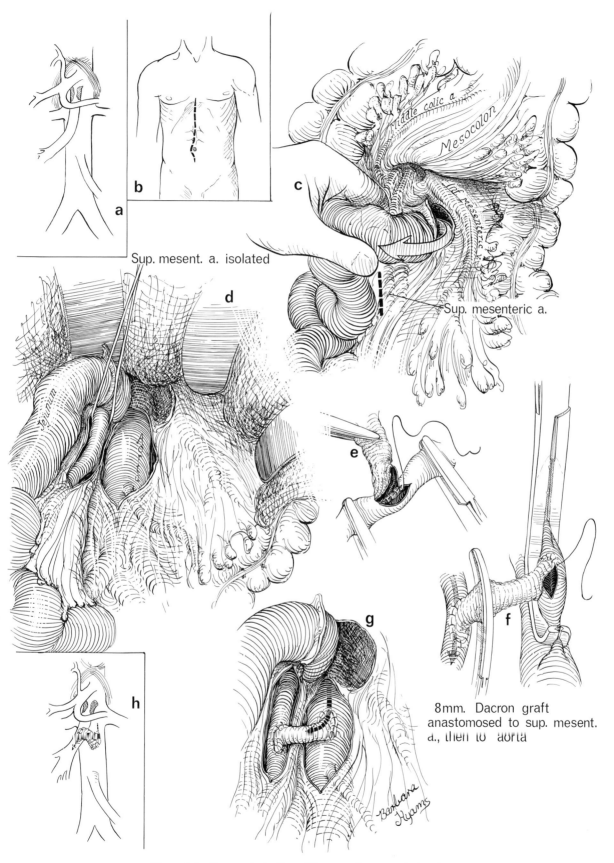

Sup. mesent. a. isolated

Sup. mesenteric a.

8mm. Dacron graft anastomosed to sup. mesent. a., then to aorta

Figure 8–3 Revascularization of the superior mesenteric artery.

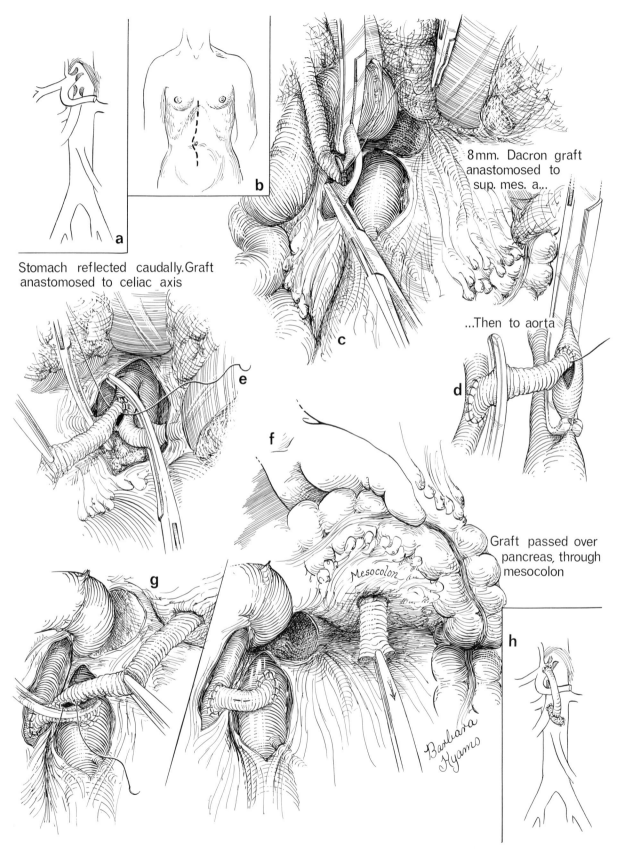

Stomach reflected caudally. Graft anastomosed to celiac axis

8 mm. Dacron graft anastomosed to sup. mes. a...

...Then to aorta

Graft passed over pancreas, through mesocolon

Mesocolon

Barbara Hyams

Figure 8–4   Operative technique for occlusion of the celiac and superior mesenteric arteries.

The superior mesenteric end-to-side anastomosis was done by proximal and distal total occlusion of the artery with a braided polyester suture (Fig. 8–3, c). A partial occlusion clamp was applied to the abdominal aorta and the proximal anastomosis was performed by using a similar suture technique (Fig. 8–3, f). When the clamps were removed, a normal vigorous pulsatile flow was restored in the mesenteric artery (Fig. 8–3, g and h). The length of the graft should be carefully estimated for this procedure because an excessively long graft may lead to kinking and subsequent thrombosis and occlusion. Indeed, in cachexic patients a side-to-side anastomosis is technically feasible without kinking the mesenteric artery; therefore, the graft may need to be no longer than 3 to 4 cm.

Occlusion of the Celiac and Superior Mesenteric Arteries

Not infrequently, patients who have abdominal angina demonstrate more than one visceral arterial occlusion. In the patient depicted in Figure 8–4, both the celiac and superior mesenteric arteries were shown to be stenotic by lateral aortography (Fig. 8–4, a). Operation was performed through a standard upper midline incision (Fig. 8–4, b). The superior mesenteric artery was first revascularized by using the technique demonstrated in Figure 8–3. A double velour 8.0 mm knitted Dacron graft was anastomosed end-to-side to the artery and abdominal aorta (Fig. 8–4, c and d). The celiac artery was dissected by the technique described in Figure 8–2. A 7.0 mm knitted Dacron tube was then interposed between the side of the celiac artery and the previously placed mesenteric graft by using an end-to-side technique (Fig. 8–4, e to h). In this case, the graft to the celiac artery was placed ventral to the pancreas and passed through the mesocolon. Another route could have been selected dorsal to the body of the pancreas, creating a tunnel by digital partial dissection. An anastomosis to branches of the celiac artery (namely, the hepatic or splenic arteries) may accomplish the same purpose for celiac revascularization.

Usually, isolated occlusions of the inferior mesenteric artery cause no symptoms owing to extensive collateral blood supply. Implantation of the artery into an abdominal graft can be done readily, and we have used this technique frequently after resection of aneurysms of the abdominal aorta.

Multiple Occlusions of the Visceral Arteries

Multiple occlusions of the visceral arteries may require extensive and complex revascularization techniques. Usually, surgical correction taxes the ingenuity of the surgeon, but, fortunately, with the present availability of synthetic vascular substitutes in many sizes and configurations, a satisfactory solution to any technical problems may be achieved.[23]

In the case depicted in Figure 8–5, all the major abdominal visceral arteries were severely stenotic, but the abdominal aorta was relatively normal. A 12 mm × 7 mm knitted Dacron double velour graft was used as the source for a five-vessel revascularization. The first anastomosis was made between the end of the main stem of the bifurcation graft and the infrarenal abdominal aorta, and the branches were connected end-to-side to the right and left renal arteries. The black guidelines assisted in placing the grafts without twisting or kinking. Additional side branches were then connected to the source graft and to the superior mesenteric and celiac arteries, respectively. Final revascularization was accomplished when the stenotic inferior mesenteric artery was detached from the aorta and anastomosed to the source graft. It has been our observation that direct anastomosis between an artery

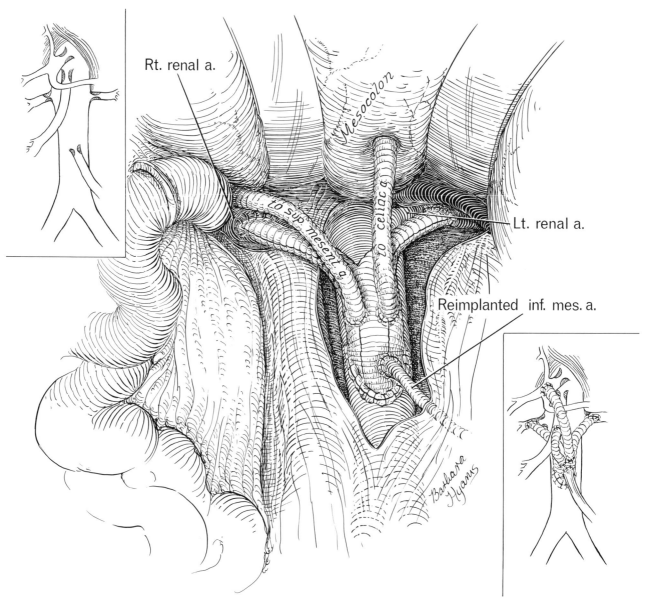

Figure 8–5 Revascularization in multiple occlusions of the visceral arteries.

and synthetic graft develops and maintains a larger flow than when the artery is reanastomosed to the parent vessel.

Arterial Bypass for Aortic, Iliac, Celiac, and Superior Mesenteric Occlusion

Challenging technical exercises are often encountered in patients who have aortoiliac occlusive disease.[24] In the case illustrated in Figure 8–6, the patient, a 64-year-old woman, presented with symptoms of both intestinal ischemia with angina and intermittent claudication of the lower extremities. Aortographs had confirmed the presence of aortic, iliac, celiac, and superior mesenteric arterial occlusion. The operation was performed using a midline abdominal incision and a bilateral femoral incision (Fig. 8–6, b). A 12 mm × 7 mm knitted velour Dacron bifurcation graft was first anastomosed end-to-side to the abdominal aorta (Fig. 8–6, c and d). The aortic partial occlusion clamp was released after the graft was occluded proximally with a stronger graft clamp. The next anastomosis was made between a 7 mm knitted tube and the main celiac artery (Fig. 8–6, e). The graft was then tunneled through the mesocolon ventral to the body of the pancreas (Fig. 8–6, f), where it was anastomosed to the main source graft (Fig. 8–6, g). Another similar tube graft was used to connect the superior mesenteric artery with the source graft (Fig. 8–6, h and i). After arterial flow was restored to the visceral vessels, the operation was completed by tunneling the limbs of the bifurcation graft into the femoral incision, where the ends were anastomosed to the side of the common femoral arteries (Fig. 8–6, j to l). Various combinations of visceral and limb grafts may be fashioned to fulfill the needs of a specific clinical problem.

VISCERAL ARTERY ANEURYSMS (EXCLUDING RENAL)

Aneurysms of major arteries may result from many causes, although the etiologic factors are often difficult to identify except for conjecture. When aneurysms occur in abdominal vessels, they may be congenital, with localized elastic tissue deficits, or they may be arteriosclerotic, mycotic associated with sepsis,[25] or due to multiple other causes, including sharp or blunt trauma.[26] Usually, the lesions do not cause symptoms and are discovered when abdominal aortography or sonography reveals their presence as an incidental finding. Rarely do they grow to such size that they become palpable as a physical finding. Surgical intervention is indicated to prevent ischemia, or to relieve symptoms of visceral ischemia. Of course, when acute symptoms appear, indicating thrombosis or rupture, operation is mandatory.[27, 28]

The patient depicted in Figure 8–7 was a 28-year-old woman who complained of postprandial abdominal pain centered in the mid- and upper abdomen. The presence of an upper abdominal bruit led to performance of abdominal aortography that revealed the presence of an aneurysm of the main trunk of the celiac artery (Fig. 8–7, a). At laparotomy, the aneurysm was exposed through a midline incision (Fig. 8–7, b). The aorta was clamped above and below the origin of the celiac artery (Fig. 8–7, c), and the aneurysm was excised (Fig. 8–7, d). Restoration of flow was obtained by interposition of a segment of reversed autologous saphenous vein (Fig. 8–7, e). Although the patient recovered from the operation without complication, three months later symptoms recurred and aortography revealed occlusion of the vein graft. Viability of the liver and other organs was maintained through rich collateral vessels from the superior mesenteric artery, mostly the pancreatic and gastroduo-

Text continued on page 127.

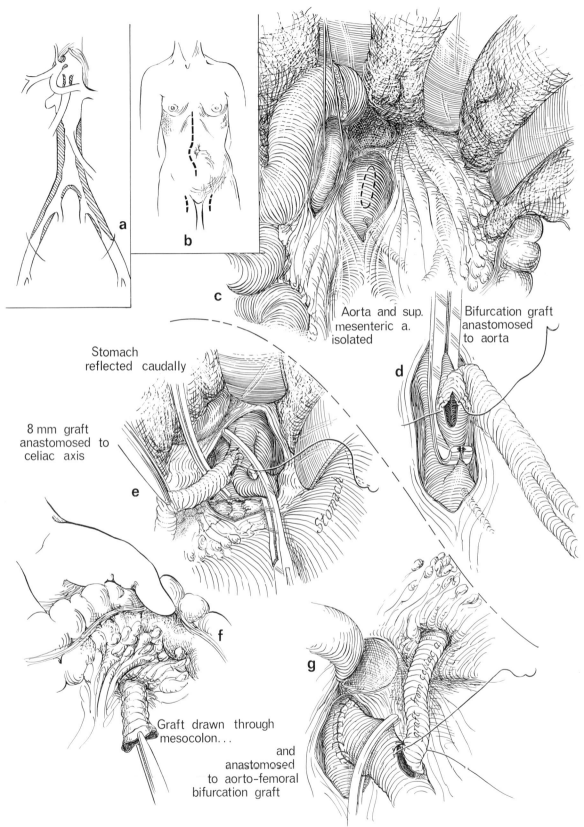

a

b

c

Aorta and sup. mesenteric a. isolated

Bifurcation graft anastomosed to aorta

d

Stomach reflected caudally

8 mm graft anastomosed to celiac axis

e

f

Graft drawn through mesocolon...

and anastomosed to aorto-femoral bifurcation graft

g

Figure 8–6   Arterial bypass for aortic, iliac, celiac, and superior mesenteric occlusion.

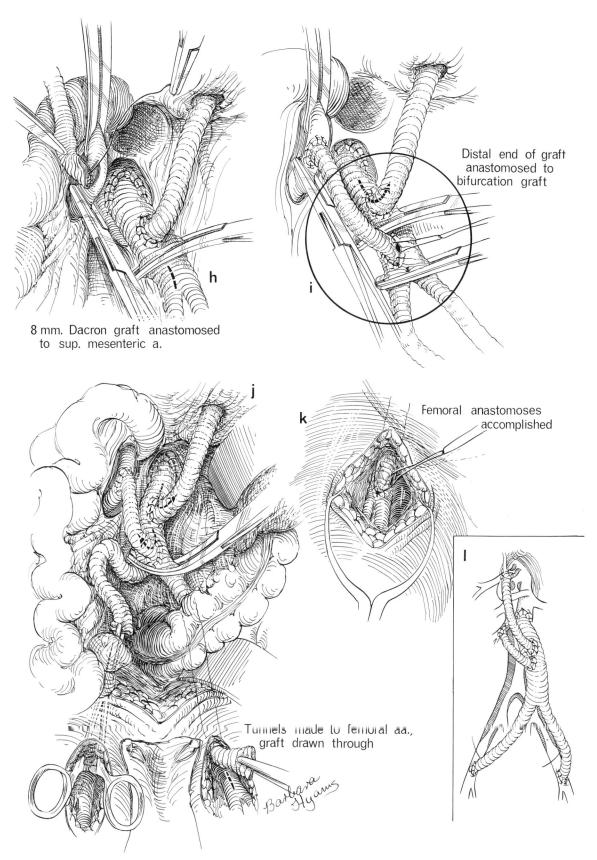

8 mm. Dacron graft anastomosed
to sup. mesenteric a.

Distal end of graft
anastomosed to
bifurcation graft

Femoral anastomoses
accomplished

Tunnels made to femoral aa.,
graft drawn through

Figure 8–6 *Continued.*

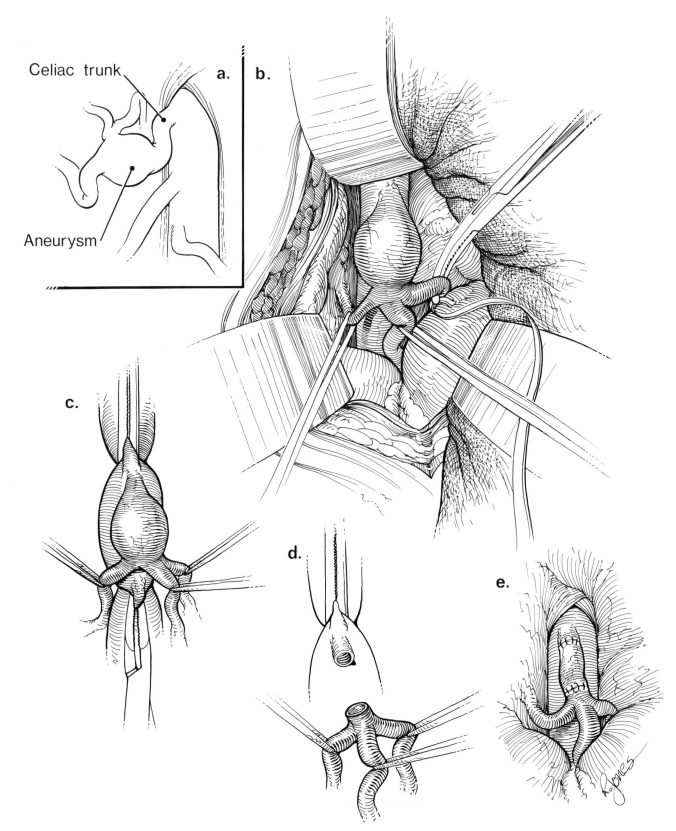

Celiac trunk

Aneurysm

a.
b.
c.
d.
e.

Figure 8–7 Repair of aneurysm of the main trunk of the celiac artery.

denal connections. If symptoms are not relieved by further natural development of collateral vessels, another operation, with grafting of the individual branches of the celiac artery, may be necessary.

HEPATIC ARTERY ANEURYSMS

Aneurysms of the hepatic artery are relatively common in comparison to those of other visceral arteries. As they increase with size, they may encroach upon the common bile duct or the head of the pancreas. Rupture of hepatic aneurysms has been reported, and for these reasons, the lesions should be resected when the diagnosis is made. In the case depicted here (Fig. 8–8), an aneurysm in the proximal segment of the common hepatic artery was resected and replaced with a 6 mm double velour Dacron graft. The patient recovered uneventfully.

SPLENIC ARTERY ANEURYSMS

When aneurysms are discovered in the splenic artery, the need for restoration of flow following resection of the lesion is not as vital as for other major visceral arteries because the spleen is an expendable organ.[29, 30] Thus, resection of an aneurysm of the distal artery and spleen is a relatively satisfactory procedure (Fig. 8–9). Recently, however, emphasis has been placed on preservation of the spleen for its vital or useful role as the major organ in the reticuloendothelial and lymphatic systems. Thus, *the organ should not be sacrificed, particularly in young patients, unless it*

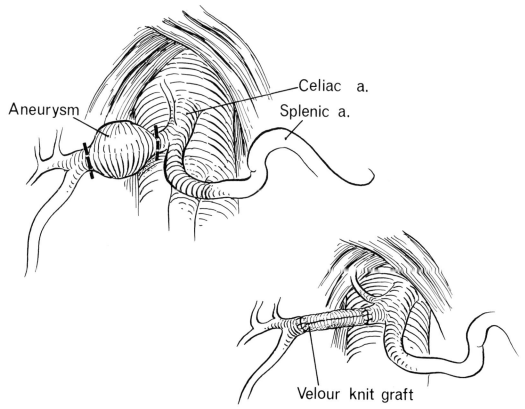

Figure 8–8 Repair of aneurysm of the hepatic artery.

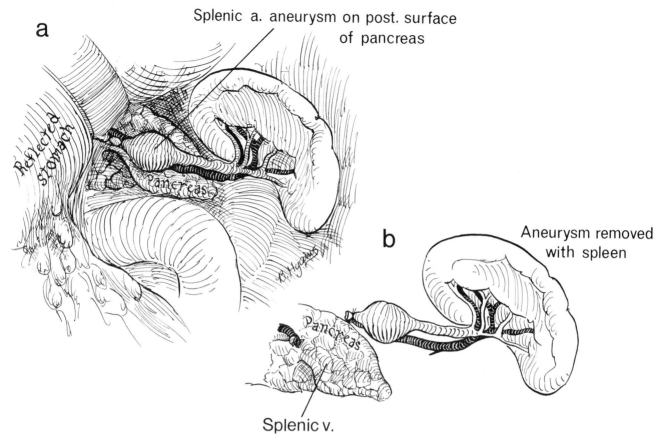

a

Splenic a. aneurysm on post. surface
of pancreas

b

Aneurysm removed
with spleen

Splenic v.

Figure 8–9 Repair of aneurysm of the splenic artery.

becomes a technical necessity because of damage during dissection of the aneurysm. Ligation of the splenic artery is well tolerated by the spleen, since it derives an adequate blood supply from the short gastric arteries. Therefore, ligation of the splenic artery proximal and distal to the aneurysm, with excision or marsupialization of the sac, may be the procedure of choice. Excision of asymptomatic splenic aneurysms should be done because of the possibility of acute rupture and also because of the low operative risk.

REFERENCES

Acute Occlusive Lesions

1. Bergan JJ: Recognition and treatment of intestinal ischemia. Surg Clin North Am 47:109, 1967.
2. Wilson GSM, Block J: Mesenteric vascular occlusion. Arch Surg 73:330, 1956.
3. Atwell RB: Superior mesenteric artery embolectomy. Surg Gynecol Obstet 112:257, 1961.
4. Baue, AE, Austen WG: Superior mesenteric artery embolism. Surg Gynecol Obstet 116:474, 1963.
5. Marston A: Causes of death in mesenteric arterial occlusion. II. Observations on revascularization of the ischemic bowel. Ann Surg 158:960, 1963.
6. Pierce GE, Brockenbrough ED: The spectrum of mesenteric infarction. Am J Surg 119:233, 1970.
7. Jordan PH Jr, Boulafendis D, Guinn GA: Factors other than major vascular occlusion that contribute to intestinal infarction. Ann Surg 171:189, 1970.
8. Johnson WC, Nabseth DC: Visceral infarction following aortic surgery. Ann Surg 180:312, 1974.
9. Hallman GL, Jordan GL Jr, Cooley DA: Massive intestinal infarction. Survival after resection and superior mesenteric embolectomy. Am J Surg 112:770, 1966.
10. Connolly JE, Stemmer EA: Intestinal gangrene as the result of mesenteric arterial steal. Am J Surg 126:197, 1973.
11. Bole PV, Munda RT, Carbonaro T, Lande A, Purdy RT: Aortofemoral steal: Hemodynamic deprivation in mesenteric artery. J Cardiovasc Surg 15:486, 1974.

12. Rutledge RH: Superior mesenteric artery embolectomy. Ann Surg 159:529, 1964.
13. Zuidema GD: Surgical management of superior mesenteric arterial emboli. Arch Surg 82:267, 1961.

Chronic Occlusive Lesions

14. Bergan JJ: Recognition and treatment of intestinal ischemia. Surg Clin North Am 47:109, 1967.
15. Dardik H, Seidenberg B, Parker JG, Hurwitt ES: Intestinal angina with malabsorption treated by elective revascularization. J Am Med Assoc 194:1206, 1965.
16. Shingleton WW, Woods LP: Malabsorption syndrome. Surgery 59:886, 1966.
17. Morris GC Jr, DeBakey ME, Bernhard V: Abdominal angina. Surg Clin North Am 46:919, 1966.
18. Mikkelsen WP: Intestinal angina. Its surgical significance. Am J Surg 94:262, 1957.
19. Watt JK, Watson WC, Haase S: Chronic intestinal ischaemia. Br Med J 3:199, 1967.
20. Dunphy JE: Abdominal pain of vascular origin. Am J Med 192:109, 1936.
21. Reul GJ Jr, Wukasch DC, Sandiford FM, Chiariello L, Hallman GL, Cooley DA: Surgical treatment of abdominal angina: Review of 25 patients. Surgery 75:682, 1974.
22. Buxton B, Reul GJ Jr, Cooley DA: Transdiaphragmatic approach to the descending thoracic aorta for proximal control during surgery on the abdominal aorta. Bulletin of the Texas Heart Institute 4(#3):290, 1977.
23. Reul GJ Jr, Wukasch DC, Sandiford FM, Chiariello L, Hallman GL, Cooley DA: Surgical treatment of abdominal angina: Report of 25 patients. Surgery 75:682, 1974.
24. Rob C: Surgical diseases of the celiac and mesenteric arteries. Arch Surg 93:21, 1966.
25. Farooki MA: Aneurysms in the United States and the United Kingdom. Int Surg 58:475, 1973.
26. Mattox KL: Traumatic aneurysms. In *Vascular Surgery* (edited by Rutherford RB), W. B. Saunders Company, Philadelphia, 1977, pp 723–730.
27. Stoney RJ, Wylie EJ: Recognition and surgical management of visceral ischemic syndromes. Ann Surg 164:714, 1966.
28. DeBakey ME, Cooley DA: Successful resection of mycotic aneurysms of superior mesenteric artery; case report and review of literature. Am Surg 19:202, 1953.
29. Owens JC, Coffey RJ: Aneurysm of the splenic artery, including a report of 6 additional cases. Int Abstr Surg 97:313, 1953.
30. Bedford PD, Lodge B: Aneurysm of the splenic artery. Gut 1:312, 1960.

CHAPTER 9

Aortoiliac Occlusive Disease

Claudication, a term applied to the classic symptom of aortoiliac occlusive disease (AIOD), is derived from the Latin word *claudicare,* meaning to limp. This symptom was first described by Bouley in 1831,[1] a French veterinary student, who determined that one cause of limping in horses was muscle pain, resulting from thrombosis of the femoral artery. The syndrome produced by AIOD was described in 1923 by Leriche[2] as *aortitis terminalis.* Leriche prescribed bilateral sympathectomy for this condition, but predicted that the ultimate treatment would be restoration of circulation by means of an arterial graft. The concept of carotid artery endarterectomy was described by dos Santos in 1947,[3] applied to the abdominal aorta and iliac arteries by Wylie in 1952,[4] and extended to gas endarterectomy by Sobel and coworkers in 1966.[5] In our opinion, inversion endarterectomy, as described by Connolly in 1970,[6] has not been a practical solution to the problem.

In 1948, Gross and his colleagues[7] demonstrated the feasibility of using aortic homografts for the correction of coarctation, and homografts were later used for the treatment of AIOD. The major advance in the treatment of this disease, however, was the introduction of a synthetic Vinyon graft by Voorhees, Jaretzki, and Blakemore in 1952.[8] This new concept of synthetic grafts, combined with the technique of bypassing obstructive lesions as conceived by Kunlin of Paris in 1948,[9] led to the successful treatment of AIOD.

GENERAL CONCEPTS

BYPASS AS OPPOSED TO ENDARTERECTOMY

Although endarterectomy is the technique of choice for treating carotid artery occlusive disease, fabric bypass grafts have proven superior to endarterectomy of the abdominal aorta and iliac arteries. The bypass technique allows for preservation of collateral branches and the main channels above and below the site of occlusion. A disadvantage of endarterectomy in the region of an aortic bifurcation is that it destroys sympathetic fibers in this area, resulting in a high incidence of sexual impotency in males.

ADVANTAGES OF END-TO-END PROXIMAL ANASTOMOSIS

The end-to-end proximal anastomosis for aorta-to-iliac or femoral bypass is usually preferred to an end-to-side proximal anastomosis for several reasons: (1) The entire blood flow through the graft prevents stagnation and thrombosis; (2) the superior hemodynamics achieved by this method result in less turbulence and diminished recurrent atheroma formation; (3) visualization and inspection of the renal artery orifices is allowed in case of possible renal artery stenosis; and (4) the likelihood of microembolization or "trash foot" is minimized by complete endarterectomy and cleaning of the aorta below the renal arteries. This last point is emphasized because complete removal of debris within the aorta is difficult when a partial occluding clamp is placed for an end-to-side proximal anastomosis. An exception may occur when complete occlusion of both common or external iliac arteries would prevent retrograde flow to the inferior mesenteric and internal iliac arteries. Under these conditions, to preserve circulation to the sigmoid colon, an end-to-side proximal anastomosis is preferred. When the occlusion is localized and confined to the aortic bifurcation or common iliac arteries, a proximal end-to-side anastomosis may also be preferred.

Numerous techniques have been developed for preventing embolization of debris from the aorta proximal to the occluding clamp. The most commonly used method of flushing the aorta through the graft ("external flushing") results in significant blood loss, sometimes necessitating blood transfusion. External flushing also requires multiple clamping of the aorta, causing greater disruption of debris and more likelihood of microembolism. We have developed the technique of "internal flushing" to prevent microembolism while avoiding the above disadvantages. By this technique, loose debris in the proximal aorta is flushed into the pelvic region or thigh, where it can be tolerated without the disastrous effects (amputations) which often result from microemboli to the feet or toes. The proximal clamp is not released until the graft is in place and all anastomoses are completed; then the most proximal clamp is removed from one of the distal anastomoses, followed by gradual release of the proximal aortic clamp (Fig. 9–1, a to c). In the case of an aorta–common femoral artery bypass, this maneuver directs initial blood flow and loose debris retrograde up the common femoral artery into the internal iliac artery. The profunda femoral artery clamp is then removed, directing blood and debris into the thigh. The superficial femoral artery clamp is the last to be released. This technique may be applied during aorta-external iliac artery bypass by first releasing the proximal external iliac artery clamp, thus directing initial blood flow retrograde into the internal iliac artery rather than distally into the extremity. This technique has reduced the incidence of peripheral microembolism ("trash foot") in our cases.[10]

INDICATIONS AND CONTRAINDICATIONS

Where aortoiliac occlusive disease (AIOD) is revealed by aortography, revascularization is indicated when the following symptoms are present: intermittent claudication that interferes with the life style of the patient, pain at rest, or severe ischemia of the lower extremity that threatens viability of the limb. Operation is contraindicated in the absence of threatened tissue loss if the patient is sedentary or unable to walk for other reasons, such as paralysis, advanced age, and general debility. Significant extracranial carotid artery or coronary artery occlusive disease should be evaluated and treated prior to or concomitantly with revascularization of the lower extremities.

TREATMENT OF ASSOCIATED CONDITIONS

Cholecystectomy or gastric resection may be safely performed during surgery for AIOD after careful reperitonealization over the graft.[11] However, procedures that require opening of the small bowel or colon, such as elective appendectomy or colon resection for diverticulitis, are contraindicated because of the danger of graft infection.

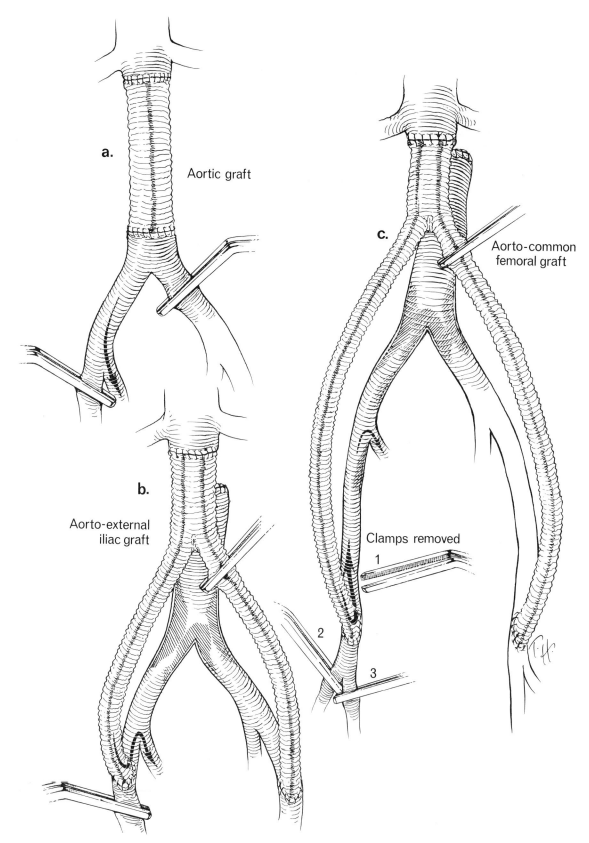

a. Aortic graft

b. Aorto-external iliac graft

c. Aorto-common femoral graft

Clamps removed

1

2

3

Figure 9–1 Clamping techniques (end-to-end anastomosis).

PREOPERATIVE MANAGEMENT

Angiographic evaluation of carotid artery and coronary artery occlusive disease should be performed if the patient has a history of findings suggestive of such lesions. Coagulation defects should be identified and corrected if possible. Acutely infected lesions in the lower extremities should be treated prior to surgery unless surgical delay would jeopardize viability of a foot or leg.

The patient should not undergo operation in a dehydrated condition. If a patient remains *nulla per os* (NPO) all day prior to arteriography and also prior to surgery the following day, the resulting state of dehydration will increase the risk of postoperative renal insufficiency. Routine antibiotics, usually 1 gm of cephalothin preoperatively and every six hours postoperatively, are indicated whenever arterial surgery is performed, and especially when prosthetic graft material is used.

STANDARD OPERATIVE PROCEDURES

AORTA–EXTERNAL ILIAC OR FEMORAL BYPASS

The symptom complex now referred to as the Leriche syndrome[1] results from occlusive disease in the terminal aorta, in the iliac arteries, and often in the femoral arteries (Fig. 9–2, a). Aortography is necessary in all cases to delineate the location and extent of the occlusive process and to assist in selecting the appropriate operative procedure. Distal anastomoses may be made to either the external iliac arteries or the common femoral arteries, depending upon the extent of disease in the iliac arteries. By using the external iliac arteries, an incision in the groin is avoided, and the chances of graft infection are decreased. In the majority of patients, however, the disease will extend into the external iliac or femoral arteries, necessitating distal anastomosis to the common or profunda femoris arteries. Particular attention must be given to stenosis at the origin of the profunda femoris artery. Profundoplasty should be performed in such instances. Distal anastomosis to the common iliac arteries is rarely indicated, because of the risk that subsequent distal disease will develop.

The abdomen is entered through a midline incision, care being taken not to "key hole" the umbilicus (Fig. 9–2, b). After exploration of the intra-abdominal organs and assurance that the nasogastric tube is properly positioned, the aorta is exposed by incising the peritoneum between the duodenum and inferior mesenteric vein (Fig. 9–2, c). When dissecting the duodenum from the aorta, it is important to leave a small cuff of peritoneum for later reperitonealization as a graft covering and to avoid placing sutures into the duodenum itself, predisposing to aortic duodenal fistula.

The external iliac arteries are exposed immediately cephalad to the inguinal ligaments, taking care to avoid injury to the ureters, which cross the arteries proximal to the site of dissection. The external iliac arteries may be elevated with tapes, but this is optional. A tunnel is then made with the index finger proximally beneath the posterior peritoneum under the sigmoid colon and mesocolon on the left.

Following systemic heparinization (2 mg/kg of body weight) and preclotting of the graft with blood, usually drawn from the inferior vena cava, the aorta is cross-clamped immediately below the renal arteries (Fig. 9–2, d). It is not necessary to pass a tape around the aorta, as doing so may tear a lumbar vein posterior to the aorta. The aortic clamp is applied at a point just distal to the origin of the renal arteries. If endarterectomy of the renal arteries is required, the aortic clamp is placed above the renal arteries after systemic injection of 25 gm of mannitol. A vascular clamp is placed on the distal aorta immediately proximal to the origin of the inferior mesenteric artery, thus preserving blood supply to the sigmoid colon. The aorta is then transected; approximately 3 cm is excised, and the distal aorta is oversewn with a 3–0

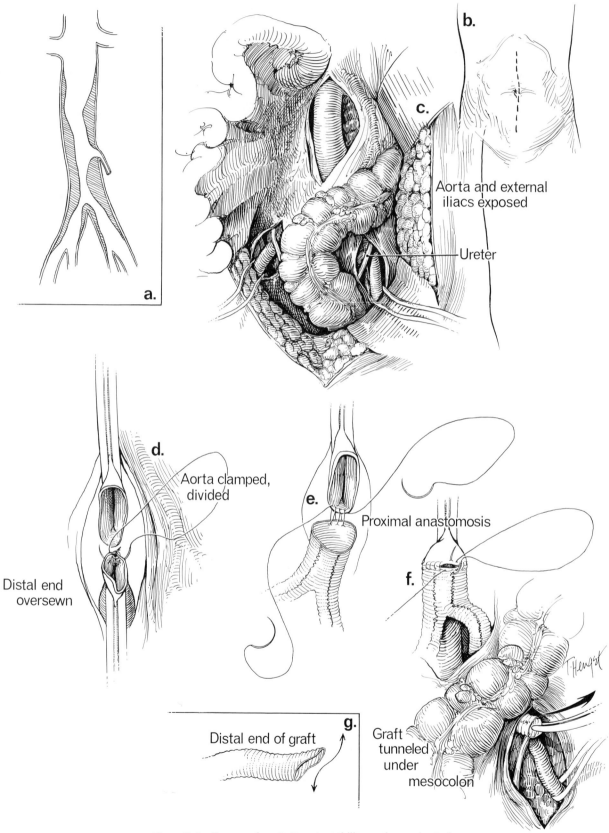

Figure 9–2 Bypass of aorta to external iliac or femoral arteries.

Illustration continued on opposite page.

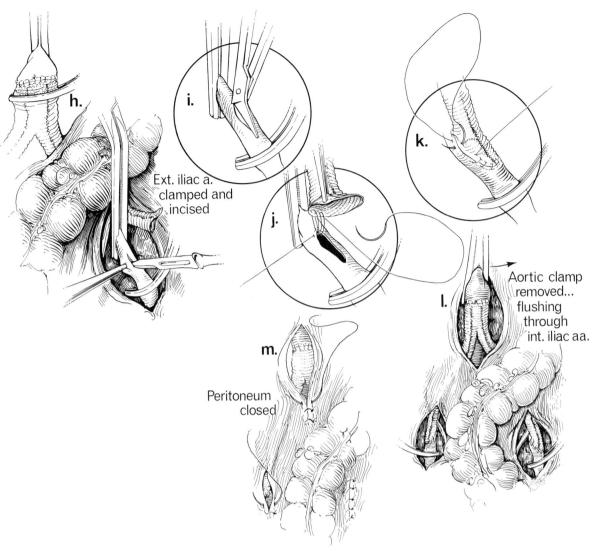

Figure 9–2 *Continued.*

polyester suture — even if it is completely occluded. A complete endarterectomy of the proximal aorta is performed, extending to the adventitial layer if necessary. An appropriate-sized double velour Dacron graft (usually 14 × 8 mm, or possibly a 12 × 7 mm for female patients) is then anastomosed end to end to the proximal aorta with a continuous 3–0 polyester double-ended suture (Fig. 9–2, e). The distal ends of the graft are then passed through the previously made retroperitoneal tunnels, under the mesocolon on the left (Fig. 9–2, f), and they are tailored by means of an S-shaped incision to ensure a rounded rather than a sharply pointed end (Fig. 9–2, g). After clamping the external iliac artery, a vertical arteriotomy is made with a No. 15 blade scalpel (Fig. 9–2, h), and extended with Potts scissors (Fig. 9–2, i). The distal anastomoses are made with running 4–0 polyester sutures (Fig. 9–2, j and k).

After completion of both anastomoses, it is important to remove the clamps in proper sequence to prevent debris from the aorta proximal to the clamp from being directed into the lower extremities and producing microembolization or "trash foot." The proximal iliac clamps are removed first, followed by gradual removal of the aortic clamp (Fig. 9–2, l). In this manner, the initial blood flow and possible debris from the proximal artery are directed retrograde into the internal iliac arteries where the debris may be less harmful. If possible, the aortic clamp should be applied and removed only once, thereby minimizing dislodgement of debris in the proximal aorta. Flow is finally restored to the lower extremities by removing the distal iliac clamps, and the effects of heparin are reversed by giving systemic protamine, 1.5 mg for each 1.0 mg of previously given heparin. The peritoneum is closed over the graft with meticulous care to avoid penetrating the duodenum or inferior mesenteric vein proximally and injuring the ureters distally (Fig. 9–2, *m*).

In rare cases where both external iliac arteries are completely occluded and retrograde flow to the pelvis by way of the internal iliac or inferior mesenteric arteries is prevented, an end-to-side proximal aortic anastomosis should be made (Fig. 9–3, *a*).

AORTOFEMORAL BYPASS

To perform an aortofemoral bypass, the common femoral arteries are exposed through vertical incisions in the groins (Fig. 9–3, *b*). A retroperitoneal tunnel is made under the inguinal ligament by careful blunt dissection with the use of both index fingers. A pointed instrument should never be used, as it may cause injury to the ureters, colon, or bladder. If the tunnel is too tight, constriction and occlusion of the graft can result. Adequate tunnel size in some patients may be obtained by cutting a portion of the inferior aspect of the inguinal ligament. In our observation, postoperative inguinal or femoral herniation has not resulted from this maneuver. The completed tunnel should allow easy passage of the surgeon's index finger. The distal limbs of the graft are then passed distally through the tunnel by means of a curved ring forceps.

The distal anastomoses to the common femoral arteries just proximal to the bifurcation are made in the same fashion as in the external iliac arteries. The sequence of releasing the distal clamps to prevent microembolization should be

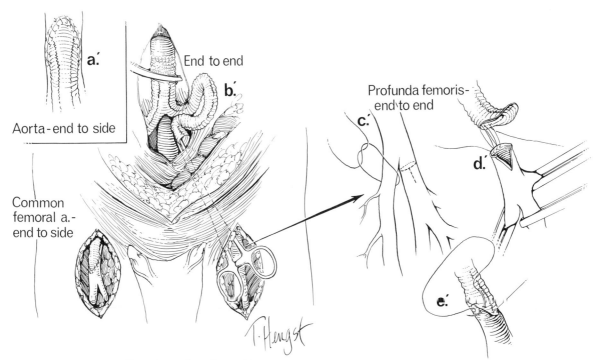

Figure 9–3 Aortofemoral bypass and reconstruction of profunda femoris.

used. First, the proximal common femoral artery clamp is removed, followed by gradual removal of the aortic clamp, thus directing the initial blood flow retrograde into the internal iliac arteries. The profunda femoris artery clamp is removed next, allowing any remaining debris to be washed into the musculature of the thigh rather than into the toes. The superficial femoral artery clamp is removed last, and protamine is administered.

PROFUNDA FEMORIS ARTERY RECONSTRUCTION

Not infrequently, both the common and superficial femoral arteries will be completely stenosed at the origin of the profunda femoris artery. In these situations, it is imperative to dissect distally down the profunda femoris artery as far as is necessary to obtain a favorable location for the anastomosis (Fig. 9–3, c).

Although it is occasionally necessary to dissect past the third or fourth branches, as many of these branches should be saved as possible. In cases of dissection past the third or fourth branches, the distal limb of the graft often must be anastomosed end-to-end to the profunda femoris artery (Fig. 9–3, d and e). "Blind" endarterectomy of the profunda femoris artery should be avoided. Even a moderate restoration of flow to the profunda femoris arteries should provide enough circulation to the lower extremities to prevent limb loss even though the superficial femoral artery is completely occluded. In such cases, femoral popliteal bypass may be deferred for at least three months to assess the degree of symptomatic improvement. The majority of such patients do not return for further femoral popliteal revascularization. In patients with extensive peripheral occlusive disease involving the superficial femoral, popliteal, and tibial arteries, a concomitant lumbar sympathectomy should be done, removing one or two ganglia. Routine sympathectomy in AIOD is not performed in our patients, however, because it is usually unnecessary, may cause impotency in male patients, and may cause troublesome postsympathectomy neuralgia.

FEMORAL-TO-FEMORAL-ARTERY BYPASS

Although iliac artery occlusive disease is often symmetrical, some patients present with unilateral iliac artery disease, with a bounding femoral pulse on one side and none on the other (Fig. 9–4, a). Such patients, especially those of advanced age or those who are extremely obese and in whom intra-abdominal surgery may be undesirable, will benefit from femoral-to-femoral-artery bypass. This procedure provides satisfactory long-term results, and avoids the necessity of entering the abdomen.

Both common femoral arteries are exposed through vertical groin incisions (Fig. 9–4, a). A subcutaneous tunnel is made just above the pubis by digital dissection anterior to the pubic fascia (Fig. 9–4, b). Following systemic heparinization (2 mg/kg of body weight) and clamping of the arteries, vertical arteriotomies are made in both common femoral arteries (Fig. 9–4, c). An 8 mm Dacron double velour graft is used. After completion of the proximal anastomosis with running 4–0 polyester suture (Fig. 9–4, d), the graft is passed through the suprapubic tunnel with a curved ring forceps (Fig. 9–4, e); the distal anastomosis is made in a similar fashion (Fig. 9–4, f and g). If the superficial femoral artery is completely occluded or stenosis of the proximal profunda femoris artery exists on the side of the distal anastomosis, as is frequently the case, the anastomosis should be extended distally down the profunda femoris artery, past the site of obstruction. Alternatively, the distal anastomosis may be made end-to-end to the profunda femoris artery.

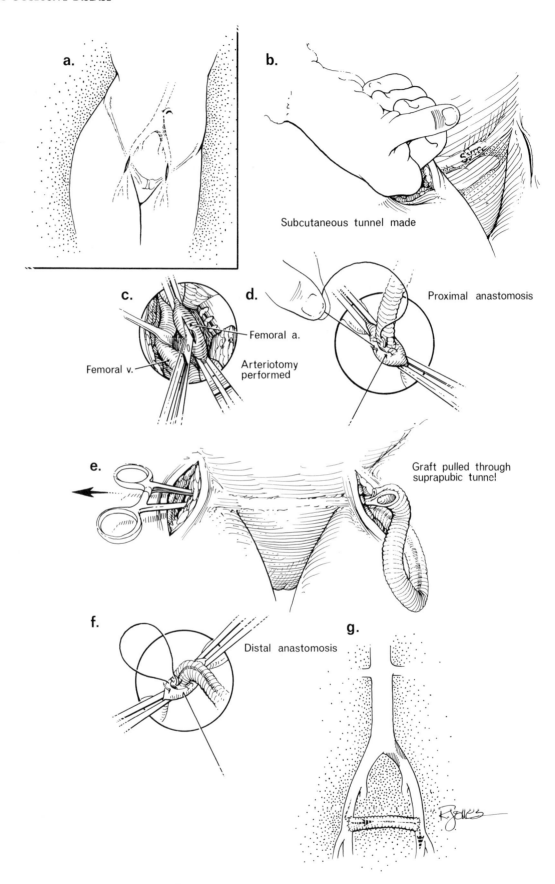

a.

b.

Subcutaneous tunnel made

c.

Femoral a.

Femoral v.

Arteriotomy performed

d.

Proximal anastomosis

e.

Graft pulled through suprapubic tunnel

f.

Distal anastomosis

g.

Figure 9–4 Femoral-to-femoral artery bypass.

RECURRENT DISEASE AND "REDO" PROCEDURES

INTRODUCTION

Reoperation for late thrombosis of a graft often precludes a standard surgical procedure and necessitates innovation in overcoming technical problems. The patient with recurrent aortoiliac occlusive disease (AIOD) who has had one or more previous vascular anastomoses may benefit from one of three surgical approaches: (1) standard removal of the previous graft with replacement by a new graft, (2) end-to-side placement of a new proximal anastomosis to the supraceliac abdominal aorta at the level of the diaphragm (see Chapter 8, Fig. 8–1, a and b), or (3) ascending aorta-to-femoral-artery bypass.[12]

STANDARD "REDO" AORTOFEMORAL BYPASS

In patients who require reoperation because of late graft thrombosis, revascularization can usually be accomplished by removal and replacement of the previously placed graft. The abdomen is entered through the old incision, and the skin scar is excised. After the graft in the abdomen has been exposed to the left of the duodenum, its fibrous encasement is incised, allowing the graft to be peeled away. Clamping of the aorta below the renal arteries may be difficult because of scar tissue surrounding the proximal anastomosis; often, therefore, the aorta may be more easily clamped above the renal arteries or at the level of the diaphragm. The latter is accomplished by dissecting the aorta at this level, to the right of the esophagus.

Rather than entirely removing the old graft, the previous proximal anastomosis is left in place, along with a 1-cm cuff, to which the new graft is anastomosed. Dissection of the aorta in the area of the old anastomosis is avoided because of its friability and difficulty of repair in an area of previous dissection.

The distal anastomoses are exposed through the earlier groin incisions. The tedious dissection required to obtain proximal and distal control of an old anastomosis may be avoided by dissecting downward on the old graft and entering the anastomosis directly, with control of back-bleeding by Fogarty catheters. It is usually desirable, however, to obtain control by dissecting the artery proximally and distally prior to opening the anastomoses.

As a general rule, it is desirable to redo the distal anastomoses instead of replacing the graft limb and leaving a cuff. Since the cause of graft thrombosis is usually unknown, it seems theoretically desirable to change as many factors as possible. This line of reasoning emphasizes the importance of making a *new* tunnel between the abdomen and groin. After removal of the thrombosed graft limb, the new tunnel should be formed by gentle finger dissection from above and below. Use of any instrument in this maneuver is *absolutely contraindicated* to prevent injury to the ureter, bladder, or colon. *Gradual constriction by scar tissue within the tunnel is, most likely, a principal cause of graft thrombosis; therefore, the temptation to use the old tunnel, which may have caused the graft failure in the first place, should be avoided.)*

Another important decision is necessary when one limb of a bifurcation has become thrombosed but the other remains patent. The surgeon must determine whether or not to replace the patent limb. The easy way is to leave it alone; however, the factors that caused the thrombosis of one limb — whether pseudointima build-up or constriction within the tunnel — may be developing bilaterally and may result in thrombosis of the other limb at a later date if not corrected. Therefore, consideration should be given to replacing the patent limb as well, particularly if thick pseudointima build-up is present at the time of operation. If the decision is made to replace only one limb of the graft, the bifurcation of the old graft should be resected and replaced.

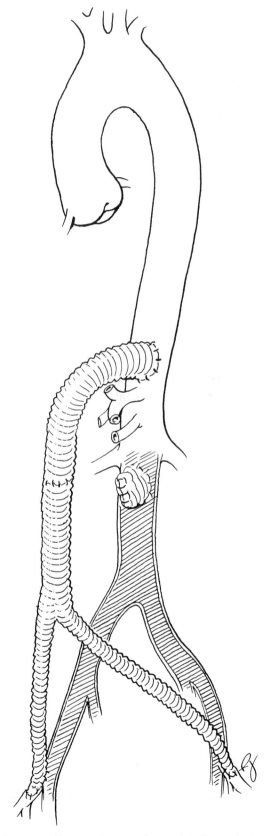

Figure 9–5 Bypass of supraceliac aorta to femoral artery.

SUPRACELIAC AORTA-TO-FEMORAL-ARTERY BYPASS

In complex situations that preclude the standard operative approach, such as inaccessibility of the infrarenal aorta because of adhesions or pseudoaneurysm formation, proximal anastomosis to the supraceliac aorta at the level of the diaphragm is a practical solution.[12] The previous graft is transected, and the distal end is oversewn, leaving the proximal anastomosis in place (Fig. 9–5). When a false aneurysm of the proximal anastomosis is present, the entire graft must be removed and the aorta itself oversewn.

The supraceliac abdominal aorta is exposed by retracting the left lobe of the liver cephalad and the stomach in a caudad direction. The posterior peritoneum is incised above the upper margin of the pancreas. The right crus of the diaphragm is incised, exposing a 6-cm length "bare area" of the abdominal aorta proximal to the celiac axis (see Chapter 8, Fig. 8–1, a). After heparinization, this segment of the aorta is clamped with either a partially occluding clamp or two vascular clamps (see Chapter 8, Fig. 8–1, b). The proximal end of a 14 × 8 mm Dacron double velour knitted graft is anastomosed to the aorta end-to-side with a continuous suture of 3–0 polyester. The graft is placed anterior to the pancreas, to the left of the third portion of the duodenum, along the aorta retroperitoneally into the groin, where distal anastomoses are made (Fig. 9–5).

Use of the supraceliac "bare area" of the abdominal aorta appears to offer a new and practical solution to otherwise difficult situations.[12] Several characteristics make this segment of the aorta an ideal site for proximal anastomosis. It is of adequate length to accommodate the graft and is the portion of aorta least likely to be affected by atherosclerosis. In addition, the aorta is relatively free of tributaries at this site, lessening the potential of spinal cord devascularization.

ASCENDING AORTA–FEMORAL ARTERY BYPASS

In rare cases when the supraceliac aorta is extensively diseased and unsatisfactory for anastomosis, the ascending thoracic aorta may be used as the site of the proximal anastomosis.[12] In any "redo" vascular procedure, the patient is prepped and draped so that his chest is exposed, in the event that use of the ascending aorta becomes necessary. In addition to recurrent aortoiliac occlusive disease (AIOD) (Fig. 9–6, e), the ascending aorta may be used for proximal anastomosis in other complex conditions, including recurrent coarctation of the thoracic aorta with or without infection (Fig. 9–6, a),* coarctation of the thoracic aorta with associated intracardiac conditions requiring concomitant treatment (Fig. 9–6, b), interruption of the aortic arch in infants (Fig. 9 6, c), and coarctation of the abdominal aorta (Fig. 9–6, d).*

Several ingenious bypass procedures for managing such difficult situations have been reported: Axillofemoral bypass for AIOD (Blaisdell and Hall, 1963);[13] innominate artery–distal abdominal aorta bypass for coarctation (Inokuchi and colleagues, 1971);[14] descending thoracic aorta–femoral artery bypass for AIOD (Nunn and Kamal, 1073);[15] and aortic arch or proximal descending thoracic aorta–distal descending thoracic aorta bypass for recurrent coarctation (Weldon and associates, 1973).[16]

Use of the ascending aorta for proximal anastomoses was reported in 1968 by Shumacker and coworkers[17] in a patient who had a mycotic aneurysm after repair of coarctation of the thoracic aorta. In this case, a graft was extended from the ascend-

---

*See Chapter 12, Coarctations of the Thoracic and Abdominal Aorta.

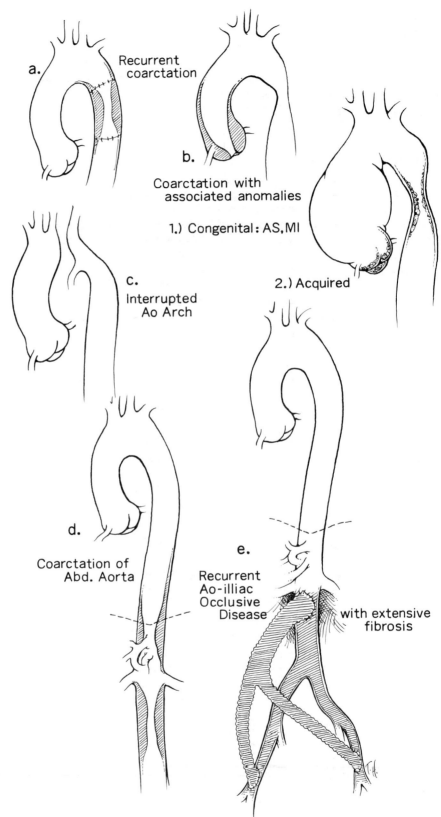

a. Recurrent coarctation

b. Coarctation with associated anomalies

1.) Congenital: AS, MI

2.) Acquired

c. Interrupted Ao Arch

d. Coarctation of Abd. Aorta

e. Recurrent Ao-illiac Occlusive Disease with extensive fibrosis

Figure 9-6 Some conditions requiring ascending aorta–abdominal aorta bypass.

ing aorta to the infrarenal abdominal aorta. In 1972, Robinson and colleagues[18] reported treatment of a dissecting descending thoracic aortic aneurysm by means of a graft from the ascending aorta to the infrarenal abdominal aorta. In 1974, Siderys and associates[19] reported a successful bypass graft from the ascending aorta to the infrarenal abdominal aorta in a patient with coarctation of the thoracic aorta that was inaccessible because of a fibrothorax. The same year, Frantz and associates[20] reported a case in which an ascending aorta–femoral bypass was performed in a patient with severe AIOD. Twelve cases in which the ascending aorta was used for proximal anastomosis were reported from our institution in 1977.

OPERATIVE TECHNIQUE

When the ascending aorta is to be used for proximal anastomosis, the midline abdominal incision is extended cephalad to become a standard median sternotomy. The ascending aorta is exposed by dividing the mediastinal tissues, leaving the pericardium intact; systemic heparinization is instituted after the grafts have been preclotted. A partially occluding clamp is then placed on the ascending aorta, and a preclotted 16-mm Dacron double velour graft is anastomosed end-to-side to the aorta with 3–0 polyester suture (Fig. 9–7). The graft is passed to the right of the right atrium, ventral to the inferior vena cava, and then through a T-shaped opening made in the fibrous portion of the diaphragm.

Because standard grafts are not long enough for this procedure, a second preclotted 16 × 8 mm Dacron double velour graft is anastomosed end-to-end to the first graft, thus affording the required length (Fig. 9–7). After traversing the diaphragm, the graft is passed through the gastrohepatic ligament, posterior to the stomach, into the retroperitoneum, anterior to the pancreas, and along the course of the abdominal aorta and iliac arteries. The femoral anastomoses are constructed as described previously. *The importance of maintaining retrograde flow through at least one external iliac artery into the pelvis and abdomen is emphasized. When this is not accomplished, gangrene of the entire lower abdomen and pelvis can occur, with otherwise successful revascularization of the lower extremities.* The wounds are closed in standard fashion, with a single tube placed to drain the mediastinum.

AVOIDING IMPOTENCY

Sexual dysfunction in males is frequently associated with aortoiliac occlusive disease (AIOD) and surgical treatment. Disorders of sexual function are generally classified as impotency (inability to achieve and maintain an erection) and retrograde ejaculation.[21] These disorders may be due to either the basic disease process, i.e., diminished blood flow to the penis via the internal iliac arteries, or to iatrogenic surgical intervention, most frequently by disruption of the sympathetic innervation of the genitalia, but occasionally by shunting previously adequate blood flow away from the internal iliac arteries.

After revascularization for AIOD, the incidence of impotence has been reported by May and coworkers[22] to be 34 percent and the incidence of postoperative abnormalities of ejaculation 49 percent. In postoperative resection of abdominal aortic aneurysm, the incidence of impotency is 21 percent and retrograde ejaculation 63 percent.[22] Weinstein and Machleder[21] found similar results: 20 percent of their patients who underwent aortofemoral bypass for AIOD experienced postoperative impotence, and none complained of retrograde ejaculation. Among their abdominal aortic-aneurysm resection patients, 8 percent experienced postoperative impotence and 50 percent complained of postoperative retrograde ejaculation. Lumbar sympathectomy with bilateral excision of the L1 ganglia will increase the risk of impo-

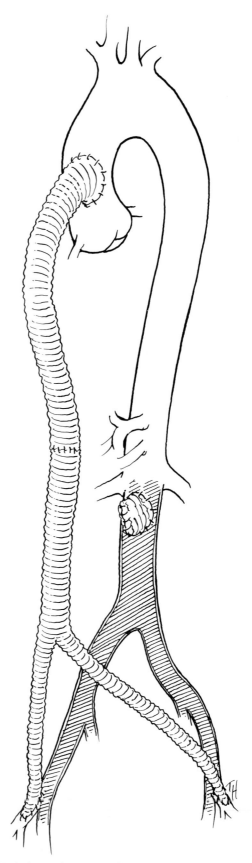

Figure 9–7 Operative technique when ascending aorta is to be used for proximal anastomosis. A second preclotted 16 × 18 mm Dacron double velour graft is anastomosed end-to-end to the first graft for increased length.

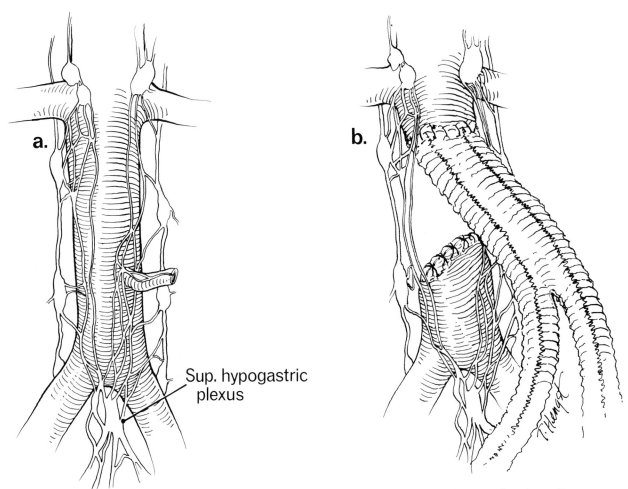

Sup. hypogastric
plexus

Figure 9-8 Aortofemoral bypass and preservation of the sympathetic plexi surrounding the aortic bifurcation.

tency.[23] Resection of the superior hypogastric plexus at the aortic bifurcation (Fig. 9-8, a) results in retrograde ejaculation.[21, 24] Therefore, high sympathetic denervation (L1–L2 level) produces impotency, whereas lower denervation (L2–L3 level, or at presacral and hypogastric plexi) results in retrograde ejaculation.[21]

To avoid impotency, several principles should be followed:

(1) When performing lumbar sympathectomy, the L1 ganglia should be preserved.

(2) The hypogastric plexus (Fig. 9-8, a), which is formed immediately distal to the aortic bifurcation, lies over the left common iliac vein, and extends above the level of the inferior mesenteric artery, must not be removed unless absolutely necessary. In our opinion, aortoiliac endarterectomy is more likely to result in disruption of the sympathetic plexus than is the bypass technique. For this reason, we prefer aortofemoral bypass and preservation of the sympathetic plexi surrounding the aortic bifurcation rather than aortoiliac endarterectomy (Fig. 9-8, b). Preservation of the hypogastric sympathetic plexus during abdominal aortic aneurysm resection is more difficult. Whenever possible, the aortic bifurcation is preserved and a tube graft is used, even in the presence of significant calcification of the common iliac arteries. Because the hypogastric plexus usually is situated over the left lateral aspect of the aorta surrounding the inferior mesenteric artery, the aneurysm should be incised along its right lateral aspect. When a bifurcation graft is necessary, the left common iliac artery wall and overlying sympathetic plexus can be preserved by passing the left limb of the graft through the intact segment of the common iliac artery.[21]

(3) It is important to remember that during construction of an aortofemoral bypass graft, blood flow to at least one internal iliac artery must be preserved.

REFERENCES

1. Bouley J: Claudication intermittente des membres posterieurs determinee par l'obliteration des arteres femoralis. Rec de Med Veter 8:517–527, 1831.
2. Leriche R: Des obliterations arterielles hautes (obliteration de la terminaison de l'aorte) comme causes des insutlisances circulatories des membres inferieurs. Bull Mem Soc Chir Paris 49:1904, 1923.
3. dos Santos, JC: Sur la deobstruction des thromboses arterielles anciennes. Mem Acad Chir 73:409, 1947.
4. Wylie EJ.: Thromboendarterectomy for atherosclerotic thrombosis of major arteries. Surgery 32:275, 1952.
5. Sobel S, Kaplitt MJ, Reingold M, Sawyer PN: Gas endarterectomy. Surgery 59:517, 1966.
6. Connolly JE, Stemmer EA: Eversion endarterectomy of the aortoiliofemoral arteries. Arch Surg 100:461, 1970.
7. Gross RE, Bill AH Jr, Peirce CE II: Methods of preservation and transplantation of arterial grafts; observations on arterial grafts in dogs; report of transplantation of preserved arterial grafts in nine human cases. Surg Gynec Obstet 88:689, 1949.
8. Voorhees AB, Jaretzki A, Blakemore AW: The use of tubes constructed from Vinyon "N" cloth in bridging arterial defects. Ann Surg 135:332, 1952.
9. Kunlin J: Le traitement de l'arterite obliterante par la greffe veinuse. Arch Mal Coer 42:371, 1949.
10. Wukasch DC, Cooley DA, Bennett JG, Trono R: Results of a new Meadox-Cooley double velour Dacron graft for arterial reconstruction. J Cardiovasc Surg (Torino) 1979 (in press).
11. Tompkins WC Jr, Chavez CM, Conn JH, Hardy JD: Combining intra-abdominal arterial grafting with gastrointestinal or biliary tract procedures. Am J Surg 126:598, 1973.
12. Wukasch DC, Cooley DA, Sandiford FM, Nappi G, Reul GJ Jr: Ascending aorta–abdominal aorta bypass: Indications, techniques, and report of 12 patients. Ann Thorac Surg 23:442, 1977.
13. Blaisdell FW, Hall AD: Axillofemoral artery bypass for lower extremity ischemia. Surgery 54:563, 1963.
14. Inokuchi K, Kusaba A, Ono K, Sugimachi K: Innomino-abdominal aortic bypass graft: a safe alternative for coarctation of aorta. Jpn J Surg 1:161, 1971.
15. Nunn DB, Kamal MA: Bypass grafting from the thoracic aorta to femoral arteries for high aortoiliac occlusive disease. Surgery 72:749, 1972.
16. Weldon CS, Hartman AF, Steinhoff NG, Morrissey JD: A simple, safe and rapid technique for the management of recurrent coarctation of the aorta. Ann Surg 15:510, 1973.
17. Shumacker HB Jr, King H, Nahrwold DL, Waldhausen JA: Coarctation of the aorta. Curr Probl Surg 1968, pp. 16–48.
18. Robinson G, Siegelman S, Attai L: Recurrent dissecting aneurysm of aorta. NY State J Med 72:2328, 1972.
19. Siderys H, Graffs R, Hallbrook H, Kasbeckar V: A technique for management of inaccessible coarctation of the aorta. J Thorac Cardiovasc Surg 67:568, 1974.
20. Frantz SL, Kaplitt MJ, Beil AR Jr, Stein HL: Ascending aorta-bilateral femoral artery bypass for the totally occluded infrarenal abdominal aorta. Surgery 75:471, 1974.
21. Weinstein MH, Machleder HI: Sexual function after aorto-iliac surgery. Ann Surg (June) p 787, 1975.
22. May AG, DeWeese JA, Rob CG: Changes in sexual function following operation on the abdominal aorta. Surgery 65:41, 1969.
23. Whitelaw GP, Smithwick RH: Some secondary effects of sympathectomy. N Engl J Med 245:121, 1951.
24. Leiter E, Brendler H: Loss of ejaculation following bilateral retroperitoneal lymphadenectomy. J Urol 98:375, 1967.

CHAPTER 10

Femoropopliteal Occlusive Disease

INTRODUCTION AND GENERAL CONCEPTS

Since the first femoropopliteal bypass was reported by Kunlin in 1949,[1] surgical treatment of femoropopliteal occlusive disease (FPOD) has proven effective for relief of ischemic symptoms and limb salvage in properly selected patients. Several general principles of treatment for this condition have evolved from our experience.

Femoropopliteal bypass procedures (FPB) should be restricted to patients in whom claudication interferes with their quality of life or in whom loss of limb is threatened. Reversed saphenous vein grafts appear to be the material of choice; however, if a suitable vein is not available (or in certain selected elderly patients with satisfactory above-the-knee popliteal artery segments), Dacron material, particularly the newly developed Cooley-Meadox Dacron double velour fabric,* has proven to be an acceptable arterial substitute. Bangash and coworkers[2] have reported excellent results in 54 patients in whom this material was used for below-the-knee anastomosis. Although bovine heterografts have provided satisfactory immediate results, long-term follow-up in our own experience with this material has not been satisfactory. Long-term results reported by the Dardik brothers concerning use of the Dardik Biograft** (an umbilical vein homograft) have been encouraging. This material holds promise for use in patients requiring distal tibial or peroneal artery anastomoses, in whom autogenous saphenous vein grafts (SVG) are not available.[3] Others have reported successful use of grafts fabricated from expanded Teflon (polytetrafluoroethylene),† but long-term results are not available.

Because disease is frequently present in the proximal popliteal artery, even when not discernible by arteriography, below-the-knee popliteal anastomosis is usually preferable to anastomosis above the knee, especially if a suitable SVG is available.

When visualized with oblique arteriographic views, many patients with occluded superficial femoral arteries will demonstrate stenosis of the proximal profunda femoris artery, and their symptoms will be significantly relieved by patch profundaplasty rather than by FPB, with its inherent failure rate.[4, 5] In applying the former approach, one should consider the possibility of extending the endarterectomy and patch arterioplasty beyond the third muscular branch of the profunda femoris artery.[6]

Arteriography for visualization of the distal popliteal runoff should be performed (or supervised) if possible by the surgeon responsible for making the anatomic decisions for operative therapy. *Surgeons who have had to make critical intraopera-*

---

*Available from Meadox Medicals, Oakland, New Jersey.
**Obtainable from Meadox Medicals, Oakland, New Jersey.
†Available from W. L. Gore & Associates, Inc., Newark, Delaware.

tive decisions with inadequate arteriograms will appreciate this point. Facilities for intraoperative arteriograms should always be available, although it is not always necessary to employ them routinely.

TECHNIQUE OF SAPHENOUS VEIN PREPARATION

After the leg has been shaved, treated with cleansing and antiseptic solution, and draped appropriately to expose the inner aspect of the groin, thigh, and leg to the ankle, the saphenous vein is removed. We use multiple 4 to 6 cm incisions parallel to the course of the vein. This multiple incision technique appears to reduce postoperative complications, adds to the comfort of the patient, and enhances healing. The initial incision is usually in the groin where the entrance of the vein into the common femoral vein is identified (Fig. 10–1, *a*). From there, multiple skin incisions are made along the course of the vein, and the tributaries are identified and divided (Fig. 10–1, *b*). If a long length of graft is needed, the vein may be mobilized to the ankle. We usually divide the tributaries as they are encountered, placing a hemoclip distally and removing the vein from the extremity before ligating the branches next to the vein.

When the vein has been removed, a plastic disposable cannula of small diameter is tied into the distal end (Fig. 10–1, *c*). The cannula will be used to inject and distend the vein. For this purpose, blood is removed from either the femoral vein or artery

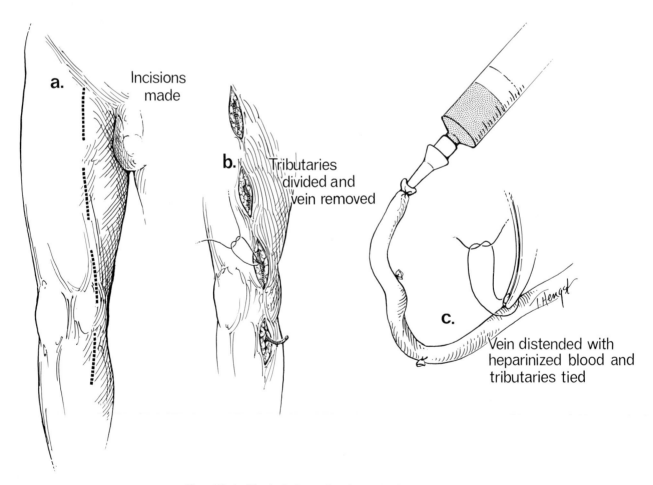

a. Incisions made

b. Tributaries divided and vein removed

c. Vein distended with heparinized blood and tributaries tied

Figure 10–1 The technique of saphenous vein preparation.

Antero-medial view-Rt. leg

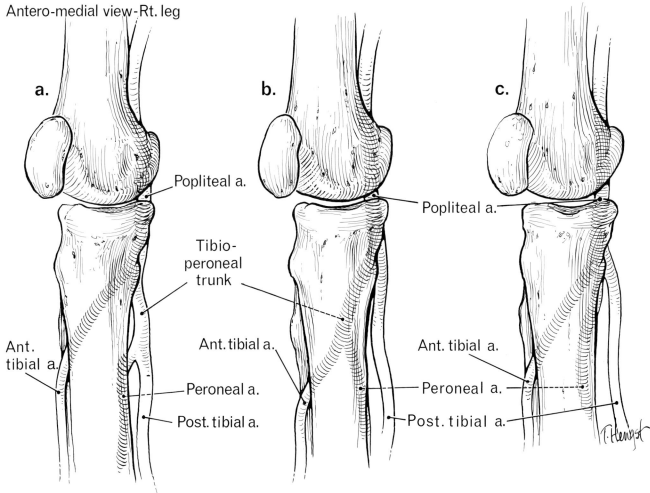

Figure 10–2 Anatomic variations of the popliteal artery.

into a syringe containing heparin. We are of the opinion that blood is the best medium for distending the vein because it will not diffuse into the wall of the vein as would electrolyte solutions, thus causing mechanical damage to the cellular structures. The vein is gently distended, just enough to overcome smooth muscle spasm. Overdistention, which may be injurious, is avoided. Tributaries are identified, grasped with small hemostatic forceps, and ligated with a 3–0 ligature, usually of silk. If the stump of the branch vessel is short, the ligature may compromise the lumen of the saphenous vein. Under these circumstances, dissection of adventitia may relieve the constriction. If not, the branch vessel should be oversewn with a 5–0 or 6–0 monofilament polypropylene suture. Once the vein has been prepared by distention with blood and all leaks closed, the blood should be removed by injecting a balanced salt solution (preferably cold) and put aside in a cup containing the cold solution until it is inserted.

ANATOMIC VARIATIONS OF THE POPLITEAL ARTERY

The popliteal artery normally divides into the anterior tibial and tibioperoneal trunk, which, after 3 to 4 cm, bifurcates into the peroneal and posterior tibial arteries (Fig. 10–2, *a*).[7] Most anatomy books incorrectly describe the popliteal artery as dividing into three branches and do not even mention the "tibioperoneal trunk." Two major variations in popliteal artery division have been described by Morris and associates[8]; they are (1) a high origin of the posterior tibial, which occurs in 2 percent of persons (Fig. 10–2, b), and (2) a true trifurcation, which occurs in 2.9 percent (Fig. 10–2, c).

FEMOROPOPLITEAL BYPASS WITH SAPHENOUS VEIN

Femoropopliteal bypass with below-the-knee anastomosis and the use of an autogenous saphenous vein is the procedure of choice for patients with occlusion of the superficial femoral artery but no significant stenosis at the origin of the profunda femoris artery (Fig. 10–3, a). The patient is placed in the supine position with the involved leg prepped to the ankle and the entire lower extremity mobilized so that it may be flexed at the knee or straightened as required during the procedure (Fig. 10–3, b). Folded towels placed under the knee facilitate exposure of the saphenous vein and popliteal artery. Dissection of the saphenous vein is performed through four separate incisions over the length of the vein, thus avoiding an incision which crosses the flexion crease of the knee. Adequate skin bridges should be left. Side branches of the vein are ligated with hemoclips at least 0.5 cm away from their origin and are transected. To assure that ligation with 3–0 silk will not constrict the vein lumen, ligation of the branches on the vein side is deferred until the entire vein has been removed and distended (Fig. 10–3, c). Heparinized blood drawn from the femoral vein is used in distention because solutions with less osmolarity, such as saline, may diffuse into the vessel wall, resulting in edema and possible late fibrosis. During dissection, care is taken to *prevent* crushing of the vein with forceps, which can produce intimal damage.

Exposure of the common femoral and popliteal arteries is carried out through upper and lower incisions (Fig. 10–3, d), avoiding injury to the femoral nerve, which lies immediately lateral to the femoral artery. Injury to this nerve results in severe pain and partial paralysis of the musculature at its distribution, including the quadriceps. It is most commonly caused by improper placement of a pointed retractor or a too deeply placed suture around the nerve during closure of the wound. This complication is rarely recognized until after surgery. Should it become evident postoperatively, early re-exploration of the nerve should be performed along with neurolysis to determine whether a closing suture was placed around the nerve. Exposure of the popliteal artery below the knee may be facilitated by dividing the tendons of the semitendinosus and semimembranosus muscles and repairing them during wound closure (Fig. 10–3, d).

A tunnel is made through the popliteal space by blunt finger dissection under the medial head of the gastrocnemius muscle and under the sartorius muscle (Fig. 10–3, e). Following administration of systemic heparin (2 mg/kg of body weight), distal anastomosis between the vein graft and the popliteal artery is performed end-to-side with running 6–0 polypropylene suture (Fig. 10–3, f) and (Fig. 10–3, g and h). After completion of the distal anastomosis, the clamps are removed from the popliteal artery and then the vein graft is gently clamped (Fig. 10–3, i). To obtain proper determination of length and to prevent twisting, the graft is distended with heparinized blood and is then passed cephalad through the previously made tunnel.

Prior to final estimation of vein length, the folded towels are removed from behind the knee, which is then straightened. Failure to perform this maneuver will result in a vein graft which is too short when the leg is subsequently straightened. The surgeon checks each portion of the tunnel by passing his fingers through to assure that it is not too tight.

A vertical arteriotomy is made over the *common femoral artery* and the proximal anastomosis is made end-to-side in a similar fashion (Fig. 10–3, *j*). *The profunda femoris artery should always be identified to assure that the proximal anastomosis is made to the common femoral artery and not to the superficial femoral artery.* If stenosis of the proximal profunda femoris exists, a patch profundaplasty should be performed concomitantly. The vein graft is gently clamped and the arterial clamps are removed to assure that any loose debris will be flushed down the profunda femoris artery rather than down the vein graft (Fig. 10–3, *k* and *l*). Circulation is restored through the graft (Fig. 10–3, *m*), and systemic heparin is reversed with protamine sulfate in a ratio of 1.5/1.0 to the previous heparin dose. The completed graft is demonstrated in Figure 10–3, *n*.

BYPASS TO DISTAL BRANCHES OF THE POPLITEAL ARTERY

Due to recent improvements in surgical techniques for small vessel bypass procedures, limbs can often be salvaged, even when the popliteal artery is completely occluded and only one of the distal branches of the popliteal artery is patent.[9, 10, 11] The following sections will describe surgical exposure of the peroneal, anterior tibial, and posterior tibial arteries.

SURGICAL APPROACH TO PERONEAL ARTERY

Herbert and Irving Dardik, who have obtained acceptable early patency rates with anastomoses to the distal peroneal and tibial arteries (86 percent at 3 months and 67 percent at 1 year) describe a simplified technique for exposing the peroneal artery. Our procedure is adopted from their technique.[12]

The peroneal artery arises from the tibioperoneal trunk (Fig. 10–4, *a*) and lies deep in the posterior lateral aspect of the leg, medial to the fibula. The artery is contained in a fibrous sheath and courses adjacent to the soleus and posterior tibial muscles proximally and along the flexor hallucis longus muscle distally.

With the hip and knee flexed and rotated medially, a lateral incision is made over the fibula (Fig. 10–4, *b*). The peroneal muscles are reflected medially, the gastrocnemius and soleus muscles are reflected posteriorly, and the soft tissue attachments, including the interosseus membrane, are dissected with a cautery (Fig. 10–4, *c*). An 8 cm segment of fibula is resected with a Gigli saw, and the peroneal artery is mobilized (Fig. 10–4, *d*). A distal anastomosis is made end-to-side and the graft (saphenous vein or Dardik Biograft*) is tunneled through the popliteal space and anastomosed to the common femoral artery as described in the previous section (Fig. 10–4, *e*).

SURGICAL APPROACH TO ANTERIOR TIBIAL ARTERY

Exposure of the anterior tibial artery is facilitated by straightening the knee, with the foot dorsiflexed and internally rotated to relax the anterior compartment muscles. A skin incision is made approximately 2 cm lateral to the tibia in the groove between the anterior tibial and extensor hallucis muscles (Fig. 10–4, *f*). Following incision of the deep fascia, these two muscles are separated to expose the anterior

Text continued on page 155.

*Available from Meadox Medicals, Oakland, New Jersey.

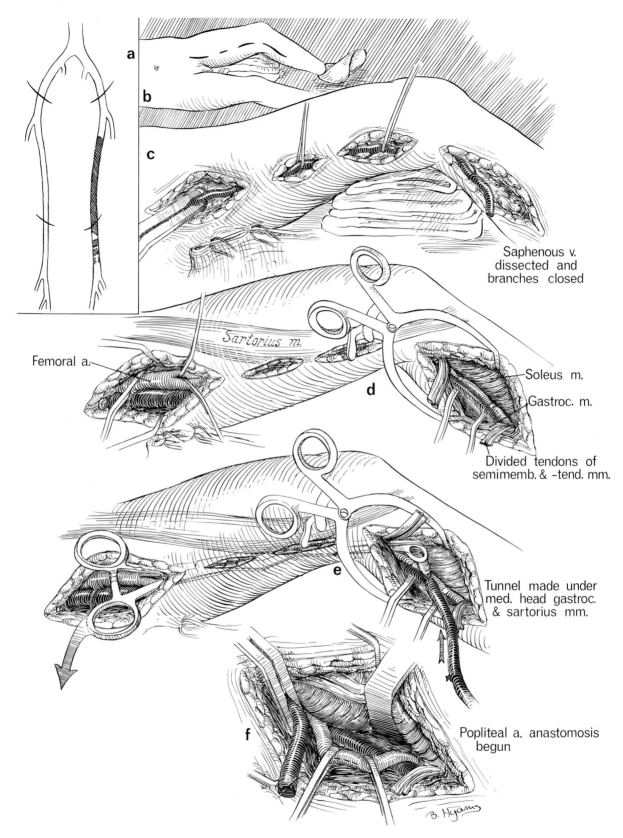

Saphenous v. dissected and branches closed

Femoral a.

Sartorius m.

Soleus m.

Gastroc. m.

Divided tendons of semimemb. & -tend. mm.

Tunnel made under med. head gastroc. & sartorius mm.

Popliteal a. anastomosis begun

B. Hyams

Figure 10–3 Femoropopliteal bypass with the use of autogenous saphenous vein and below-the-knee anastomosis.

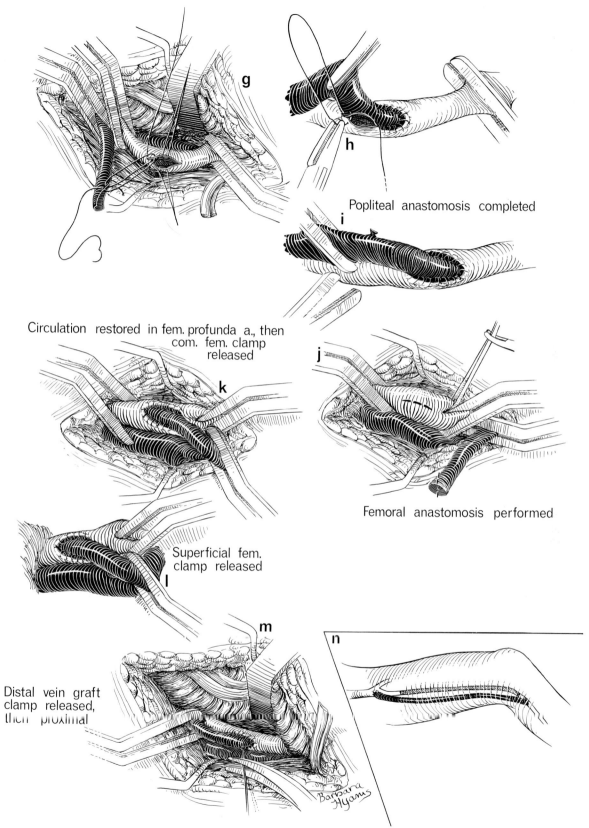

g

h

Popliteal anastomosis completed

i

Circulation restored in fem. profunda a., then com. fem. clamp released

k

j

Femoral anastomosis performed

Superficial fem. clamp released

l

m

n

Distal vein graft clamp released, then proximal

Barbara Hyams

Figure 10–3 *Continued.*

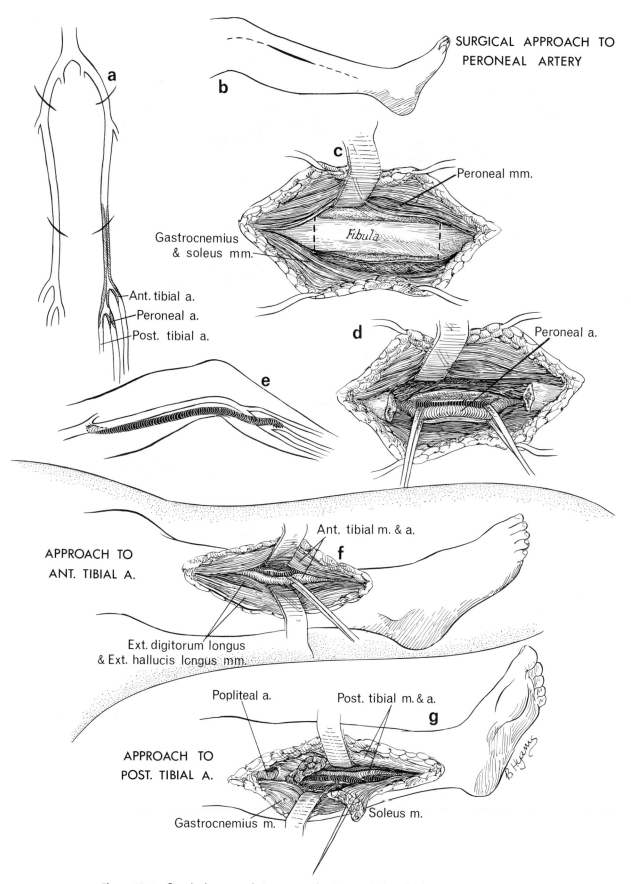

SURGICAL APPROACH TO
PERONEAL ARTERY

a

b

c

Peroneal mm.

Gastrocnemius
& soleus mm.

Fibula

Ant. tibial a.

Peroneal a.

Post. tibial a.

d

Peroneal a.

e

APPROACH TO
ANT. TIBIAL A.

Ant. tibial m. & a.

f

Ext. digitorum longus
& Ext. hallucis longus mm.

Popliteal a.

Post. tibial m. & a.

g

APPROACH TO
POST. TIBIAL A.

Gastrocnemius m.

Soleus m.

B. Hyams

Figure 10–4 Surgical approach to peroneal artery, anterior tibial artery and posterior tibial artery.

tibial artery lying on the anterior surface of the interosseous membrane. A distal anastomosis is made (as previously described) and tunneled through the popliteal space by following the course of the anterior tibial artery proximally to where it passes through an anatomic defect in the cephalic end of the interosseous membrane. Dilatation of this defect should be done by blunt finger dissection but can be facilitated by inserting and gently spreading the tips of a large hemostat.

SURGICAL APPROACH TO POSTERIOR TIBIAL ARTERY

A medial skin incision is made along the posterior border of the tibia and extended through the musculofascial attachment of the soleus muscle to the tibia. The gastrocnemius muscle is retracted posteriorly; if necessary, fibers of the soleus muscle may be transected (Fig. 10–4, g). A distal anastomosis is made as previously described. A tunnel is then created by gentle blunt finger dissection along the posterior tibial artery beneath the soleus muscle into the popliteal space.

PROFUNDA FEMORIS ARTERY RECONSTRUCTION

The importance of the profunda femoris artery has long been recognized; however, only recently has profundaplasty become emphasized as an alternative to femoral popliteal bypass in patients with complete occlusion of the superficial femoral artery associated with significant stenosis of the proximal profunda femoris artery.[4, 5, 6] Three basic techniques of restoring flow are described.

We condemn the use of "blind" endarterectomy, i.e., removal of distal plaque without direct visualization of its extent. It is important to dissect the profunda femoris artery as far as necessary distally (even to the mid thigh level) to obtain a suitable segment of vessel for anastomosis. Even if the vessel is of small caliber, the extensive runoff is such that the vessel will usually dilate to accommodate the restored flow, which is distributed to the entire extremity. Although as many muscular branches as possible should be preserved, the first several branches can be sacrificed if they are diseased.

Profundaplasty is most commonly indicated in cases of aortofemoral grafting for correction of aortoiliac occlusive disease (AIOD) associated with complete occlusion of the superficial femoral arteries and disease in the profunda femoris arteries (Fig. 10–5, a). The vast majority of patients in these cases will experience satisfactory results if adequate circulation is restored to the profunda femoris arteries. A decision as to the need for femoral popliteal bypass usually can be deferred until at least three months following aorta–profunda femoral bypass. Most patients will then be so improved that they will not require femoral popliteal bypass.

In patients who have developed completely occluded proximal common femoral and external iliac arteries, end-to-end anastomosis to the profunda femoris artery is the technique of choice (Fig. 10–5, b). In such situations, where occlusion of both common femoral arteries precludes retrograde flow to the pelvis, the proximal aortic anastomosis should be made end-to-side rather than end-to-end to the aorta, in order to preserve as much flow to the pelvis, rectum, and sigmoid colon as possible.

If one common femoral artery is even partially patent (Fig. 10–5, c), the distal profunda anastomosis should be made end-to-side in order to preserve some retrograde flow into the pelvis. Again, it is emphasized that the arteriotomy should be

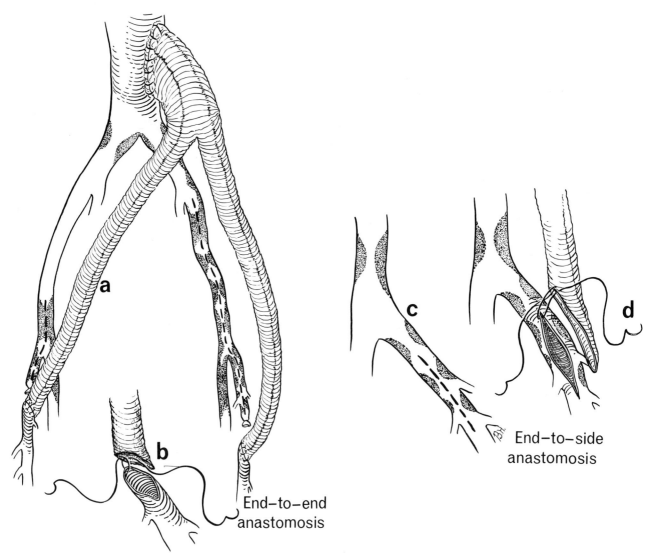

Figure 10–5 Profunda femoris artery reconstruction: (a and b) end-to-end anastomosis; (c and d) end-to-side anastomosis.

extended distally as far as necesssary to obtain good quality profunda artery (Fig. 10–5, *d*). In patients with no significant AIOD, this technique may be varied by applying a vein or Dacron patch arterioplasty to the profunda femoris artery as an alternative to femoral popliteal bypass. If the common femoral artery is the only artery diseased proximally, the patch arterioplasty can be extended from the common to the profunda femoris artery.

POPLITEAL ARTERY ENTRAPMENT

The syndrome of popliteal artery occlusion due to the artery's abnormal relationship to the medial head of the gastrocnemius muscle was first described by Stuart in 1879.[13] Delaney[14] has classified four variants of the syndrome into types; of these, Types I and II comprise 75 percent of cases.

In Type I, the medial head of the gastrocnemius muscle arises normally from the posterior aspect of the medial condyle of the femur, resulting in a characteristic medial deviation of the proximal popliteal artery as seen arteriographically. The Type II anomaly results when the medial head of the gastrocnemius muscle arises more laterally than normal from the medial femoral condyle, with the popliteal artery abnormally coursing medially as in Type I. Because of the muscle's abnormal lateral location, the popliteal artery is not displaced so far medially and therefore does not usually demonstrate the characteristic arteriographic medial deviation. In Type III variants of the syndrome, the artery courses normally between the heads of the gastrocnemius muscle but is entrapped and compressed by an abnormal accessory slip of muscle or tendon from the medial head of the gastrocnemius, which originates more laterally than normal (Fig. 10–6, *a* and *b*). Type IV anomalies result from entrapment of the popliteal artery by the popliteus muscle[15] or a fibrous band.[16] The popliteal artery may course either normally between the heads of the gastrocnemius muscle, or medial to its medial head.

The syndrome has been observed most frequently in men under 30 years of age. Approximately 25 percent of cases are bilateral. The entrapment syndrome can produce constriction of the artery, with mural thickening, fibrosis, thrombosis or post stenotic aneurysmal formation. Claudication may result from constriction of the artery but usually does not develop until complete thrombosis has occurred.

The syndrome should be suspected in young men with claudication, in whom atherosclerosis is unlikely. Arteriographic confirmation is made by demonstrating the characteristic medial "looping" and deviation or isolated segmental occlusion of the proximal popliteal artery.

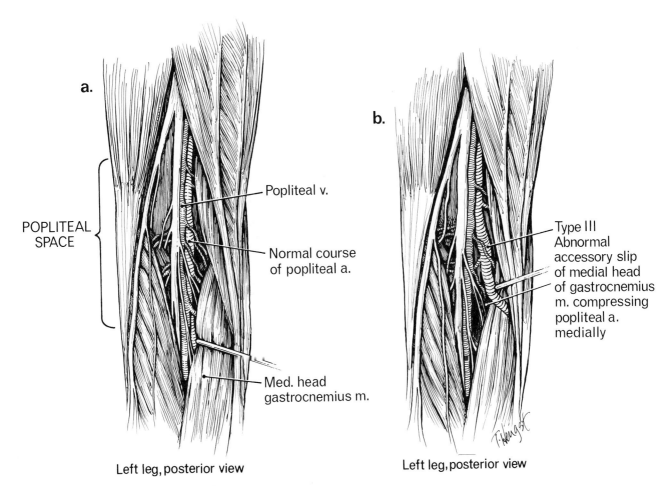

Figure 10–6 *a,* Normal course of popliteal artery; *b,* Type III variant of popliteal artery occlusion with entrapment of the artery.

OPERATIVE TREATMENT

Operation and release of the constricting structure is indicated whether or not the artery has become completely occluded. The surgical approach of choice is a direct posterior incision into the popliteal space. An S-shaped incision is made, with the cephalad aspect medial to and the transverse aspect across the posterior popliteal skin crease. Dissection is carried down to the deep fascia, which is incised longitudinally into the popliteal space. The tibial nerve and medial sural cutaneous branch are identified and retracted laterally. The popliteal artery, which lies posterior-medial to the vein, is identified as it exits with the popliteal vein from Hunter's canal under the semimembranosus muscle. The popliteal artery is dissected distally until it passes medial to and beneath the medial head of the gastrocnemius muscle (Types I and II), which is then divided.

If the popliteal artery is demonstrated to be normal arteriographically and visually at operation, it may not require further surgical correction after being restored to its normal anatomic position. When the artery is fibrotic or thrombosed, as is most frequently the case, the involved segment should be resected and replaced with a Dacron double velour graft, or preferably an autogenous saphenous vein graft. Reapproximation of the medial head of the gastrocnemius muscle is not necessary.

REFERENCES

1. Kunlin J: Le traitement de l'arterite obliterante par la greffe veinuse. Arch Mal Coer 42:371, 1949.
2. Bangash M, Zaorski Jr. Iradj S, Gammas M: Selection of arterial grafting material: A report of two hundred cases. Cardiovascular Diseases, Bulletin of the Texas Heart Institue 1(#5):449, 1974.
3. Dardik I, Ibrahim I, Dardik H: Femoral popliteal bypass employing modified human umbilical cord vein: An assessment of early clinical results. Cardiovascular Diseases, Bulletin of the Texas Heart Institute 3(#3):314, 1976.
4. Martin P, Frawley JE, Barabas AP,Rosengarten DS: On the surgery of atherosclerosis of the profunda femoris artery. Surgery 71(#2):182, 1972.
5. Vollmar J, Frede M, Laubach K: Principles of reconstructive procedures for chronic femoro-popliteal occlusions: A report of 546 operations. Ann Surg 168:215, 1968.
6. DeWeese JA, Barner HB, Mahoney EB, Rob CG: Autogenous vein bypass grafts and thromboendarterectomies for atherosclerotic lesions of the femoropopliteal arteries. Ann Surg 163:205, 1966.
7. Warwick RW, Williams PL: *Gray's Anatomy, 35th British Edition.* Churchill Livingstone, London, 1973. Available in United States from W. B. Saunders, Philadelphia.
8. Morris GC, Edwards W, Cooley DA: Surgical importance of profunda femoris artery: Analysis of 102 cases with combined aorto-iliac and femoral popliteal disease treated by revascularization of the deep femoral artery. Arch Surg 82:32, 1961.
9. Leeds FH,Gilfillan RS: Revascularization of the lower limb: Importance of profunda femoris artery. Arch Surg 82:25, 1961.
10. Blaisdell FW, Hall AD: Axillary femoral artery bypass for lower extremity ischaemia. Surgery 54:563, 1962.
11. Cohn LH, Trueblood W, Crowley LG: Profunda femoris reconstruction in the treatment of femoropopliteal occlusive disease. 103:475, 1971.
12. Dardik I, Dardik H: Peroneal artery bypass: technical film. From Meadox Medicals, Oakland, New Jersey (1976).
13. Stuart TPA: Note on a variation in the course of the popliteal artery. J Anat 13:162, 1879.
14. Delaney TA, Gonzalez LL: Occlusion of popliteal artery due to muscular entrapment. Surgery 69:97, 1971.
15. Love JW, Whelan TJ: Popliteal artery entrapment syndrome. Am J Surg 109:620, 1965.
16. Haimovici H, Sprayregen S, Johnson F: Popliteal artery entrapment by fibrous band. Surgery 72:789, 1972.

CHAPTER 11

Peripheral Aneurysms

POPLITEAL ANEURYSMS

Surgical treatment of popliteal aneurysms dates back almost 200 years to John Hunter's ligation of such a lesion in 1786.[1] The technique of endoaneurysmorrhaphy, introduced by Rudolph Matas in 1888, involved ligating the aneurysm, opening the sac, and ligating the branches from within.[2] This method was later modified to allow restoration of vascular continuity and, as such, it forms the basis of techniques currently in use. Resection of a popliteal aneurysm and replacement with a segment of popliteal vein was performed by Goyanes in 1906.[3]

RESECTION OF POPLITEAL ANEURYSMS

Popliteal aneurysms occasionally rupture but more often cause ischemia of the lower extremity, resulting from either multiple emboli to the distal circulation, or complete distal occlusion. Diagnosis can usually be made by palpation of the pulsating (or thrombosed) mass in the popliteal space. Femoral arteriography should be performed to ascertain the status of the distal arterial tree and to assure that sufficient distal circulation is present to allow re-establishment of circulation. If the distal circulation is completely thrombosed, sympathectomy and amputation are the only alternatives — should the former prove ineffective, amputation becomes necessary.

The surgical technique of choice for this condition is endoaneurysmorrhaphy with ligation of branches from within the aneurysm and re-establishment of circulation with a saphenous vein or Dacron double velour graft, using end-to-end anastomoses proximally and distally. Complete excision of the aneurysm should be avoided, as damage to the closely adherent popliteal veins may predispose deep vein thrombophlebitis, thrombosis, or pulmonary emboli. Bypass of the evacuated aneurysm by means of a graft may be used in some instances.

Although exposure of a popliteal aneurysm can be obtained by either a posterior or lateral approach, a medial approach is the most satisfactory (Fig. 11–1, a). With the patient placed in the supine position, the lower extremity is draped to the ankle and flexed at the knee, supported by folded towels. An incision is made over the medial aspect of the knee along the posterior aspect of the sartorius muscle, which is reflected anteriorly. The aneurysm is exposed by transecting the gracilis, semitendinosus, and semimembranosus muscles and the medial head of the gastrocnemius muscle. After clamps are placed proximally and distally to the aneurysm and the thrombus evacuated, the aneurysm is incised longitudinally and collateral vessels are ligated from within the sac (Fig. 11–1, c). The network of popliteal veins surrounding and closely adhering to the aneurysmal sac are not dissected from the aneurysm. A saphenous vein or Dacron graft is anastomosed end-to-end to the proximal and distal popliteal artery. If recent embolization distal to the aneurysm is suspected, a Fogarty catheter should be passed down the distal artery prior to completion of the anastomosis. The trimmed wall of the aneurysm is then reapproximated around the

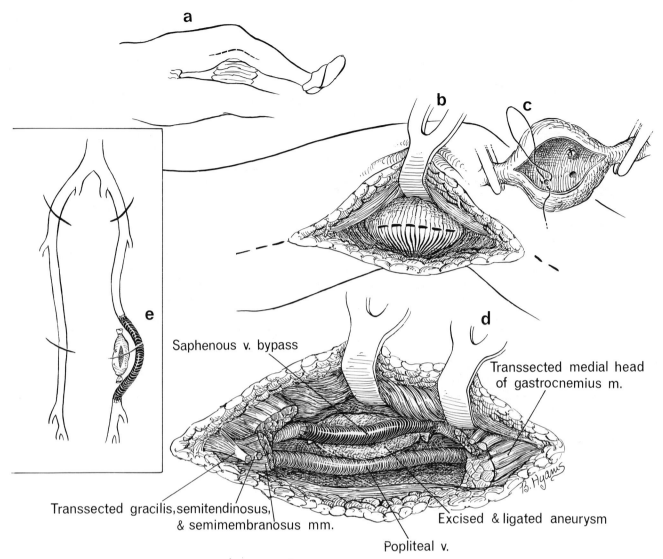

Saphenous v. bypass

Transsected medial head
of gastrocnemius m.

Transsected gracilis,semitendinosus,
& semimembranosus mm.

Excised & ligated aneurysm

Popliteal v.

Figure 11–1 Resection of popliteal aneurysm.

graft (Fig. 11–1, *d*). The transected muscles are repaired and the wound is closed with interrupted sutures.

FALSE ANEURYSMS OF FEMORAL POPLITEAL BYPASS

False aneurysms of the anastomoses of femoropopliteal bypass grafts are usually associated with prosthetic graft materials rather than with autogenous saphenous vein grafts. The most common cause of these aneurysms is the type of suture material used (usually silk suture, which deteriorates after five to seven years). Use of the silk suture for prosthetic graft anastomoses is now universally contraindicated. Many vascular surgeons still believe that monofilament polypropylene suture is acceptable for anastomosing prosthetic graft materials; however, in an anastomosis between a prosthetic graft and an artery, the bond will always be dependent upon continued integrity of the suture material. Therefore, the use of monofilament suture, which has an inherent propensity for material fatigue and eventual breakage is, in our opinion, contraindicated for anastomosis of prosthetic graft material. Infrequent causes of false aneurysms include infection and faulty surgical techniques.

A false popliteal aneurysm (Fig. 11–2, *a, b,* and *c*) is exposed by means of a

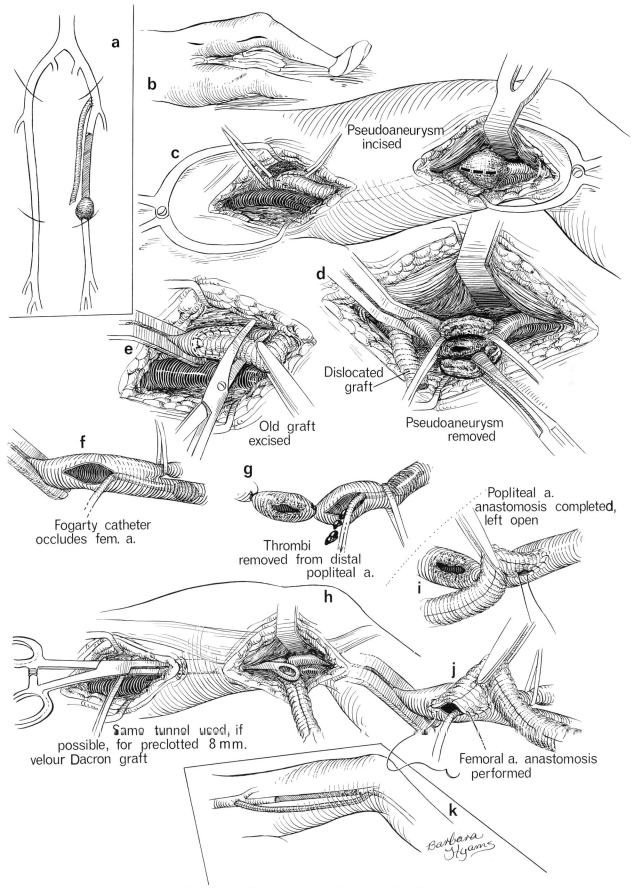

a

b

Pseudoaneurysm
incised

c

d

Dislocated
graft

Pseudoaneurysm
removed

e

Old graft
excised

f

Fogarty catheter
occludes fem. a.

g

Thrombi
removed from distal
popliteal a.

Popliteal a.
anastomosis completed,
left open

i

h

Same tunnel used, if
possible, for preclotted 8 mm.
velour Dacron graft

j

Femoral a. anastomosis
performed

k

Barbara
Hyams

Figure 11–2   False aneurysm of femoral popliteal bypass.

medial approach, as previously described. Even though a false aneurysm may be apparent only in the distal anastomosis, conditions predisposing to aneurysm formation (i.e., type of suture material) will also be present at the site of proximal anastomosis, and both anastomoses should be redone to preclude subsequent similar complications. The distal popliteal false aneurysm is removed (Fig. 11–2, *d*), and the proximal anastomosis secured, with complete removal of the old graft. Because of fibrous tissue ingrowth around old anastomoses, it is rarely necessary to obtain proximal and distal control by tedious dissection prior to opening the false aneurysm or old anastomosis. Bleeding from within the artery is easily controlled by inserting and inflating a Fogarty catheter from within the vessel (Fig. 11–2, *f*). Thrombi are removed from the distal popliteal artery by the same method (Fig. 11–2, *g*). The previous tunnel can often be dilated and reused unless it is constricted by scar tissue or infection is present. A new tunnel should then be made (Fig. 11–2, *h*). A new popliteal anastomosis is constructed either at the previous site or more distally, depending upon the quality of the vessel, and the suture line is left open for later flushing of the distal artery (Fig. 11–2, *i*). With completion of anastomosis (Fig. 11–2, *j*), the reconstruction is concluded (Fig. 11–2, *k*).

Whenever a second procedure is performed (or a procedure is redone), the wounds should be irrigated with an antibiotic solution and the entire wound closed with interrupted sutures.

MYCOTIC PERIPHERAL ANEURYSMS

In 1885, Osler[4] first applied the term *mycotic aneurysm* in describing aneurysms that resulted from bacterial infection of the arterial wall. In 1923, Stengel and Wolferth[5] described mycotic aneurysms involving peripheral arteries and suggested that they were secondary to infected emboli from bacterial endocarditis. Before the advent of antibiotic therapy, these aneurysms usually resulted in abscess formation around the arterial wall, with eventual rupture and fatal hemorrhage.[6]

CAUSES AND PREVENTION

Four known causes of mycotic aneurysms are: (1) septal embolization from bacterial endocarditis, which accounts for at least 50 percent of cases; (2) infection by septicemia of a previously formed aneurysm; (3) spread of infection by direct extension, or indirectly via the lymphatics from an area of abscess or cellulitis; and (4) traumatic injury and contamination of an artery wall.[7] The most common causative organisms are Staphylococcus, Streptococcus, and Pneumococcus.[8] The aorta, mesenteric, intracranial, and popliteal arteries are the most frequently involved.[9]

Although the incidence of these aneurysms has decreased because of antibiotic treatment of bacterial endocarditis, knowledge of the principles of surgical treatment is essential to the cardiovascular surgeon. Bacterial infection of cardiac valve prostheses is particularly likely to cause septic emboli and mycotic aneurysm formation despite intensive intravenous antibiotic therapy. Because of the increased number of patients undergoing cardiac valve replacement and the relatively stable incidence of postoperative prosthetic infection, it appears likely that mycotic aneurysms will continue to require treatment.

We have recently treated several such lesions resulting from bacterial endocarditis or prosthetic cardiac valve infection. In one of these patients, an aneurysm developed in the popliteal artery 14 days after aortic valve replacement for acute endocarditis. Cultures demonstrated *Streptococcus faecalis* despite intensive intravenous antibiotic treatment; cultures from the wall of the resected aneurysm were negative. In another patient, mycotic aneurysms occurred in both the posterior tibial and brachial arteries two months following mitral valve replacement of a previous mitral valve prosthesis infected with Staphylococcus; there were no organisms grown from the wall of either aneurysm.

During operation for valvular bacterial endocarditis, awareness of predisposing conditions for development of mycotic aneurysms is essential in preventing their occurrence. Two critical events to avoid are disruption of vegetations from the involved cardiac valve and trauma to an artery from positioning of an extremity. To prevent the former, the heart should not be manipulated during cannulation or before the cross-clamp has been applied. Trauma to a peripheral artery, which may predispose it to seeding during an episode of transient bacteremia, must be prevented by careful positioning of the patient and cushioning all extremities during operation.

PRINCIPLES OF DIAGNOSIS AND TREATMENT

The diagnosis of mycotic aneurysm should be suspected in a patient who complains of pain, tenderness, heat, or redness in an extremity after an episode of bacterial endocarditis or its surgical treatment. Arteriography should be performed to confirm the diagnosis and establish the status of the distal circulation.

Mycotic aneurysms are associated with morbidity from distal embolization and a high mortality rate from rupture; therefore, emergency surgical treatment should be instituted. Adequate treatment requires complete resection of the infected aneurysm wall in contrast to that of ordinary aneurysms, the posterior walls of which are often best left in place. Restoration of vascular continuity should be performed in major vessels. Autogenous saphenous veins are the preferred graft material in small or medium-sized arteries, although Dacron may be used when necessary. Distal peripheral arteries, such as the posterior tibial, may be ligated following excision of the aneurysm.

OPERATIVE TREATMENT

Mycotic Aneurysm of Popliteal Artery. The aneurysm in the popliteal artery is exposed either above or below the knee, depending on its location as determined arteriographically (see Chapter 10). Following systemic heparinization (2 mg/kg body weight), the artery is clamped proximally and distally to the aneurysm. The aneurysm is carefully dissected from the popliteal vein, which will most likely be involved in the inflammatory process. The importance of preserving continuity of the popliteal vein is emphasized because the entire venous circulation from the leg may be channeled through this vessel in the area of the knee. The aneurysm is excised completely, and care is taken to avoid leaving any residual infection. A segment of autogenous saphenous vein or Dacron graft is used to restore arterial continuity, as described in Chapter 10. Prior to closure, the wound is thoroughly irrigated with a solution containing the antibiotic appropriate for the offending organism.

Mycotic Aneurysm of Brachial Artery. The lesion is exposed as described in Chapter 14 (see Fig. 14–1, a). Care is taken to ascertain complete excision of the aneurysm wall. Because of the more diffuse venous collaterals in the elbow than in the knee, veins involved in the inflammatory process may be ligated without trepidation. Ideally, arterial circulation should be restored if possible with an autogenous vein graft; however, in most cases, the brachial artery may be ligated without loss of the extremity.

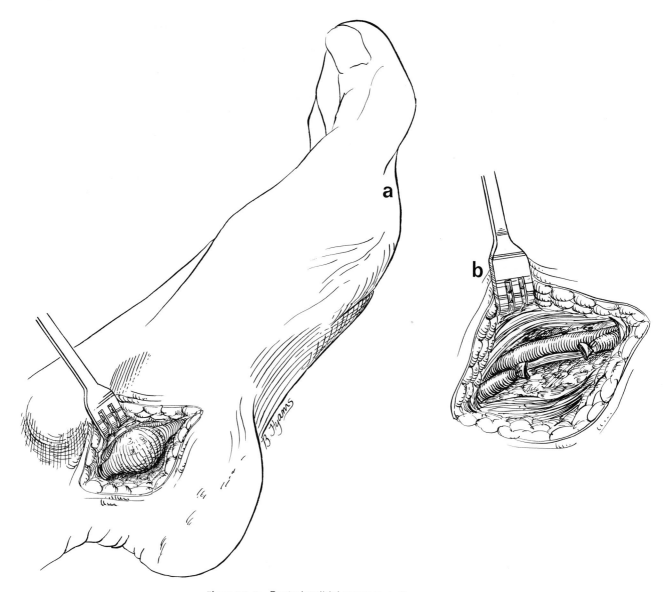

Figure 11–3 Posterior tibial artery mycotic aneurysm.

Mycotic Aneurysm of Posterior Tibial Artery. Exposure of the aneurysm is obtained by an incision overlying the involved artery (Fig. 11–3, *a*). The aneurysm is completely excised and the artery ends are doubly ligated with a permanent monofilament suture (Fig. 11–3, *b*). The wound is irrigated with the appropriate antibiotic solution. A drain is not used.

REFERENCES

1. Hunter, John: Lectures. Transactions of the Society for the Improvement of Medicine & Chirurgie, London, 1793, pp 138-181.
2. Matas, Rudolph: Traumatic aneurysm of the left brachial artery: Incision and partial excision of the sac recovery. Med News, New York 53:462, 1888.
3. Goyanes J: Nuevos trabajos de cirugia vascular, substitucion plastica de las venas o arterioplastia venosa, aplicada como nuevo metodo al tratamiento de los aneurismios. Siglo Med 53:546, 1906.
4. Osler W: Gulistonian lectures on malignant endocarditis. Br Med J 1:467, 1885.

5. Stengel A, Wolferth CC: Mycotic (bacterial) aneurysms of intravascular origin. Arch Int Med 31:527, 1923.
6. Tufnell J: On the influence of vegetations on the valves of the heart in the production of secondary arterial diseases. Dublin Quart J M Sci 15:371, 1953.
7. Smith RF, Szilagyi DE, Colville JM: Surgical treatment of mycotic aneurysms. Arch Surg 85:663, 1962.
8. Anderson CB, Butler HR Jr, Ballinger WF: Mycotic aneurysms. Arch Surg 109:712, 1974.
9. Dickman FN, Moore IB: Mycotic aneurysm: A case report of a popliteal mycotic aneurysm. Ann Surg 167:590, 1968

CHAPTER 12

Congenital Arterial Anomalies

COARCTATION OF THE THORACIC AORTA

Successful operations for repair of coarctation of the aorta were first performed in 1944 by Crafoord[1] in Sweden and in 1945 by Gross[2] in the United States. Over the intervening years, procedures for reconstructing the aorta and major arteries have been greatly improved, and today the surgeon has several methods of establishing circulatory continuity.[3] Emphasis should be placed upon producing full pulsatile flow from the proximal to the distal aorta without sacrificing major collateral vessels or the subclavian artery.

The first technique developed for repairing coarctation was resection of the coarcted segment with end-to-end anastomosis. Major complications in those early operations included hemorrhage from the suture line, late stenosis, and aneurysm formation. Such complications were caused by two factors: excessive tension on the anastomosis and the use of everting sutures, as suggested by Alexis Carrel many years before.[4] Although some surgeons still think that extensive mobilization of the distal aortic segment is necessary, there are now so many alternatives that extensive dissections can and should be avoided. It is not advisable to divide the large, dilated, often thin-walled intercostal arteries. Such dissections, with ligation and division of the collateral vessels, can lead to serious bleeding. These arteries should be avoided if possible.

RESECTION WITH END-TO-END ANASTOMOSIS

Adequate exposure is achieved through an incision in the left fourth intercostal space (Fig. 12–1, a). Large collateral vessels, particularly those passing through the latissimus dorsi muscle, should be identified, doubly clamped, and ligated. Digital compression by the surgeon and his assistants during the division of these vessels can prevent excessive bleeding. Smaller collateral arteries may be cauterized. The mediastinal dissection is centered over the vagus nerve; the best reference point is the ligamentum arteriosum, encircled by the recurrent laryngeal nerve. The superior intercostal vein is ligated and divided.

Tape ligatures are carefully passed around the aorta proximal and distal to the coarcted segment and are used for gentle traction to facilitate dissection on the posterior and medial aspects (Fig. 12–1, b). After the aorta and the left subclavian artery have been freed and the intercostal arteries have been identified proximally and distally, vascular clamps are applied (Fig. 12–1, c). The clamps should have atraumatic jaws with serrations that will hold firmly without crushing or cutting the delicate aortic wall. Heparin is not necessary in the repair of coarctation.

166

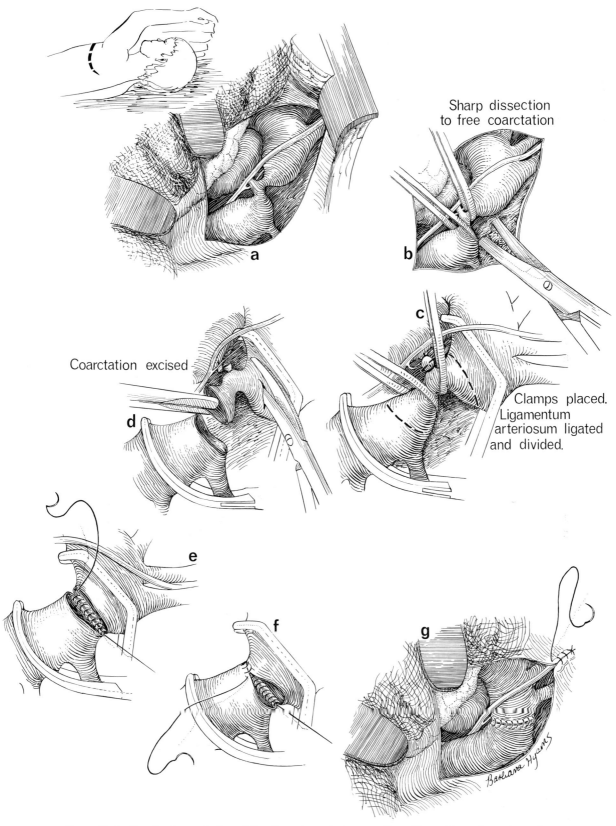

Sharp dissection to free coarctation

Coarctation excised

Clamps placed. Ligamentum arteriosum ligated and divided.

Figure 12–1 Repair of coarctation of the thoracic aorta by resection with end-to-end anastomosis.

After application of the proximal clamp, the arterial peak systolic pressure may rise above 150 mm Hg. If this occurs, the anesthesiologist should lower the pressure by administering additional anesthetic agents or vasodilator drugs to prevent damage to the aortic wall during the period of cross-clamping. Nitroprusside is currently being used for this purpose. *(The aorta may be seriously lacerated proximally with the use of a poorly designed vascular clamp.)*

The proximal clamp usually occludes both the proximal aorta and the subclavian artery to make the proximal opening as large as possible. The suture line should extend to the subclavian artery. Distally, the line of excision is placed obliquely to preserve the ostia of the dilated intercostal arteries (Fig. 12–1, *d*).

If the two ends of the aorta are *easily* approximated (as they usually are in infants and children), the surgeon may decide to fashion a direct end-to-end anastomosis. Since the proximal aortic wall is often very thin, noncutting needles with a suture no larger than 3–0 should be used, but usually a 4–0 suture is preferred.

A circumferential suture line made with nonabsorbable material may not enlarge as the patient grows and, consequently, may lead to late stenosis. This can be avoided by using interrupted braided sutures on a part or all of the anastomosis in infants.[5]

In our experience, double-armed Dacron sutures treated with Teflon have been very satisfactory because they pass through the aortic wall easily and produce small needle holes without tearing. We have recently used 4–0 polypropylene monofilament sutures in a continuous over-and-over technique, suturing from inside the lumen on the posterior circumference (Fig. 12–1, *e*). The everting mattress suture technique has been discarded because it seems to give a weaker suture line than the simple continuous suture. After the posterior suture line is made and drawn taut, the anastomosis is completed anteriorly with the second needle (Fig. 12–1, *f*). After completion, the suture ends are tied (Fig. 12–1, *g*). Before closing the mediastinal pleura, the repair should be carefully inspected. If chyle is encountered during the procedure, the thoracic duct should be identified behind the aorta, doubly ligated *(not sutured)*, and divided. After hemostasis is secured, the mediastinal pleura is approximated with a continuous suture.

The chest is closed, using underwater seal drainage with a plastic tube. Injury to the large intercostal arteries on the thoracic cage must be avoided during insertion of the pericostal sutures, and the lower rib margin must be given a wide berth. The standard rib approximator may injure the intercostal vessels and cause a large hematoma. The assistant may approximate the ribs either manually or by crossing the ends of adjacent sutures while the knots on the pericostal sutures are tied.

RESECTION WITH FABRIC GRAFT REPLACEMENT

Excision with graft replacement has greatly simplified coarctectomy and rendered the operation far safer than when end-to-end anastomosis was the only option. Fabric grafts of Dacron have proved to be highly satisfactory, with few early or late complications. They are available in either knitted or woven form, and bleeding through the interstices may be controlled by preclotting with the patient's blood. Because of the availability of fabric grafts, an end-to-end anastomosis should not be attempted if excessive longitudinal tension on the suture line would result, or if the extent of the resection would be limited because of the desire for direct anastomosis. Extensive resection may be necessary if the coarcted segment extends several centimeters in length, if the intercostal arteries are aneurysmal, or if the aortic wall is calcified or damaged during the dissection. In these instances, synthetic grafts should be used. Satisfactory repair requires a large unobstructed anastomosis without tension.

The surgical approach to the coarctation (Fig. 12–2, *a* to *d*) is identical to that

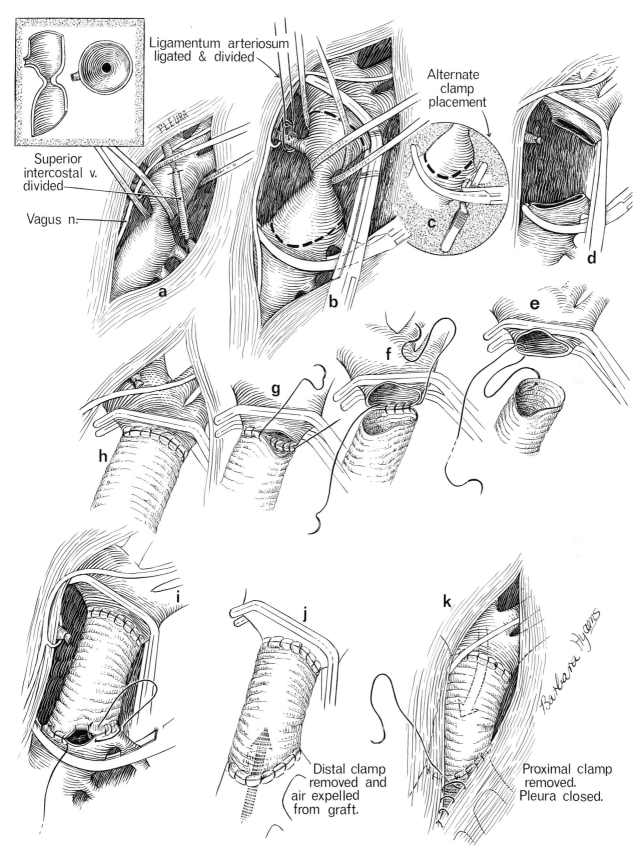

Ligamentum arteriosum
ligated & divided

Alternate
clamp
placement

Superior
intercostal v.
divided

Vagus n.

PLEURA

a

b

c

d

e

f

g

h

i

j

k

Distal clamp
removed and
air expelled
from graft.

Proximal clamp
removed.
Pleura closed.

Barbara Hyams

Figure 12–2   Resection of aortic coarctation with fabric graft replacement.

shown in Figure 12–1. A graft of suitable diameter (usually 12 to 14 mm) is selected, and the anastomosis is performed with a 4–0 double-armed Dacron polyester suture. The sequence of placement (Fig. 12–2, *d* to *h*) is the same, and care is taken not to tear the delicate aortic wall as the sutures are drawn through. After completion of the distal anastomosis (Fig. 12–2, *i*), the distal clamp is released (Fig. 12–2, *j*). If both suture lines are secure and there is no unusual bleeding, the proximal clamp may be released gradually. We use aortic clamps with long ratchets so that they may be set at the preferred opening and released only partially. While the patient's circulatory volume readjusts and the needle holes and interstices of the fabric are being sealed by platelets and fibrin, the chest tube may be inserted. Full release of the clamp may consume 5 to 10 minutes if necessary to avoid excessive blood loss (Fig. 12–2, *k*). In the illustration, note the oblique direction of the distal anastomosis, which preserves the large intercostal arteries posteriorly, thus permitting a large anastomotic opening.

AORTOPLASTY WITH PATCH GRAFT

Aortoplasty with a patch graft of Dacron polyester fabric is a useful alternative technique for the correction of coarctation.[6] This method is used successfully in patients of all ages and seems particularly useful in small infants. One advantage is the avoidance of a circumferential suture line, theoretically permitting subsequent enlargement of the anastomosis. Other advantages include the avoidance of extensive dissection and mobilization of the aorta. At present in our operations for coarctation this method of repair is used almost exclusively. In infants it is superior to standard techniques that use end-to-end anastomosis, and the late appearance of stricture is rare indeed. Apparently, the aortic segment that is not resected has the ability to enlarge as the body size increases, and although the fabric patch remains unchanged, the overall aortic diameter increases with the patient's growth.

The usual left thoracotomy incision is made and dissection of the aorta is performed (Fig. 12–3, *a*). Vascular clamps are applied to the proximal and distal aortic segments (Fig. 12–3, *b*). A suture ligature may be passed around the ligamentum arteriosum. A longitudinal incision is made in the aorta, beginning on the distal segment, crossing the coarcted area, and extending up the proximal segment into the subclavian artery. A ring or membrane of hypertrophied intima is usually found at the coarcted point adjacent to the ligamentum arteriosum. This ring of tissue is excised to enlarge the aortic lumen (Fig. 12–3, *c*). A woven or knitted elliptical patch of Dacron is then sewn into the longitudinal defect (Fig. 12–3, *d*), enlarging the coarcted area to a diameter greater than the distal aortic arch (Fig. 12–3, *e* and *f*). To restore circulation with minimal bleeding from the patch, the clamps are released gradually.

BYPASS GRAFT FOR COARCTATION

Several techniques are available for correction of complicated or recurrent coarctation. Dissection of the aorta after a previous repair of coarctation can be difficult and dangerous.[7-10] The fibrous tissue is dense and the aorta may be soft and easily torn. For this reason, we do not recommend that the aorta be mobilized in such instances (Fig. 12–4, *a* and *b*). A safer and equally effective repair may be obtained by dissecting only enough of the lateral surface of the distal aorta and left subclavian artery to permit application of a partial-occlusion vascular clamp (Fig. 12–4, *a*). A fabric graft (12 to 14 mm in diameter) is anastomosed proximally and distally, restoring circulation without disturbing the underlying cicatricial tissues and intercostal vessels (Fig. 12–4, *b*).

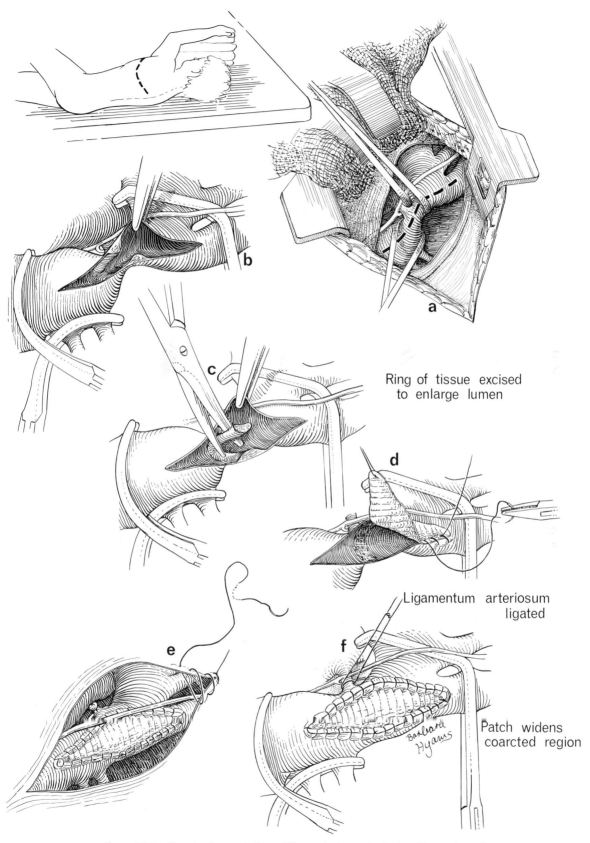

Ring of tissue excised to enlarge lumen

Ligamentum arteriosum ligated

Patch widens coarcted region

Figure 12–3 Repair of coarctation of the aorta by aortoplasty with patch graft.

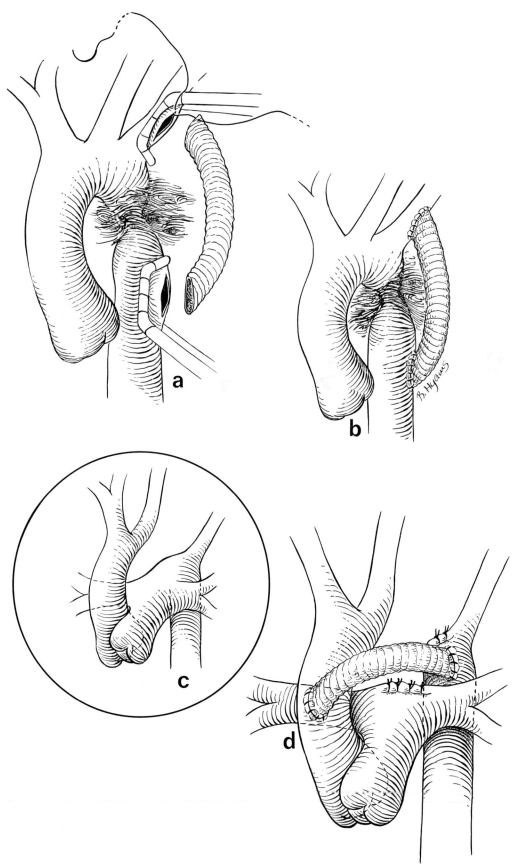

Figure 12–4 Bypass graft for aortic coarctation.

A similar technique may be employed in patients with an interrupted aortic arch or recurrent coarctation when the left subclavian artery is obstructed (Fig. 12–4, c). A partial-occlusion clamp may be applied at the base of the left common carotid artery, occluding that vessel for a short period if necessary. If the ascending aorta is large enough to permit application of a partial-occlusion clamp without excessively compromising aortic flow, the proximal anastomosis is made more proximally, or on the ascending aorta. A clamp may then be placed on the graft; the vascular clamp on the vessel is proximally released after that anastomosis is completed (Fig. 12–4, d). This permits full flow through the aorta or carotid artery while the distal anastomosis is being completed.

Another technique, which may be used in unusual situations, involves a midline sternotomy and upper midline abdominal incision to expose the ascending aorta and proximal or supraceliac segment of the abdominal aorta. The pericardium is opened in the midline. A knitted or woven Dacron graft, 14 to 16 mm in diameter, is sutured to the ascending aorta with the use of a 4–0 braided polyester suture. This may be done with a partial-occlusion vascular clamp applied to the aorta. The aortic clamp is released and another clamp is placed on the graft, and the end-to-side anastomosis is tested for adequacy. An incision is made in the membranous portion of the diaphragm ventral and to the left of the inferior vena cava. The graft is passed through the diaphragm, where it is anastomosed to the side of the proximal abdominal aorta.

This technique is useful in patients with recurrent coarctation after previous repair, in extensive complex aortic anomalies with stenosis, or in patients with associated cardiac valvular disease requiring sternotomy for the open heart procedure.

COARCTATION OF THE ABDOMINAL AORTA

The first case of coarctation of the abdominal aorta was described by Quain in 1846.[11] The defect comprises approximately 2 percent of all aortic coarctations,[12, 13] which may be either localized or diffuse, and can affect the distal thoracic and abdominal aorta in many locations, with or without visceral and renal involvement. The incidence of renal artery involvement, however, is generally greater than 50 percent.[14] There is a female predominance of 3:1, and the patient's age at presentation is often early in the third decade, although the condition can develop at any time during the first to the sixth decades.

The major symptom is severe, labile, uncontrollable hypertension with decreased distal pulses, and, as noted, the patient is often relatively young. Intermittent claudication, leg cramps, and manifestations of abdominal angina occasionally are present. Patients may develop congestive heart failure or have a cerebrovascular accident, which is the major cause of death in untreated patients.

The etiology of abdominal coarctation is essentially unknown. Maycock[15] attributes the condition to a faulty fusion of the dorsal aortas, with resultant hypoplasia and atresia. Abdominal coarctation has been reported in von Recklinghausen's disease[16] after abdominal irradiation,[17] and also in association with active tuberculosis.[18] Inada[19] has shown that an inflammatory aortitis, such as that associated with Takayasu's pulseless disease, may affect the distal aorta. The pathologic presentation of abdominal coarctation in the United States, however, usually involves hypoplasia, subinternal fibrosis, and nonspecific aortitis.[18, 20] The routine use of angiography in young patients with hypertension leads to an occasional diagnosis of this condition.

SURGICAL APPROACHES

The first successful repair, reported by Glenn in 1952,[21] utilized a splenic artery bypass from the thoracic aorta to the abdominal aorta, circumventing a suprarenal coarctation. The surgical approach to coarctation of the abdominal aorta depends upon the site or sites of the lesion and the degree of visceral involvement. Various procedures have been used, including resection with graft replacement,[22] angioplasty, and bypass grafting. Although we formerly performed resection and graft replacement, we found that the technique was applicable only for an isolated area of obstruction above the celiac areas or below the inferior mesenteric artery — a pattern that is uncommon.

AORTIC ANGIOPLASTY

An area of limited stenosis may be repaired expeditiously by Dacron patch angioplasty, particularly if the visceral arteries are not involved (Fig. 12–5, a). A vertical incision is made over the area of stenosis, and the involved aorta is enlarged by placement of a preclotted Dacron double-velour patch. To prevent iatrogenic stenosis at either end of the patch, the aortotomy incision must extend both above and below the obstructed area. Associated stenosis of the origin of the inferior mesenteric artery may be relieved by resecting the stenotic area and reimplanting the inferior mesenteric artery into the Dacron patch (Fig. 12–5, b).

BYPASS GRAFT

In patients with extensive coarctation of the abdominal aorta or involvement of the renal, celiac, or superior mesenteric arteries, the bypass graft technique has proved to be the most straightforward and effective method of revascularization (Fig. 12–15, c). This approach precludes extensive dissection in the area of coarctation, which is often surrounded by fibrosis, and allows for selective individual grafts to obstructed visceral arteries. The proximal end of a 14-mm Dacron double-velour graft is anastomosed end-to-side to the supraceliac abdominal aorta at the level of the diaphragm, as described in Chapter 8 (Occlusion of the Celiac and Superior Mesenteric Arteries). Individual autogenous saphenous vein or 7-mm Dacron double velour grafts are anastomosed end-to-side to the visceral arteries, as indicated, and end-to-side to the aortic graft (Fig. 12–5, c).

THORACOABDOMINAL BYPASS GRAFT

The patient with combined coarctation of the descending thoracic and abdominal aorta and renal artery stenosis (Fig. 12–6, a) may be satisfactorily revascularized by means of the bypass graft technique (Fig. 12–6, j). Two incisions are used to expose the descending thoracic and abdominal aorta (Fig. 12–6, b). The descending thoracic aorta is dissected through a left anterior lateral incision at the level of the seventh intercostal space (Fig. 12–6, b). The parietal pleura is incised posterior to the vagus nerve (Fig. 12–6, c). After systemic heparinization (2 mg/kg of body weight) has been achieved, a partial-occlusion clamp is applied to the descending thoracic aorta, and the graft is anastomosed end-to-side (Fig. 12–6, d). An opening is made in the left diaphragm, and the graft is drawn retroperitoneally along the left colic gutter into the abdomen (Fig. 12–6, e). It is anastomosed to the left lateral aspect of the abdominal aorta well beyond the area of coarctation (Fig. 12–6, f), and flow to the lower extremities through the graft is re-established.

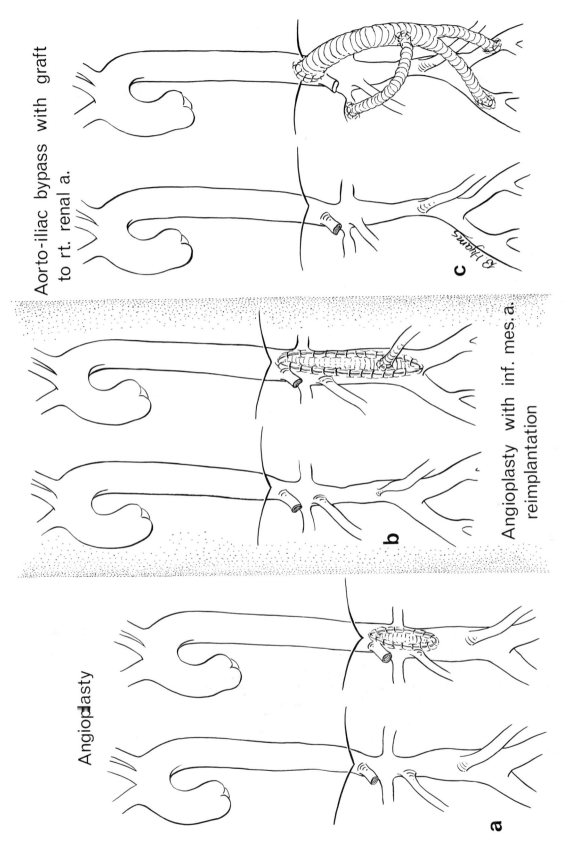

Angioplasty

Angioplasty with inf. mes.a.
reimplantation

Aorto-iliac bypass with graft
to rt. renal a.

Figure 12–5   Aortic angioplasty and bypass graft for coarctation of the abdominal aorta.

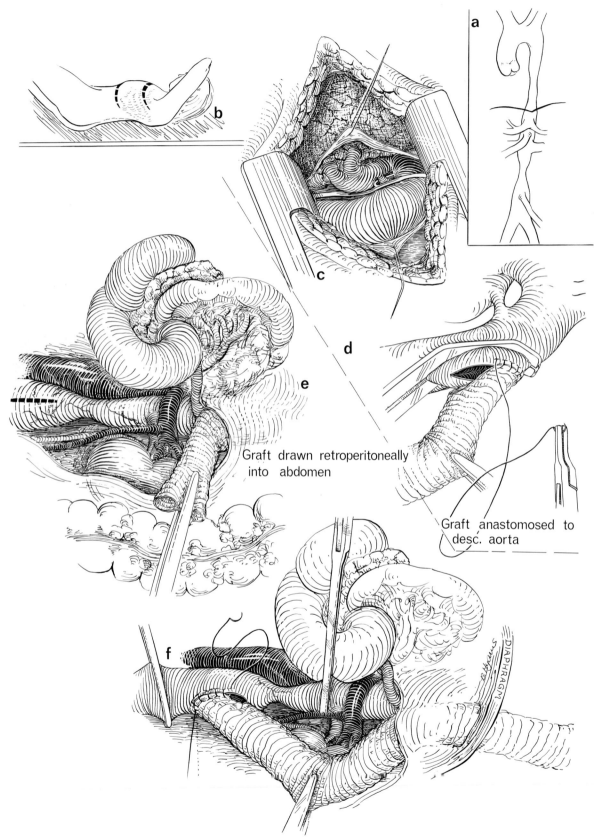

Graft drawn retroperitoneally into abdomen

Graft anastomosed to desc. aorta

Figure 12–6 Thoracoabdominal bypass graft for coarctation of the aorta.

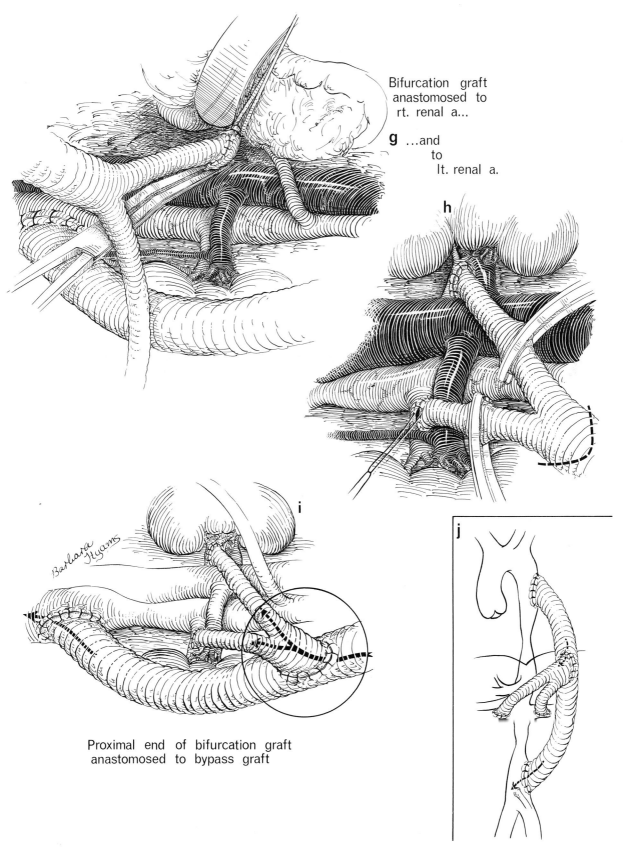

Bifurcation graft anastomosed to rt. renal a...

g ...and to lt. renal a.

h

i

Proximal end of bifurcation graft anastomosed to bypass graft

j

Figure 12–6 *(Continued)*

The right renal artery is isolated lateral to the inferior vena cava, and one limb of a preclotted 14 × 7 mm Dacron double-velour bifurcation graft is anastomosed end-to-side (Fig. 12–6, g). The remaining limb of the bifurcation graft is anastomosed end-to-side to the left renal artery (Fig. 12–6, h). The proximal end of the bifurcation graft is anastomosed to the thoracoabdominal graft (Fig. 12–6, i), thus completing the revascularization (Fig. 12–6, j).

ASCENDING AORTA TO ABDOMINAL AORTA BYPASS

An alternate approach in the patient with coarctation involving both the descending thoracic and abdominal aorta is the use of a bypass graft from the ascending thoracic aorta to the abdominal aorta (Fig. 12–7).[23] The advantage in this approach is that the entire procedure may be performed through a midline incision extended as a median sternotomy. Entry into the pleural cavities is thus avoided. This technique provides a desirable degree of flexibility during the operative management of complex situations. For example, when it is impossible to judge preoperatively whether or not a thoracoabdominal approach will be required, only a midline abdominal incision need be made. If revascularization can be achieved through the abdomen, nothing further need be done. If more proximal access to the aorta is required, however, the midline abdominal incision can be extended to a median sternotomy, and a graft can be brought from the ascending aorta. (The reader is referred to the section on Recurrent Disease and "Redo" Procedure in Chapter 9 for technical details of anastomosing the graft to the ascending aorta and passing it into the abdomen through the diaphragm. Exposure of the supraceliac aorta is described in Chapter 8.)

AORTIC ARCH ANOMALIES (VASCULAR RING)

Anomalies of the aortic arch are interesting from a developmental and embryological standpoint. They result from failure of the embryonic vascular arches to fuse and regress in the usual manner during the formation of the pulmonary artery and aortic arch system. A description of these anomalies and the application of techniques for repair may be credited largely to Robert Gross.[24, 25] These lesions may cause serious symptoms in newborn infants due to esophageal or tracheal obstruction. Thus, the vascular ring should be suspected in any newborn infant with stridor, respiratory distress, or inability to feed properly. Diagnosis is usually established by esophagogram or bronchogram, but aortography is often useful.[26-28]

DOUBLE AORTIC ARCH

The most common type of vascular ring that causes symptoms during infancy is a double aortic arch surrounding the trachea and esophagus; this causes respiratory distress and stridor, and, in some patients, regurgitation of food (Fig. 12–8, a). The double arch system usually presents with the larger arch passing to the right of the trachea and the smaller arch to the left. Therefore, most of these anomalies may be approached by a left posterolateral incision entering the fourth intercostal space (Fig. 12–8, b). The anatomy may be confusing in some cases, but the vagus and its recurrent laryngeal nerve, which always encircles the ductus arteriosus or ligamentum, should be the reference point to follow. The recurrent laryngeal nerve must be carefully preserved during subsequent dissection and mobilization of the esopha-

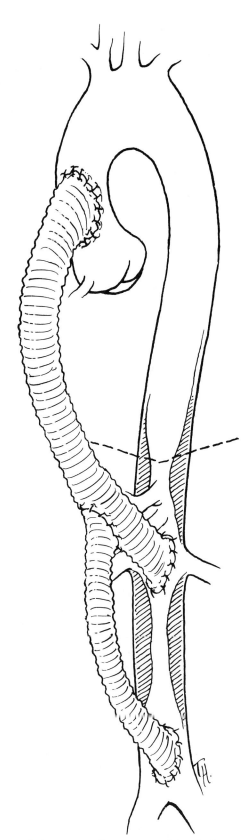

Figure 12–7 Bypass graft from ascending aorta to abdominal aorta to repair coarctation.

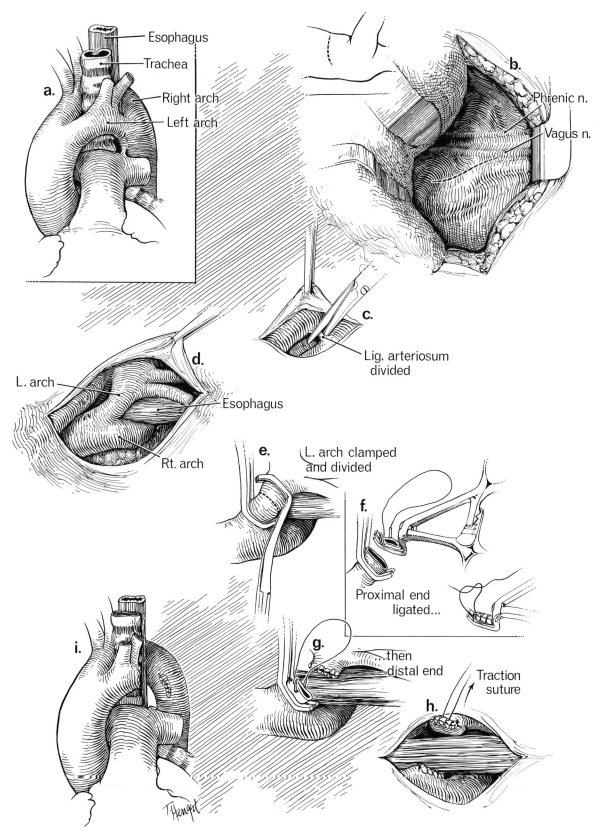

Figure 12–8 Repair of double aortic arch.

gus. After the ligamentum is divided (Fig. 12–8, c), the dissection is continued, with identification of the descending thoracic aorta, the left and right arches, and vessels arising from the arch (Fig. 12–8, d). When the smaller left arch has been identified, it may be occluded with vascular clamps and divided (Fig. 12–8, e). The ends of the arch are then oversewn and are ligated if desired (Fig. 12–8, f and g).

Many surgeons mistakenly believe that once the arch has been divided the ring will "spring open," releasing the underlying trachea and esophagus which were compressed. The trough or groove in which these structures lie remains the same after the left arch is divided; therefore, the arterial components should be dissected and freed from the attachments to the arch system. To enlarge the space occupied by the trachea and esophagus, traction sutures should be sewn to the ligated ends and attached to the endothoracic fascia anteriorly and posteriorly, thus providing maximum relief of the obstruction (Fig. 12–8, h). The pleura should not be closed over the mediastinal structures.

Infants who undergo operation for vascular ring due to double aortic arch do not always gain immediate relief from respiratory and digestive symptoms. The cartilaginous rings under the area of tracheal compression are often soft and poorly developed; therefore, the trachea may collapse during inspiration. Several weeks or months may be required for this condition to correct itself. In some patients, swallowing difficulties may persist until the esophagus resumes normal coordinated peristalsis.[28-30]

DOUBLE AORTIC ARCH (DOMINANT LEFT)

In some cases with double aortic arch, the left arch is the larger and should be preserved to relieve the compression (Fig. 12–9, a). This anomaly may also be approached by way of a left thoracotomy. Dissection is begun on the vagus nerve, which identifies the ligamentum arteriosum. Dissection along the posterior aspect of the esophagus demonstrates the obstructing element which, in this case, is the smaller right arch (Fig. 12–9, b). With the use of tapes encircling the left arch and descending aorta, the aorta is retracted to the left so that an adequate length of the right arch can be visualized. Vascular clamps are placed on the right arch, and the vessel is divided and oversewn. This should be done with particular care because the right arch retracts toward the right after release and may be difficult to retrieve if bleeding occurs. After the posterior arch is divided, the trachea and esophagus should be freed from the remaining left arch and traction sutures applied to eliminate any residual compression (Fig. 12–9, c).

RETROESOPHAGEAL SUBCLAVIAN ARTERY

This is the most common of all vascular rings. Since the ring is only partial and does not completely encircle the trachea and esophagus, symptoms are often mild or absent during infancy and childhood. Symptoms of dysphagia (dysphagia lusoria) may appear during adolescence and become progressively worse. Respiratory symptoms are unusual. The retroesophageal artery has a tendency to become aneurysmal later in life, and fatal hemorrhages have been reported.

RIGHT ARCH — RETROESOPHAGEAL LEFT SUBCLAVIAN ARTERY

In this anomaly, the subclavian artery arises on the posterior aspect of the proximal descending aorta near to the point of attachment of the ligamentum arterio-

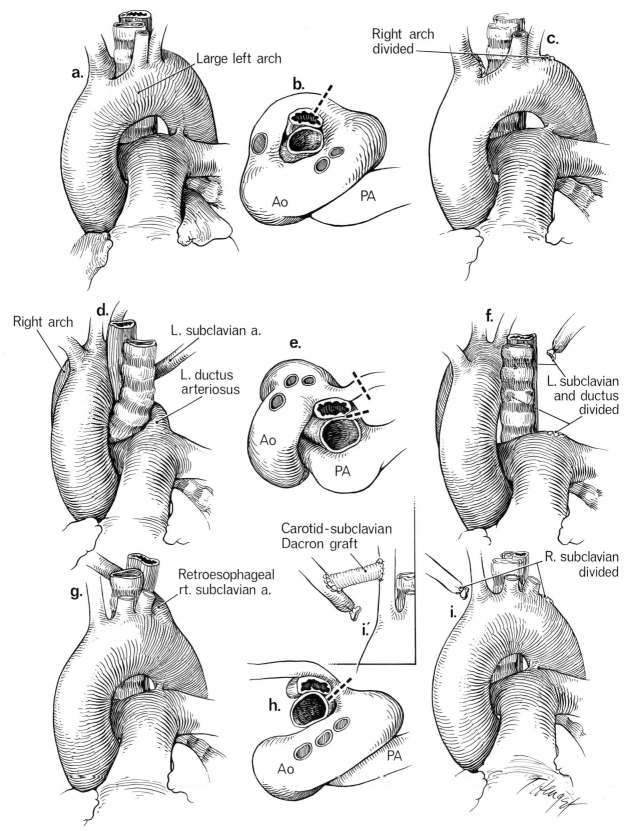

a. Large left arch

b. Ao PA

c. Right arch divided

d. Right arch — L. subclavian a. — L. ductus arteriosus

e. Ao PA

f. L. subclavian and ductus divided

g. Retroesophageal rt. subclavian a.

Carotid-subclavian Dacron graft

i'.

h. Ao PA

i. R. subclavian divided

Figure 12–9 Repair of double aortic arch.

sum (Fig. 12–9, d). The ligamentum is also involved in the formation of the vascular ring. Operation is performed through a left thoracotomy. The vagus and recurrent laryngeal nerve help to identify the ligamentum arteriosum, which is divided and partially releases the ring (Fig. 12–9, e). The anomalous left subclavian artery is then dissected back to the point where it joins the descending limb of the aortic arch. The artery is divided and the ends are oversewn or ligated (Fig. 12–9, f). The trachea and esophagus are dissected free of the surrounding vascular structures.

LEFT ARCH — RETROESOPHAGEAL RIGHT SUBCLAVIAN ARTERY

In comparison with other vascular deformities of the aortic arch, this anomaly is relatively common (Fig. 12–9, g). Using the left thoracotomy approach, the descending limb of the aortic arch is encircled with tape ligatures for traction. The subclavian artery is also encircled with tape ligatures. The subclavian artery, which may be extremely thin-walled, is dissected and divided (Fig. 12–9, h). The ends are oversewn or ligated (Fig. 12–9, i).

After closure of the subclavian artery, young patients seldom experience significant disability except for a cool hand, which may cause some discomfort during winter months, or ischemic symptoms such as weakness during strenuous arm and shoulder exercise. If the subclavian artery is not revascularized, they may also develop symptoms of "subclavian steal," such as dizziness during shoulder exercise. Revascularization of the subclavian has become a relatively simple procedure that can be done immediately or at any time following the operation. A small transverse lateral collar incision is made on the side of the subclavian insufficiency, and the common carotid and subclavian arteries are dissected for anastomosis. An 8-mm Dacron tube graft about 4.0 cm in length is then used as a bypass from the carotid to the subclavian artery (Fig. 12–9, i).

RESTORATION OF VASCULAR CONTINUITY IN THE DIVIDED SUBCLAVIAN ARTERY

In recent years we have elected to restore vascular continuity in the divided subclavian artery at the time of the initial thoracotomy (Fig. 12–10, a to e). After the subclavian artery is divided and freed from the esophagus, a Dacron graft (7 or 8 mm in diameter) is used to connect the subclavian artery stump to the ascending aorta. A partial-occlusion clamp is placed on the aorta for the proximal anastomosis (Fig. 12–10, d). The graft should be placed lateral and anterior to the vena cava to prevent venous obstruction (Fig. 12–10, e). We have seen no complications after this technique, and late circulatory problems have been avoided.

ABERRANT LEFT PULMONARY ARTERY (PULMONARY ARTERY SLING)

In most vascular anomalies that cause tracheal and esophageal obstruction, compression is produced by arteries having systemic arterial pressure; in this anomaly, however, compression is caused by the relatively low-pressure pulmonary artery. First described by Glaevecke and Doehle in 1897,[31] this rare anomaly occurs embryologically when the two lung buds derive their blood supply from the right sixth vascular arch. As the lungs develop, the origin of the pulmonary blood supply to the

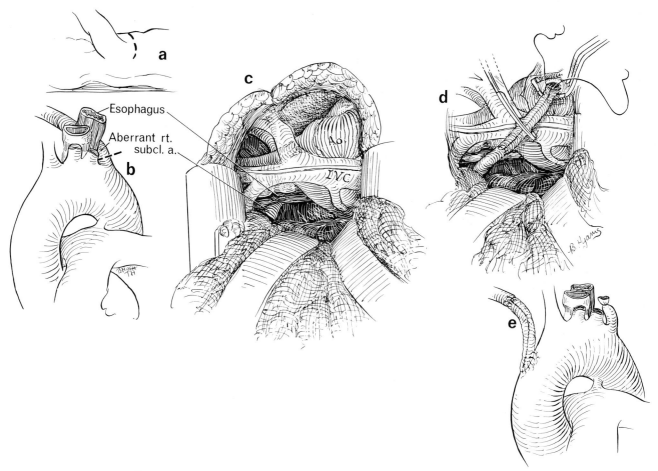

Figure 12–10 Restoration of vascular continuity in the divided subclavian artery.

left lung traverses the midline in the mediastinum, passing between the trachea and esophagus, compressing both structures. In all reported cases, a patent ductus arteriosus or ligamentum arteriosum has been present. The ligamentum attaches to its usual site on the aortic arch and to the main pulmonary trunk — not to the anomalous left pulmonary artery.[32-35] Theoretically, a similar origin of the right pulmonary artery from the left is a possibility, in which case a similar compression of the tracheobronchial tree could occur. To our knowledge, such an anomaly has not been described clinically.

The anomalous left pulmonary artery originates at a point just over the right main stem and right upper lobe bronchus, producing hypoplasia and arresting the growth of the cartilaginous rings. Collapsibility of the right bronchial system results in a ball-valve effect that prevents the right lung from decompressing during expiration and causes the overly distended lung to appear emphysematous on chest roentgenograms. When the trachea is also affected, overdistension of both lungs results, usually predominating on the right. The infant develops dyspnea and stridor, feeds poorly, and may be in acute distress. Diagnosis should be suspected on physical examination, and an esophagogram with a non-oily medium should reveal anterior compression of the esophagus, suggesting the correct diagnosis. For positive identification, a pulmonary arteriogram cautiously performed may be more revealing and safer for an infant than a bronchogram, which aggravates the respiratory distress.

SURGICAL CORRECTION

Successful surgical treatment was first described in 1954 by Potts and his associates,[35] who operated upon a newborn infant and divided the anomalous left pulmonary artery at its origin and anastomosed the artery to the same stump — anterior and to the left of the trachea. Respiratory stridor continued in that patient for several weeks after operation, demonstrating the effect of pulmonary sling upon underlying tracheobronchial structures. This emphasizes the need for careful surveillance by the critical care staff during the postoperative support of all patients, particularly newborn infants, after surgical treatment of vascular rings.

Several techniques of surgical correction have been described in the literature. Among these are: (1) the technique of Potts, in which the artery is moved from behind the trachea and reanastomosed to the stump; (2) division and closure of the site of origin and removal of the artery to a new site of anastomosis on the main pulmonary trunk; or (3) simply a division of the ligamentum arteriosum (a technique that is not recommended). Removal of the mechanical obstruction to the tracheobronchial structures, with full dissection and release of adherent bands and fibers, is vital. Dissection and mobilization should be performed with the greatest care to prevent perforation of the extremely thin membranous part of the trachea and right main stem bronchus.

Before the decision is made to reanastomose the left pulmonary artery to either its natural stump or the main pulmonary trunk, the surgeon should determine if the patient will tolerate temporary partial occlusion of the trunk with a special infant-sized vascular partial-occlusion clamp. If partial occlusion appears to be tolerated, we prefer to divide the artery, ligate or oversew the stump, and then anastomose the left artery into the main pulmonary trunk (Fig. 12–11). Otherwise, the point of division should be made so that the stump will be sufficiently long to permit anastomosis anterior to the trachea without interfering with circulation to the right lung, as in Potts' technique.[35]

The optimal surgical approach is by way of a left posterolateral thoracotomy, ordinarily through the third intercostal space. An approach through a median sternotomy or right thoracotomy may be acceptable, but both lack the important exposure of the trachea, esophagus, and left pulmonary hilum. The usual dissection of the

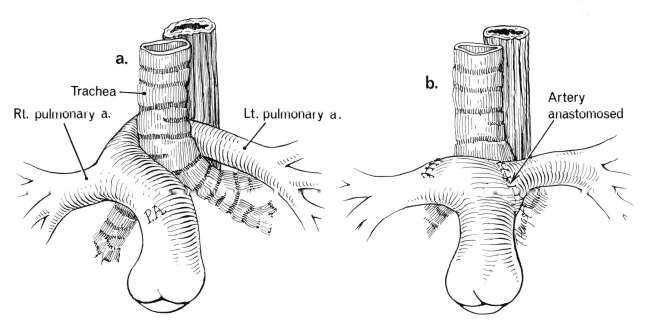

Figure 12–11 Surgical correction of aberrant left pulmonary artery.

vagus and recurrent laryngeal nerves should be done for orientation and to identify the ligamentum arteriosum and other vascular structures. The ligamentum is then divided. Dissection of the left pulmonary artery behind the trachea and to its origin from the right pulmonary artery is performed. The pericardium is opened to mobilize the main pulmonary artery for the subsequent manipulation. Once the decision is made to divide the anomalous artery and the site is chosen for anastomosis, the actual anastomosis may be performed with a 6–0 or 5–0 monofilament suture. The final step involves dissection of the trachea and right bronchus, as already described. Upon completion of the operation, the thoracotomy incision is closed in the usual manner with a small-caliber tube for underwater seal drainage.

REFERENCES

1. Crafoord C, Nylin G: Congenital coarctation of the aorta and its surgical treatment. J Thorac Cardiovasc Surg 14:347, 1945.
2. Gross RE, Hufnagel CA: Coarctation of the aorta. N Engl J Med 233:287, 1945.
3. Cooley DA, Hallman GL, Hammam AS: Congenital cardiovascular anomalies in adults. Results of surgical treatment in 167 patients over age 35. Am J Cardiol 17:303, 1966.
4. Carrel A: The surgery of blood vessels. Bull Johns Hopkins Hosp 18:18, 1907.
5. Hallman GL, Yashar JJ, Bloodwell RD, Cooley DA: Surgical correction of coarctation of the aorta in the first year of life. Ann Thorac Surg 4:106, 1967.
6. Reul GJ Jr, Kabbani SS, Sandiford FM, Wukasch DC, Cooley DA: Repair of coarctation of the thoracic aorta by patch graft aortoplasty. J Thorac Cardiovasc Surg 68:696, 1974.
7. Reid HC, Dallachy R: Infarction of ileum following resection of coarctation of the aorta. Br J Surg 45:625, 1958.
8. Glenn F, Stewart HJ, Engle MA, Lukas DS, Artusio J, Steinberg IS, Holswade GR: Coarctation of the aorta complicated by bacterial endocarditis and an aneurysm of the sinus of Valsalva. Circulation 17:432, 1958.
9. Mays ET, Sergeant CK: Postcoarctectomy syndrome. Arch Surg 91:58, 1965.
10. Hurt RL, Hanbury WJ: Intestinal vascular lesions simulating polyarteritis nodosa after resection of coarctation of the aorta. Thorax 12:258, 1957.
11. Quain R: Partial contraction of the abdominal aorta. Trans Path Soc London 1:244, 1846.
12. Wood PH: *Disease of the Heart and Circulation*, Second Edition. London, Eyre and Spottiswoode, 1956.
13. Pyorala K, Heinonen O, Koskelo P, Heikel PE: Coarctation of the abdominal aorta. Review of twenty-seven cases. Am J Cardiol 6:650, 1960.
14. DeBakey ME, Garrett HE, Howell JF, Morris GC: Coarctation of the abdominal aorta with renal arterial stenosis: Surgical considerations. Ann Surg 165:838, 1967.
15. Maycock WA: Congenital stenosis of the abdominal aorta. Am Heart J 13:633, 1937.
16. Bloor K, Williams RT: Neurofibromatosis and coarctation of the abdominal aorta with renal artery involvement. Br J Surg 50:811, 1963.
17. Colquhoun J: Hypoplasia of the abdominal aorta following therapeutic irradiation in infancy. Radiology 86:454, 1966.
18. Sen PK, Kinare SG, Kulharni TP, Parrilkar GB: Stenosing aortitis of unknown etiology. Surgery 51:317, 1962.
19. Inada K, Katsumura T, Hirai J, Semada T: Surgical treatment of aortitis syndrome. Arch Surg 100:220, 1970.
20. Sehiri V, Askerson RA: Arteritis of the aorta and its major branches. Quart J Med 33:439, 1964.
21. Glenn F, Keefer EB, Speer DS, Dotter CT: Coarctation of lower thoracic and abdominal aorta immediately proximal to the celiac axis. Surg Gynecol Obstet 94:561, 1952.
22. Cooley, DA, DeBakey ME: Resection of thoracic aorta with replacement by homograft for aneurysms and constrictive lesions. J Thorac Surg 29:216, 1955.
23. Wukasch DC, Cooley DA, Sandiford FM, Nappi G, Reul GJ Jr: Ascending aorta-abdominal aorta bypass: Indications, technique, and report of 12 patients. Ann Thorac Surg 23:442, 1977.
24. Gross RE: Surgical correction for coarctation of the aorta. Surgery 18:673, 1945.
25. Gross RE: Treatment of certain aortic coarctations by homologous grafts; report of 19 cases. Ann Surg 134:753, 1951.
26. Hallman GL, Cooley DA: Congenital aortic vascular ring: Surgical considerations. Arch Surg 88:666, 1964.
27. Hallman GL, Cooley DA, Bloodwell RD: Congenital vascular ring. Surg Clin N Am 46:855, 1966.
20. Galiolo FM, Bermudez-Canele R, Reitman MJ, Hallman GL, Cooley DA, McNamara DG: Congenital vascular rings. Analysis of 41 consecutive cases. Am J Cardiol 31:133, 1973.
29. Hallman GL, Cooley DA, Singer DB: Congenital anomalies of the coronary arteries: Anatomy, pathology, and surgical treatment. Surgery 49:133, 1966.
30. Ventemiglia R, Oglietti J, Wukasch DC, Hallman GL, Cooley DA: Interruption of the aortic arch: Surgical considerations. J Thorac Cardiovasc Surg 72:235, 1976.
31. Glaevecke and Doehle: Ueber eine seltene angeborene. Anomalie der Pulmonalarterie. Münch Med Wochenschr 44:950, 1897.

32. Contro S, Miller RA, White H, Potts WJ: Bronchial obstruction due to pulmonary artery anomalies. I. Vascular sling. Circulation 17:418, 1958.
33. Sade RM, Rosenthal A, Fellows K, Castaneda AR: Pulmonary artery sling. J Thorac Cardiovasc Surg 69 (3):333, 1975.
34. Jue KL, Raghib G, Amplatz K, Adams P Jr, Edwards JE: Anomalous origin of the left pulmonary artery from the right pulmonary artery. Am J Roentgenol 95:598, 1965.
35. Potts WL, Holinger PH, Rosenblum AH: Anomalous left pulmonary artery causing obstruction to right main bronchus: report of a case. JAMA 155:1409, 1954.

CHAPTER 13

Vascular Injuries

INTRODUCTION AND GENERAL PRINCIPLES

The management of vascular injuries is gratifying in that proper treatment will often result in the restoration of circulation and eventual recovery. On the other hand, the possibility of hemorrhage or loss of limb allows only a limited time for the initiation of aggressive, definitive treatment. More often than not, the surgeon's first attempt is his only opportunity to salvage life or limb.

The surgeon is frequently required to make irretractable decisions. The general principles of managing vascular injuries include control of hemorrhage, restoration of circulation, prevention of infection, and reduction of swelling. Fasciotomy may become necessary if vital structures are compressed. When vascular injuries are associated with fractures, stabilization of the fractures is essential to protect the repaired vessel from recurrent damage.[1] The optimal type of arterial prosthesis for use in a contaminated wound remains controversial; although autogenous saphenous veins are often recommended for these situations, we prefer Dacron grafts. In our experience, Dacron has less propensity for becoming infected in a fresh wound that has been contaminated with dirt or road grease than in a wound that has been infected with bacterial growth. Therefore, we believe Dacron is equally acceptable and possibly preferable to autogenous saphenous vein grafts in most traumatic injuries.

Damage resulting from high-velocity missiles usually extends considerably beyond the initially apparent tissue destruction. This fact is pertinent when deciding how much to debride an artery damaged by a high-velocity missile. To prevent subsequent thrombus of the artery produced by necrotic intima that may not appear damaged initially, it is better to debride too much rather than too little. Another important point is that an artery thrombosed after blunt trauma cannot be satisfactorily opened by simply removing the thrombus with a Fogarty catheter. Although circulation can often be restored for a limited time, such arteries have sustained intimal damage, and thrombus will almost always recur. Arteries so injured should be explored, and the damaged segment should be resected and replaced with a graft. The extent of intimal damage is usually apparent by external inspection, which reveals an area of bluish discoloration resulting from subintimal hemorrhage. The artery should be opened longitudinally and the arteriotomy and length of resection extended as far as necessary after inspection of the intima from within.

SUBCLAVIAN ARTERY INJURY

Injury to the subclavian artery must be suspected in connection with penetrating wounds in the area of the great vessels or blunt trauma with fracture of the clavicle. Because arteriographic visualization of these vessels is difficult and often impractical in the acutely injured patient, surgical exploration is indicated if vascular injury is suspected. Clinical findings associated with injury to the great vessels include:

diminished pulses in one upper extremity, neurological deficits, or signs of extensive hemorrhage as revealed by distortion of the anatomy or by chest x-ray film.[2, 3] It should be emphasized, however, that upper extremity pulses may remain full even with significant injury to the innominate or subclavian arteries; therefore, the presence of pulses does not exclude injury requiring exploration and repair. When clinical evidence suggests arterial injury, it is the surgeon's responsibility to disprove such evidence by either exploration or arteriography.[4]

Exposure of the great arteries arising from the aortic arch presents the major consideration in controlling hemorrhage and achieving vascular repair. The two optimal types of incision are the "trap door" and the supraclavicular (Fig. 13–1, a). When exploration is due to a penetrating injury, the "trap door" approach is preferred. This is begun as an oblique incision slightly more transverse than the medial border of the sternocleidomastoid muscle, extended caudad by splitting the upper sternum, and carried to approximately the midclavicular line on the ipsilateral side through the second or third interspace (Fig. 13–1, a). This approach allows a sizable flap of chest wall to be elevated, providing adequate exposure of the innominate, subclavian, or proximal common carotid arteries.

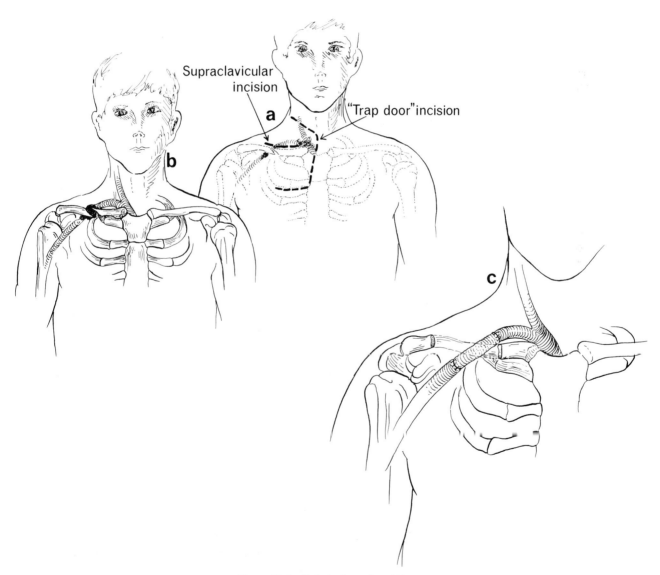

Supraclavicular incision

"Trap door" incision

Figure 13–1 Subclavian artery injury.

Subclavian arterial injuries associated with blunt trauma and fracture of the clavicle can be approached by a more limited supraclavicular incision, as detailed in Chapter 2 (under Carotid Subclavian Bypass). This incision is made 8 to 10 cm in length parallel to and approximately 2 cm above the clavicle, either over the supraclavicular fossa or centered over the fracture (Fig. 13–1, a). If more extensive exposure is required, the incision can be extended to make a "trap door" as described above. The midportion of the clavicle, including the area of fracture, is resected, and the anterior scalene muscle transected (Fig. 13–1, b). Care is taken to avoid injury to the phrenic nerve and brachial plexus. Control of the subclavian artery proximal and distal to the area of injury is obtained, and after systemic heparinization, the segment of injured artery is resected. Continuity of the artery is restored by anastomosing an appropriately sized Dacron double-velour graft end-to-end (Fig. 13–1, c). A final note of emphasis should be made regarding the necessity of resecting the fractured portion of clavicle. For successful vascular repair associated with bone fractures, either internal or external stabilization is necessary; when this is not feasible, as in the case of clavicular fracture, resection is mandatory to prevent disruption of the vascular repair.[1]

EROSION OF INNOMINATE ARTERY BY TRACHEOSTOMY

A tracheo-innominate artery fistula resulting from erosion of the innominate artery by a tracheostomy is a surgical emergency of the first order. Until recently, this complication has usually been fatal. In 1976, Jones[5] reviewed the world literature and found only ten long-term survivors among 137 recorded cases. During the past several years, however, it has been shown that this complication can be successfully managed by applying three basic concepts: (1) prompt recognition of the significance of arterial bleeding from a tracheostomy site, (2) institution of specific maneuvers to control hemorrhage and prevent aspiration, and (3) resection of the innominate artery without graft replacement in the infected field.[6–8]

Erosion of the innominate artery results from localized ischemic pressure necrosis by the tracheostomy tube or its cuff. The injury may be classified as either *extratracheal* or *endotracheal* in origin.[7] *Extratracheal* injuries are produced by erosion of the medial aspect of the innominate artery by the shank of the tracheostomy tube outside the trachea. This usually results from the technical error of placing the tracheostomy stoma too low — below the fourth tracheal ring. It can occur, however, even with correct placement of the tracheostomy, in the presence of an abnormally high innominate artery. The *endotracheal* type of erosion is caused by pressure from the cuff or tip of the tracheostomy tube.[5] This produces a true tracheo–innominate artery fistula that is directly related to cuff management.[7]

Erosion of the innominate artery must be suspected whenever arterial bleeding occurs from a tracheostomy site. If the patient is being inadequately ventilated, with poor oxygenation, the darkened arterial blood may be mistaken for venous bleeding. Innominate artery erosion typically occurs several days after tracheostomy. It is not unusual for a transient episode of hemorrhage to occur and stop spontaneously before a massive, terminal eruption.

Emergency Maneuvers: When acute arterial bleeding occurs around a tracheostomy site several days after tracheostomy, it must be presumed that erosion of the innominate artery has occurred (Fig. 13–2, a). Immediate maneuvers must be initiated if a local site of bleeding is not apparent within the tracheostomy incision. An oral or nasal endotracheal tube inserted into the trachea proximal to the tracheostomy tube allows immediate removal of the latter and advancement of the endotracheal tube should the hemorrhage become massive. In such circumstances, the digital

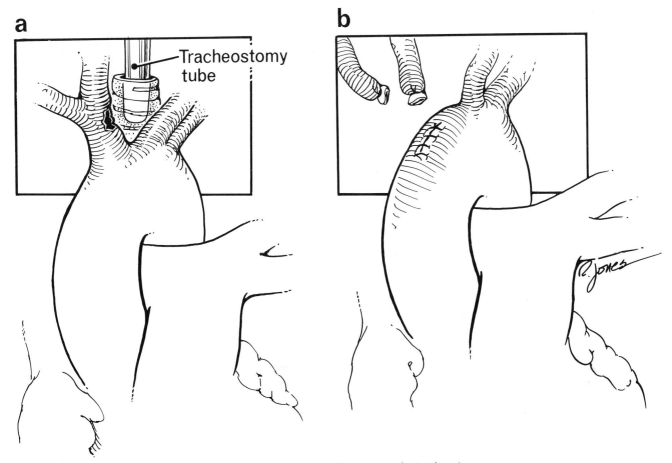

a

Tracheostomy
tube

b

Figure 13–2 Erosion of innominate artery by tracheostomy.

control technique described by Utley[8] may be lifesaving. This technique consists of dissecting the trachea and innominate artery with the index finger as in mediastinoscopy. Pressure is then applied with the finger to the posterior medial aspect of the innominate artery while the patient is being transported to the operating room.

SURGICAL TECHNIQUE

In the operating room, the oral endotracheal tube is placed with a nasal endotracheal tube by the anesthesiologist. The tracheostomy tube is removed, and the cause of hemorrhage determined by exploration of the wound after the tracheostomy has been enlarged. Should the bleeding originate from a site other than the innominate artery, ligation of the bleeding point is effected and nothing further is required.

If erosion of the innominate artery, with or without tracheo–innominate artery fistula, is confirmed, the incision is extended to provide additional exposure. The most expeditious method is to extend the tracheostomy caudad into a standard median sternotomy.[10] This provides the advantage of speed and optimum exposure but the disadvantage of a serious wound-healing problem should the incision become infected postoperatively. Alternately, the "trap door" approach (see Fig. 13–1, a) may be used. This incision consists of a partial upper sternotomy with lateral extension into the right third intercostal space. Although the approach is somewhat more cumbersome and yields less adequate exposure, it has the advantage that non-union of a partial sternotomy is a much less serious problem than in a non-union full sternotomy. We recommend either approach, depending upon the urgency of the circumstances.

During exploration of the innominate artery, the surgeon must be aware of the possible anatomic variations of the great vessels arising from the aortic arch. In approximately 10 percent of Caucasians and 30 percent of Negroes, the left common carotid artery arises from the innominate artery rather than from the aortic arch.[7] Another anatomic variation is the origin of the right vertebral artery proximal rather than distal to the right common carotid artery.[7]

The cardinal decision in planning definitive treatment is whether or not to attempt replacement with a prosthetic graft after resection of the innominate artery. The literature indicates that the risk of recurrent fatal hemorrhage associated with graft replacement is significantly higher than the approximately 5 to 10 percent incidence of neurologic deficit after resection of the innominate artery.[5-8, 11-16] Therefore, we concur that the innominate artery should be resected and the proximal innominate subclavian and right common carotid arteries oversewn with permanent monofilament suture (Fig. 13–2, b). Cooper has described a method of leaving the right common carotid-subclavian artery bifurcation intact, with complete reversal of flow to the right upper extremity, without symptoms of a subclavian steal syndrome.[6] We believe, however, that the right subclavian and common carotid arteries should be ligated separately, with division of the bifurcation so that these vessels can retract out of the contaminated area and thus lessen the likelihood of spontaneous rupture of the stumps.[7] Care must be taken to preserve the left innominate vein, which lies anterior to the innominate artery. Ligation of this vein produces severe obstruction to venous return from the head and left upper extremity.[17]

The tracheal defect is not repaired at this time. Instead, the wound is packed open with neomycin-soaked sponges, which are changed hourly until clean granulation tissue has covered the exposed arterial stumps.[6] Postoperatively, the airway is maintained by means of a nasal endotracheal tube with the cuff placed below the tracheal defect. This tube is removed after 10 to 14 days, and a new tracheostomy is performed if an airway is still required. Should tracheal stenosis develop during the late postoperative course, elective tracheal reconstruction can be performed.

As stated previously, the incidence of neurologic sequelae after resection of the innominate artery is reported to be only 5 to 10 percent.[5-8, 11-16] Should acute hemiparesis become manifest during the immediate postoperative period, however, immediate carotid-carotid bypass (see Chapter 2) can be performed. In our experience with early thrombectomy and endarterectomy for acute occlusion of the internal carotid artery, neurologic deficits are completely reversible in approximately 50 percent of patients when revascularization takes place within four hours after the occlusion (see Chapter 2). Symptoms of claudication in the right upper extremity resulting from interruption of the right subclavian artery can be relieved by elective left subclavian to right subclavian bypass.

INJURIES TO THE THORACIC AORTA

Even during peacetime, injuries to the thoracic aorta occur with moderate frequency, owing to high speed transportation, bodily assault with sharp weapons or firearms, and other forms of violence. Two broad categories of injuries occur: namely, direct penetrations or lacerations, and rupture or transection due to blunt injury — either from direct crushing of the trunk or from rapid deceleration.[18, 19] Definitive treatment of patients fortunate enough to reach the hospital emergency facility alive must combine rapid diagnosis, resuscitative measures, and immediate surgical repair when indicated.[20]

TREATMENT FOR PENETRATING WOUNDS

For penetrating wounds, the decision to perform an exploratory operation is usually not difficult, since a point of entry (and sometimes also of exit) helps to establish the trajectory of the penetrating object.[21] Diagnosis may be made by physical examination and, if time permits, may be confirmed by radiography or angiography. Exploratory thoracotomy or celiotomy should be undertaken if the slightest evidence suggests an aortic injury. Smaller penetrations may seal themselves off for a few hours or days and then reopen, resulting in exsanguinating hemorrhage. Whereas surgical exploration in a patient suspected of aortic trauma that reveals no such trauma is excusable, neglect of such an injury may be disastrous.

Repair of an aortic laceration is best accomplished by obtaining control of the vessel both proximal and distal to the lesion. In vital areas such as the ascending aorta, control may be obtained only by using temporary cardiopulmonary bypass. Usually, however, other methods may be simpler and more readily available on an emergency basis.[22, 23] A large partial-occlusion clamp may be sufficient to isolate the laceration — a technique we have found to be extremely useful is deliberately induced electrical fibrillation of the heart. For this purpose, we have available in the surgical suite a fibrillator that delivers a 10 to 50 volt current. Induced fibrillation provides a quiet, nonbleeding surgical field, with conditions that permit a rapid, precise aortic repair. After 4 to 6 minutes of circulatory arrest, cardiac action is restored by an electrical countershock, and circulation is restored, with the aid of cardiac massage if necessary. This technique may be repeated several times. We have not yet seen it result in brain damage.

Aortic repair should be accomplished without disturbing the aortic anatomy. In some instances, a fabric tube graft is necessary to prevent distortion. Abdominal tension on an aortic suture line invites disruption and subsequent development of a false aneurysm. An injury to the aortic wall produced by a bullet or metallic fragment should be debrided and repaired either with a fabric tube graft or fabric patch.

BLUNT (NONPENETRATING) INJURY

Most injuries to the aorta are caused by violent nonpenetrating trauma — more than 80 percent by automobile accidents.[20] The mechanism of aortic disruption varies and the anatomic location depends upon the areas of relative fixation and mobility of the vessel. Approximately 90 percent of injuries occur at the aortic isthmus. The remaining 10 percent are distributed almost equally between the ascending aorta, aortic arch, and distal descending aorta, with very few in the abdominal aorta.[20] (See Abdominal Vascular Injuries, Blunt Trauma to the Common Iliac Artery, p. 196.) In the abdominal aorta and iliac arteries, blunt trauma often results in thrombosis and may be accompanied by paraplegia due to spinal cord concussion or peripheral nerve shock. For thoracic lesions, several possibilities may account for the propensity of the isthmic location. Injury in this area usually consists of a transverse tear or complete transection, which could only occur if a sudden shearing force were applied. During sudden deceleration, the rather mobile descending aorta and also the ascending aorta swing forward, while the isthmus and transverse arch, which are anchored by the ligamentum arteriosum and great vessels, hold the arch in a relatively fixed position. The stress then falls upon the isthmus. A crushing injury to the chest forces the ascending aorta and transverse arch posteriorly, while the descending aorta is held in a relatively fixed position on the dorsal vertebrae, placing the stress on the isthmic zone. Longitudinal tears probably result from a sudden increase in intraluminal pressure, with rupture at susceptible points of relative weakness.

Although traumatic rupture is often difficult to diagnose, it should be suspected in any patient who survives a violent crushing injury of any type. Symbas[24] has described a triad of symptoms that his group considers diagnostic: these include hypertension in the upper extremities, hypotension (decreased pulses) in the lower extremities, and radiographic widening of the superior mediastinum. Paraplegia or paresis occurs in 10 percent of patients. In our experience, this triad is infrequently present in its entirety, and the surgeon must request aortography. Even then, the results may be inconclusive, and exploratory thoracotomy becomes necessary to rule out aortic injury.[25]

ACUTE INJURY

Many patients recover from the acute thoracic trauma without knowledge of the aortic injury. The natural tendency to heal in an aortic contusion or localized dissection is surprisingly strong. Therefore, the lesion may not be recognized until months or even years later. We have seen aneurysms in this anatomic location go unrecognized for more than 20 years before they are discovered by routine chest radiography. Usually the aneurysm has become calcified. In many such instances, however, the aneurysm begins to expand spontaneously and symptoms of pain, or even dysphagia or stridor, may appear as the lesion encroaches upon the adjacent esophagus or tracheobronchial structures. Diagnosis is confirmed by aortography.

SURGICAL TREATMENT

Once the decision has been made to explore, the choice of incision depends upon the anticipated location of the injury. For the most common type, located at the aortic isthmus, we prefer a left posterolateral incision through the fourth intercostal space. For the others, a midline sternotomy or celiotomy may be preferred, or a thoracotomy located at the sixth or seventh space may be used for a distal thoracic aortic rupture.

Upon opening the thoracic cavity and inserting the self-retaining retractor, an extensive hematoma may be found in the posterior superior mediastinum. A direct opening into the hematoma should be avoided since massive hemorrhage is often prevented only by adjacent mediastinal tissues. In some instances the intimal and medial aortic layers are transected and only the adventitia remains intact. Proximal control of the aorta between the origin of the left common carotid and subclavian arteries is the objective of mediastinal dissection. This can be accomplished most safely by first entering the pericardium, usually anterior to the phrenic nerve. The transverse aortic arch is dissected by reflecting the pericardium superiorly, and the aortic arch is mobilized by careful blunt dissection. The origin of each of the major branches of the arch should be identified. Although in the past we have used pump bypass, temporary conduits, and partial cardiopulmonary support with femoral vein and arterial cannulation, experience has convinced us that the repair can be accomplished most expeditiously and without neurologic damage by means of a straightforward aortic and subclavian cross-clamping and aortic repair, which should be easily accomplished within 30 minutes of circulatory interruption to the distal aorta.

Dissection of the aortic arch continues until the arch is encircled with a tape. Distal control is obtained with the lung retracted forward, and the subclavian artery is encircled high in the mediastinum. With vascular control secured, the proximal and distal aorta and subclavian artery are cross-clamped. We usually inject intravenously about 50 to 75 mg of heparin prior to clamping the aorta.

The hematoma is entered directly, and the aorta is exposed. In our experience, direct repair of the tear or transection should seldom be attempted because the aortic injuries may extend well beyond the laceration. Repair of the aorta should be done in undamaged tissue, and tension on the suture line must be avoided to prevent subsequent disruption or aneurysm formation. Therefore, the edges of the aortic tear should be trimmed back to healthy tissue and continuity restored with a low-porosity woven Dacron graft. For sutures, we use a 4–0 braided polyester thread with small needles to avoid lacerations of the friable aortic tissue. Occluding clamps are released gradually to avoid an abrupt fall in blood pressure. For this purpose, a vascular clamp with a long ratchet provides the most satisfactory result. Seldom will a patient suffer neurologic or cardiac sequelae if the period of occlusion does not exceed 30 to 45 minutes.[26-28]

At the conclusion of aortic repair, the heparin effect is reversed with protamine sulfate. The mediastinal pleura should be closed over the graft, the pericardium closed loosely, and the chest closed with underwater sealed drainage.

DELAYED OR CHRONIC LESION

Thoracotomy is performed for the delayed or chronic lesion in the same manner as for the acute lesion, using a left fourth intercostal space incision. Proximal and distal control of the aorta and subclavian artery is obtained by a more direct dissection because sudden rupture is not a significant threat. The excision and graft replacement are performed by the use of the same technique described for the acute lesion. We do not use shunts of any kind for removal of the late post-traumatic aneurysm.

ABDOMINAL VASCULAR INJURIES

The decision to explore injuries resulting from blunt trauma to the abdomen is probably one of the most difficult clinical judgments in surgery. In general, all penetrating wounds of the abdomen below the level of the nipples should be explored.

Even though findings of tenderness, rigidity, and distention are not progressive and a peritoneal tap for blood is negative, the abdomen that has sustained a blunt trauma injury should be under careful observation. When in doubt, surgical exploration may be the most prudent course. In this situation, an old medical adage may be appropriate: "The major hindrance to intra-abdominal diagnosis is the abdominal wall."

Injuries to intra-abdominal viscera are commonly associated with vascular injuries. Although the management of visceral injuries is beyond the scope of this book, they must be appropriately treated according to well-established surgical principles.[29] The presence of a retroperitoneal hematoma necessitates a decision as to the advisability of opening the hematoma or leaving it intact. If the hematoma is nonpulsatile and is satisfactorily tamponaded by an intact posterior peritoneum, it may be left alone. If it involves the area adjacent to the duodenum or pancreas, however, exploration by Kocher's maneuver and opening of the gastrohepatic omentum are mandatory to rule out possible injury to these structures.

AORTIC INJURIES

The urgent problem in intra-abdominal aortic or major arterial injuries is control of hemorrhage. After the abdomen has been entered, the supraceliac aorta should be cross-clamped at the level of the diaphragm. (See Chapter 8, Fig. 8–1, a and b.)

After proximal aortic control has been obtained, exposure is determined by the anticipated location of the injury relative to the midline.[30] If the injury appears to affect the proximal aorta, left renal, celiac, or superior mesenteric arteries, exposure is gained by reflecting the splenic flexure of the colon, the spleen, and the tail of the pancreas to the right. Major injuries to the inferior vena cava, portal vein, or right renal vessels located to the right of the midline are exposed by Kocher's maneuver, with reflection of the duodenum and hepatic flexure of the colon to the left. Injury of the intrahepatic inferior vena cava is discussed below.

Whether resulting from penetrating or blunt trauma, aortic injuries usually are best managed by resection and graft replacement. Injuries to the celiac, superior mesenteric, renal, or inferior mesenteric arteries are optimally treated with graft replacement. Under urgent circumstances, however, particularly in cases of associated multiple injuries, ligation of these vessels may be necessary.

BLUNT TRAUMA TO THE COMMON ILIAC ARTERY

Injuries caused by blunt trauma to the common iliac artery deserve special mention. Thrombosis of the common iliac artery without hemorrhage can result from blunt trauma. The inexperienced surgeon may attempt thrombectomy by means of a Fogarty catheter without achieving definitive repair of the intimal damage.

Acute occlusion of the common iliac artery, particularly in a young individual who has not developed collateral circulation with arteriosclerotic occlusive disease, will result in loss of the lower extremity in approximately 80 percent of patients. Therefore, revascularization is mandatory. Although the Fogarty catheter is useful for removing distal extensions of the thrombus, passage of a balloon catheter alone does not effect long-term restoration of the circulation. The damaged section of artery, which can usually be identified by the bluish discoloration resulting from subintimal hemorrhage, must be resected and replaced with a prosthetic graft.

INFERIOR VENA CAVA OR HEPATIC VEIN INJURY

Laceration of the inferior vena cava can be extremely troublesome, primarily because of the difficulty in obtaining a dry operative field. Rather than attempting to isolate and clamp the inferior vena cava or iliac veins individually, the most expeditious maneuver for obtaining hemostasis is to compress the vein proximally and distally with a ring forceps containing a folded sponge. Most vena cava injuries can be repaired primarily, but ligation of the inferior vena cava can be performed when necessary. Prosthetic graft replacement within the venous system has not proved satisfactory.

Injury to the intrahepatic vena cava or hepatic vein creates a complex situation requiring a special maneuver[31] to obtain a sufficiently dry field for repair without compromising venous return. When such an injury is identified, the abdominal incision is extended in a cephalad direction as a median sternotomy. The pericardium is opened, and a No. 34 plastic chest tube is inserted through the right atrial appendage into the inferior vena cava to the level of the renal veins. A side hole is cut in the tube approximately 20 cm from the tip prior to insertion to allow flow to be directed into the right atrium. The tube is secured by a purse-string suture held in place with a rubber tourniquet. Tapes are passed around the inferior vena cava within the pericardium and below the liver, and a vascular clamp is placed across the portal triad. This allows continuation of venous return from the lower half of the body and a dry field in which the injury can be visualized and repaired.

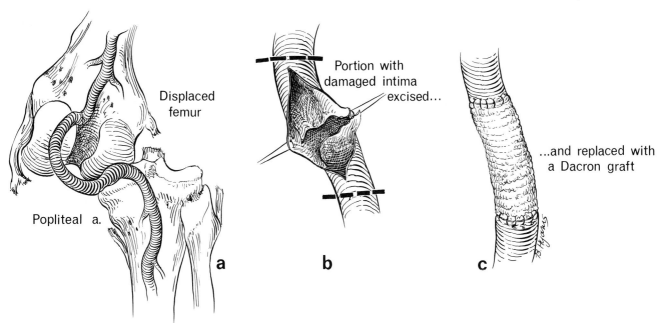

Displaced femur

Popliteal a.

Portion with damaged intima excised...

...and replaced with a Dacron graft

a   b   c

Figure 13–3 Popliteal artery crush.

POPLITEAL ARTERY CRUSH

Injury to the popliteal artery with thrombosis results in an extremely high incidence of subsequent amputation. Analysis of battle injuries during World War II, before techniques of arterial repair were generally available, reported leg amputation rate to be 78 percent following popliteal artery injury.[32] This results from the anatomic configuration of the popliteal artery in the vicinity of the knee, where minimal collateral channels exist. Even with the application of sound principles and techniques of vascular surgery during the Korean and Vietnam Wars, the incidence of amputation following popliteal artery injury was approximately 30 percent.[33, 34] This seemingly high incidence of unsuccessful revascularization results frequently from associated popliteal vein injury. The popliteal vein represents a critical area of venous return with minimal alternate collaterals. Therefore, the popliteal vein as well as the popliteal artery should be repaired with a saphenous vein graft from the opposite extremity.[35, 36]

The popliteal artery may be damaged by fractures or dislocations of the knee.[1, 37] Overlooking the possibility of this injury may result from its being masked by the swelling and more obvious deformities often associated with femoral fractures and dislocations. Diminished or absent pedal pulses are indications for emergency femoral arteriography prior to reduction of the bony injury.

The arterial injury that often accompanies knee dislocations is caused by stretching and crushing of the artery (Fig. 13–3, a), subsequently causing intimal tearing, dissection, and thrombosis (Fig. 13–3, b). Following systemic heparinization and removal of distal thrombus with a Fogarty catheter, the damaged segment of artery is resected (Fig. 13–3, b). The decision as to the extent of damaged intima to be resected may be facilitated by noting the area of bluish discoloration produced by subintimal hemorrhage or spasm that is responsive to a local injection of 2 percent papaverine. The damaged segment of artery is replaced with an appropriate sized Dacron graft (Fig. 13–3, c). In our experience, Dacron is equally as satisfactory as autogenous saphenous vein and preferable because of the expediency and ease of insertion during emergency conditions.[1] Prophylactic fasciotomy (see Chapter 16) is usually necessary to prevent additional tissue damage and necrosis from the period of limb ischemia.[38]

REFERENCES

1. DeBakey ME, Beall AC Jr, Wukasch DC: Recent developments in vascular surgery with particular reference to orthopedics. Am J Surg 109:134, 1965.
2. Flint LM, Snyder WH, Perry MO, Shires GT: Management of major vascular injuries in the base of the neck. Arch Surg 106:407, 1973.
3. Reul GJ Jr, Rubio PA, Beall AC Jr, Jordan GL Jr: Acute carotid artery injury: 25 years' experience. J Trauma 14:967, 1974.
4. Brawley RK, Murray GF, Crisler C, Cameron JL: Management of wounds of the innominate subclavian and axillary blood vessels. Surg Gynecol Obstet 131:1130, 1970.
5. Jones JW, Reynolds M, Hewitt RL, Drapanas T: Tracheo-innominate artery erosion. Ann Surg 184:194, 1976.
6. Cooper JD: Trachea-innominate artery fistula: Successful management of three consecutive patients. Ann Thorac Surg 24:439, 1977.
7. Carberry DM, Bethea MC: Intervention in tracheal fistula. Contemporary Surgery 11:9, 1977.
8. Utley JR, Singer MM, Roe BB, Fraser DG, Dedo HH: Definitive management of innominate artery hemorrhage complicating tracheostomy. JAMA 220:577, 1972.
9. Cooper HD, Grillo HC: Analysis of problems related to cuffs on intratracheal tubes. Chest 62:21 (Suppl 2), 1972.
10. Cooley DA, Norman JC: Repair through midline sternotomy. In *Techniques in Cardiac Surgery,* Texas Medical Press, Houston, Texas, 1975, p 14.
11. Biller HF, Ebert PA: Innominate artery hemorrhage complicating tracheotomy. Ann Otol Rhinol Laryngol 79:301, 1970.
12. Deslauriers J, Ginsberg RJ, Nelems JM, Pearson FG: Innominate artery rupture. Ann Thorac Surg 20:671, 1975.
13. Mathog RH, Kenan PD, Hudson WR: Delayed massive hemorrhage following tracheostomy. Laryngoscope 81:707, 1971.
14. Myers WO, Lawton BR, Sautter RD: An operation for tracheal-innominate artery fistula. Arch Surg 105:269, 1972.
15. Reich MP, Rosenkrantz JG: Fistula between innominate artery and trachea. Arch Surg 96:401, 1968.
16. Silen W, Spieker D: Fatal hemorrhage from the innominate artery after tracheostomy. Ann Surg 162:1005, 1965.
17. Fred HL, Wukasch DC, Petrany Z: Transient compression of the left innominate vein. Circulation 29:758, 1964.
18. Rittenhouse EA, Dillard DH, Winterscheid LC, Merendino KA: Traumatic rupture of the thoracic aorta: A review of the literature and a report of five cases with attention to special problems in early surgical management. Ann Surg 170:87, 1969.
19. Beall AC Jr, Arbegast NR, Ripepi AC, Bricker DL, Diethrich EB, Hallman GL, Cooley DA, DeBakey ME: Aortic laceration due to rapid deceleration. Arch Surg 98:595, 1969.
20. Reul GJ Jr, Rubio PA, Beall AC Jr: The surgical management of acute injury to the thoracic aorta. 67:272, 1974.
21. DeMeester TR, Cameron JL, Gott VL: Repair of a through-and-through gunshot wound of the aortic arch using a heparinized shunt. Ann Thorac Surg 16:193, 1973.
22. Mozingo JR, Denton IC Jr: The neurological deficit associated with sudden occlusion of the abdominal aorta due to blunt trauma. Surgery 77:118, 1975.
23. Adams HD, van Geertruyden HH: Neurologic complications of aortic surgery. Ann Surg 144:574, 1956.
24. Symbas PN, Tyras DH, Ware RE, Diorio DA: Traumatic rupture of the aorta. Ann Surg 178:6, 1973.
25. Kirsh MM, Behrendt DM, Orringer MB, Gago O, Gray LA Jr, Mills LJ, Walter JF, Sloan H: The treatment of acute traumatic rupture of the aorta: a 10-year experience. Ann Surg 184:308, 1976.
26. Cooley DA, DeBakey ME, Morris GC Jr: Controlled extracorporeal circulation in surgical treatment of aortic aneurysm. Ann Surg 146:473, 1957.
27. Bloodwell RD, Hallman GL, Cooley DA: Partial cardiopulmonary bypass for pericardiectomy and resection of descending thoracic aortic aneurysms. Ann Thorac Surg 1:46, 1968.
28. Crawford ES, Fenstermacher JM, Richardson W, Sandiford F: Reappraisal of adjuncts to avoid ischemia in the treatment of thoracic aortic aneurysms. Surgery 67:182, 1970.
29. Shirley AL, Wukasch DC, Beall AC Jr, Gordon WB, DeBakey ME: Surgical management of splenic injuries. Am J Surg 108:630, 1964.
30. Buscaglia LC, Blaisdell FW, Lim RC: Penetrating abdominal vascular injuries. Arch Surg 99:764, 1969.
31. Bricker DL, Wukasch DC: Management of an injury to suprarenal inferior vena cava. Surgical judgment in unusual surgical cases. Surg Clin North Am 50:999, 1970.
32. DeBakey ME, Simeone FA: Battle injuries of arteries in World War II; an analysis of 2,471 cases. Ann Surg 123:534, 1946.
33. Spencer FC, Grewe RB: The management of arterial injuries in battle casualties. Ann Surg 141:304, 1955.
34. Rich NM, Spencer FC: *Vascular Trauma.* Philadelphia, W. B. Saunders Company, 1978.
35. Gaspar MR, Treiman RL: The management of injuries to major veins. Am J Surg 100:171, 1960.
36. Sullivan WG, Thornton FH, Baker LH, LaPlante ES, Cohen A: Early influence of popliteal vein repair in the treatment of popliteal vessel injuries. Am J Surg 122:528, 1971.
37. Smith RF, Szilagyi E, Elliott JP Jr: Fracture of long bones with arterial injury due to blunt trauma. Arch Surg 99:315, 1969.
38. Patman RD, Thompson JE: Fasciotomy in peripheral vascular surgery. Arch Surg 101:663, 1970.

CHAPTER 14

Arterial Embolization

Arterial embolization has been recognized as a surgical emergency since before the turn of the century.[1] As early as 1895, Ssabanajeff attempted direct removal of an aortic saddle embolus.[2] Operative removal of arterial emboli, with limb salvage rates between 30 and 50 percent, was described in the early 1930's.[3, 4] Various ingenious techniques were subsequently proposed during the "pre-vascular-surgery era." Retrograde flushing with saline was suggested by Lerman and associates[5] in 1930, and successful results from the use of this technique were reported in 1956 by Crawford and DeBakey.[6] In 1960, Shaw[7] devised a corkscrew wire to remove adherent distal thrombus. Other techniques included retrograde milking with an Esmarck bandage[8] and the use of endovascular suction catheters as described by Dale.[9] The major breakthrough in the treatment of arterial emboli was the ingenious contribution of Fogarty[10] in 1963. This simple concept, which still provides the optimal treatment, consists of passing a deflated balloon past the embolus and extracting the thrombus by withdrawal of the inflated balloon.

ETIOLOGY

A definable underlying cause can usually be ascertained in patients with major arterial emboli.[1] Most major peripheral arterial emboli are cardiac in origin.[11, 12] Myocardial infarction or idiopathic hypertrophy predispose left ventricular mural thrombi. The left atrium may be the site of thrombus formation in mitral valve disease or in atrial fibrillation with or without valvular disease. Congestive heart failure from any cause is related to an increased incidence of arterial emboli. Aortic valve disease, particularly with bacterial endocarditis, can dislodge emboli. Mitral or aortic prosthetic valves are subject to the formation of thrombus, which may become dislodged. Mural thrombi on ulcerated plaques within arteriosclerotic arteries or aneurysms may shower the distal circulation with multiple small or large emboli. Although rarely associated with aortic aneurysms,[12] this is the most frequent mechanism of transient ischemic attacks in carotid artery occlusive disease and of distal occlusion of popliteal artery aneurysms. Dislodgment of the pseudointimal lining of prosthetic arterial grafts can produce distal embolization. This complication has been almost eliminated, however, by the use of recently developed Dacron double-velour grafts.*[13] Finally, the possibility of atrial myxomas or, less commonly, other growths of neoplastic origin must always be ruled out by microscopic examination of the extracted embolus.[14]

---

*Available from Meadox Medicals, Inc., P.O. Box 530, Oakland, New Jersey 07436.

DIAGNOSIS

Acute interruption of arterial inflow to any extremity produces pain and coldness in the affected part. If the ischemia persists, neuromuscular function is compromised, and numbness and weakness ensue. Physical examination reveals mottling, coldness, and cyanosis. The line of temperature demarcation is at first ill-defined but becomes more definite during the course of several hours. Visceral emboli give rise to intestinal dysfunction and infarction. Early abdominal pain and ileus are soon followed by distention and finally peritonitis, as the integrity of the intestinal wall becomes impaired by continued ischemia.

The arterial tree narrows acutely at major bifurcations; for this reason, the aortic bifurcation, iliac bifurcation, common femoral bifurcation, popliteal trifurcation, and brachial bifurcation are usual sites of embolic lodgment. Most emboli to the cerebral circulation are small and cause occlusion of intracranial branches rather than obstruction of the common carotid bifurcation.

Because of a predilection for certain areas of the arterial tree, it is fairly easy to localize the site of embolic lodgment. Emboli to the aortic bifurcation affect both legs. Femoral pulses are diminished or absent bilaterally, though not always equally reduced. There may be a bruit at the umbilicus. Pallor, cyanosis, and coldness are present to the midthigh, often to the inguinal ligament, and occasionally to the umbilicus. Iliac emboli result in a unilateral pulse deficit; pallor and cyanosis rarely extend as high as the inguinal ligament. Common femoral emboli produce physical signs of ischemia as high as the midthigh and occasionally to the knee. In these cases, the pulse is palpable at or just above the inguinal ligament. Popliteal emboli usually lodge below the knee and produce physical signs of ischemia from the midcalf down. A popliteal pulse may be palpable, but no pedal pulses can be felt. In the upper extremity along its entire course, the embolus can usually be located without difficulty.

Emboli to the cerebral circulation are best localized by means of carotid or subclavian arteriography. Neurologic symptoms usually occur on the side contralateral to the cerebral insult. These may vary considerably, however, depending upon anatomic considerations and patency of the collateral circulation.

Because most emboli can be diagnosed accurately on the basis of clinical findings alone, arteriography is rarely necessary. However, arteriography is helpful when performed in the operating room after attempts to extract the offending embolus have failed to restore distal pulses. In this situation, arteriography may demonstrate associated arteriosclerotic occlusive disease, necessitating more extensive vascular reconstruction in addition to the passage of a Fogarty catheter. As a general rule, inability to pass a Fogarty catheter is indicative of associated occlusive disease, and a bypass graft will be required to restore circulation.

GENERAL PRINCIPLES OF SURGICAL TREATMENT

Because the patient requiring embolectomy is often critically ill, the use of local anesthesia is desirable. Fortunately, the availability of the Fogarty embolectomy catheter now makes it possible to use local anesthesia for extracting emboli from all of the most common sites except the renal and other visceral arteries.

Arterial obstruction of flow by an embolus leads to the formation of thrombus, which propagates distally, thereby further compromising tissue perfusion. Full systemic heparinization is therefore advisable as soon as a diagnosis is made. Operation should be scheduled within a reasonable time, as soon as other complications can be stabilized. Cases of emboli occurring in the middle of the night may be scheduled for surgery the next morning, but delay beyond 24 hours results in a mortality five times higher than normal.[15] Preoperative arteriography is not usually necessary unless the presence of associated underlying arteriosclerotic occlusive disease must be delineated. If distal pulses are not restored after embolectomy, or if the catheter cannot be passed satisfactorily, arteriography should be performed in the operating room. The surgeon should be prepared to perform appropriate arterial reconstruction should the presence of underlying disease indicate. Therefore, even for cases of simple embolectomy, the patient should be prepared in such a fashion that other, more extensive procedures may be performed. For example, a patient about to undergo femoral embolectomy for a saddle embolus should be prepared with the abdomen and both lower extremities completely exposed.

The technique for extraction of an embolus is basically the same in all arteries, differing only in the method of exposure. A transverse arteriotomy should be made to prevent subsequent compromise of the artery. The technique of passing and withdrawing the inflated balloon is simple, but must be performed correctly to prevent intimal damage, rupture of the artery, or breakage of the balloon by overly forceful distention, with embolization of balloon fragments.[16] The exact recommended amount of fluid should be withdrawn into the syringe and the balloon tested *before* insertion into the artery. The catheter is inserted, inflated, and withdrawn *by the responsible surgeon, not by a less-experienced assistant*. Testing the balloon before insertion allows the surgeon to acquire a "feel" for the amount of resistance required to inflate the balloon prior to inserting it into the artery, at which time overly forceful inflation may rupture the artery. The catheter is inserted *gently and never forced* into the artery. *Attempts to force the catheter past arteriosclerotic plaque can perforate the artery*. If the catheter cannot be passed, an operative arteriogram should be obtained, and if indicated by the presence of arteriosclerotic obstruction, a bypass graft should be considered. *As the balloon is inflated, the catheter should be slowly withdrawn*. This important technique allows the surgeon to feel arterial resistance to the balloon and precludes damage or rupture of the artery. It must be remembered that the arterial diameter will vary, and therefore the balloon must be appropriately inflated and deflated with a sensitive finger during passage.

BRACHIAL ARTERY EMBOLECTOMY AND THROMBECTOMY FOLLOWING CARDIAC CATHETERIZATION

The brachial artery bifurcation is a common lodging site for emboli of cardiac origin. Frequently, the brachial artery becomes thrombosed after cardiac catheterization, the incidence of such cases ranging from 2 to 5 percent, depending upon the experience of the cardiologist. Because operative treatment is similar, both conditions will be discussed together. The cardinal distinction is that the site of thrombosis after cardiac catheterization must be resected rather than repaired by simple closure of the arteriotomy.

Thrombosis of the brachial artery associated with cardiac catheterization should be treated within 24 to 48 hours. If the patient is already scheduled to undergo a cardiac procedure within 48 hours, it is reasonable to defer thrombectomy and brachial artery repair until that time. If operation is to be delayed more than a day or two, however, brachial artery repair should be performed before the patient is discharged. A delay of more than 72 hours changes the character of brachial artery thrombectomy and repair from that of a simple procedure with an excellent prognosis to that of an extensive procedure, possibly requiring a vein graft, offering less certainty of a good result.

General anesthesia is preferred. The patient's arm is prepared for surgery from the axilla to the wrist and is extended on an arm board. The transverse skin incision in the flexion crease of the elbow made previously by the cardiologist is modified to

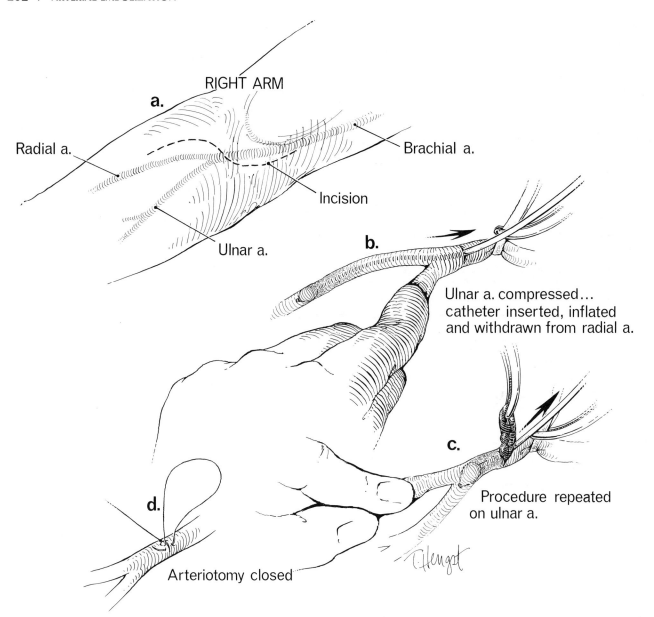

Figure 14–1 Brachial artery embolectomy and thrombectomy following cardiac catheterization.

become an S-shaped incision, extending laterally distally and medially proximally (Fig. 14–1, *a*). The brachial artery is exposed to its bifurcation so that the Fogarty catheter may be directed individually down the radial and ulnar branches (Fig. 14–1, *b* and *c*). It is a misconception that only one or the other of either the radial or ulnar branches must be made patent to ensure adequate circulation to the hand. We have seen patients with bounding pulses in the radial artery who had remaining thrombus in the ulnar artery, and experienced severe postoperative ischemia of the hand, requiring reoperation.

The brachial artery should be mobilized by ligating enough side branches so that a 1- to 2-cm segment can be resected and end-to-end anastomosis performed without tension.

After removal of the embolus, the transverse arteriotomy is repaired with a running suture of 6–0 polypropylene (Fig. 14–1, *d*). In patients undergoing thrombectomy after cardiac catheterization, the segment of artery containing the damaged intima should be resected and end-to-end anastomosis performed. In patients who have had chronic thrombosis for more than 72 hours, adherence of the organized thrombus to the intima necessitates that the entire segment of artery containing the thrombus be resected and replaced with an autogenous saphenous vein graft.

Emboli lodged more proximally in the axillary artery may be removed by exposing the artery through the axillary space.

CAROTID ARTERY EMBOLECTOMY

Emboli to the carotid bifurcation are uncommon, comprising only 4 percent of cases requiring embolectomy in our hospital.[1] Diagnosis may be made without arteriography in the patient with atrial fibrillation or other conditions involving risk of embolization, and in whom absence of the internal carotid pulse can be demonstrated by palpation posterior to the tonsillar fossa through the mouth. Although this is a reliable sign when present, it is frequently difficult to ascertain in a patient who is uncooperative because of an acute stroke. In such cases, when the location of the embolus is not clarified by physical examination, emergency carotid arteriography is indicated. Therefore, the surgeon should be able to perform percutaneous carotid arteriography when necessary in an emergency. It should be remembered that acute thrombosis of a carotid artery stenosis is far more common in older patients than are emboli, and can frequently not be differentiated arteriographically from an embolus. In these situations, the surgeon must be prepared to perform an endarterectomy. However, an attempt to remove emboli is justified up to approximately 72 hours after embolization because of the importance of maintaining collateral circulation if the return of neurologic function is not expected.

The operation may be performed under local anesthesia, although general anesthesia is preferred. An oblique incision is made over the carotid bifurcation (Fig. 14–2, a), and the carotid artery is exposed as described in Chapter 2 for carotid

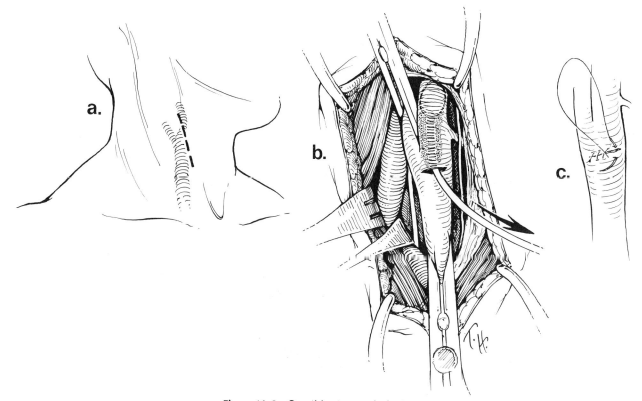

Figure 14–2 Carotid artery embolectomy.

endarterectomy (see Chapter 2, Fig. 2–1). After systemic heparinization (2.0 mg/kg of body weight) has been achieved, an arteriotomy is performed over the carotid bifurcation, and the Fogarty catheter is passed proximally and distally up both the internal and external carotid branches (Fig. 14–2, *b*). The technique of withdrawing the balloon without damaging or rupturing the vessel, as described above, is particularly critical in the internal carotid artery. After removal of all thrombus, the internal and external carotid clamps are released to flush air and any residual material out through the arteriotomy. The incision is then closed with a running suture of 5–0 polypropylene suture (Fig. 14–2, *c*), and the heparin effect is reversed with protamine.

RENAL AND VISCERAL ARTERY EMBOLECTOMY

Emboli to the renal or other intra-abdominal visceral arteries also occur infrequently, and in our series of 81 embolectomies, they represented only 2 percent.[1] However, the consequences of sudden loss of circulation to the kidneys or intestine are obviously catastrophic. The clinical manifestations of emboli to the celiac and superior mesenteric arteries are described in Chapter 8, Lesions of the Visceral Arteries. Emboli to the renal arteries may produce renal infarction manifested by flank pain and hematuria. Most often, patients experiencing renal or other visceral artery emboli will also have emboli to other major arteries. Therefore, patients presenting with symptoms of abdominal pain, tenderness, distention, or flank pain with or without hematuria, associated with embolization to a peripheral artery, should undergo appropriate selective arteriography prior to removal of the peripheral embolus.

The surgical technique is similar to that used for any peripheral artery, with exposure as described in Chapters 6 and 8 for the renal and visceral arteries, respectively. Extraction of an embolus in the right renal artery is exemplary of visceral artery embolectomy (Fig. 14–3). Through a midline incision, the renal arteries are exposed as described in Chapter 6. After systemic heparinization (2.0 mg/kg of body weight), the aorta is clamped above and below the renal arteries, and a transverse arteriotomy is made at the level of the renal arteries (Fig. 14–3, *a*). A No. 3 or 4 Fogarty catheter is used to extract the embolus (Fig. 14–3, *b*). The arteriotomy is closed with a 4–0 polypropylene running suture (Fig. 14–3, *c*).

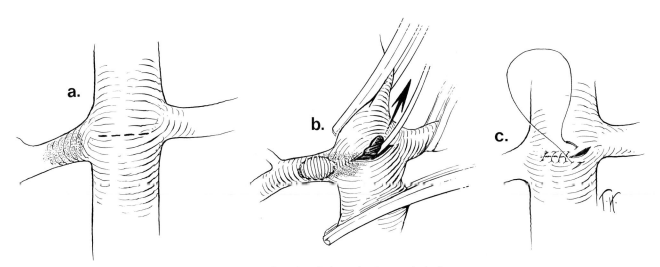

Figure 14–3   Renal and visceral artery embolectomy.

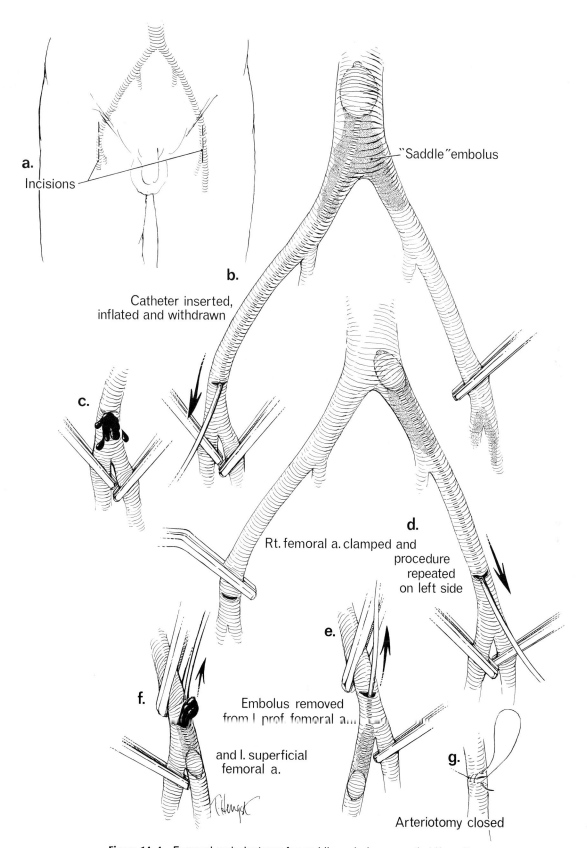

a.
Incisions

"Saddle" embolus

b.
Catheter inserted,
inflated and withdrawn

c.

d.
Rt. femoral a. clamped and
procedure
repeated
on left side

e.

f.
Embolus removed
from l. prof. femoral a....
and l. superficial
femoral a.

g.

Arteriotomy closed

Figure 14–4 Femoral embolectomy for saddle embolus or aortic bifurcation.

FEMORAL EMBOLECTOMY FOR SADDLE EMBOLUS OR AORTIC BIFURCATION

Emboli to the aortic bifurcation (saddle embolus) or common femoral bifurcation can be satisfactorily extracted via the femoral arteries. The development of the Fogarty catheter has changed what was formerly a major surgical procedure with a high death rate into a relatively simple procedure. The diagnosis is usually indicated by the sudden development of pain and coldness in the lower extremities with loss of the femoral pulses; arteriography is not required.

With the patient under either general or local anesthesia, both femoral arteries are exposed through vertical incisions (Fig. 14–4, *a*). After systemic heparinization (2.0 mg/kg of body weight), a transverse arteriotomy is made just proximal to the femoral bifurcation, and the catheter is passed proximally and distally (Fig. 14–4, *b* and *c*). Prior to proximal insertion, it is important to occlude the contralateral femoral artery and terminate flow down the opposite extremity to preclude the dislodgment of additional embolic material in that direction by the catheter. It is usually advisable to expose both femoral arteries, even though the embolus appears to occlude only one iliac artery. If only one femoral artery is exposed, however, the above maneuver can be accomplished by manual external pressure over the common femoral artery during proximal insertion of the catheter. After the first artery is occluded, the procedure is repeated on the lateral side (Fig. 14–4, *d* to *f*), and the arteriotomies are closed with running 5–0 polypropylene suture (Fig. 14–4, *g*).

Even though no embolic material is present in the common femoral artery, it is mandatory to pass the catheter down each of the superficial and profunda femoral branches, because unrecognized emboli may have passed down these arteries also. For this reason, each of these divisions should be isolated so that the catheter can be passed under direct vision. In the arteriosclerotic patient in whom the catheter cannot be passed proximally to the aortic bifurcation, or in whom unsatisfactory pulses remain after embolectomy, an aortofemoral bypass should be performed.

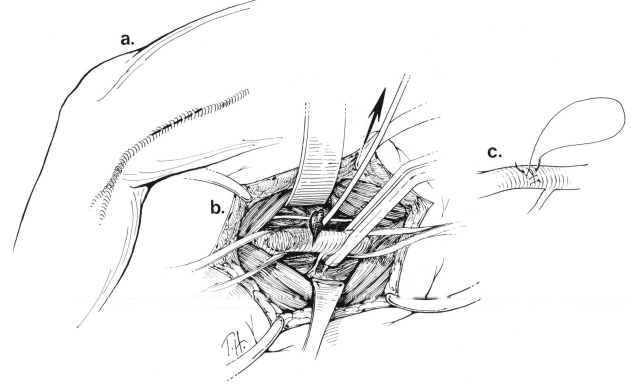

Figure 14–5 Popliteal artery embolectomy.

POPLITEAL ARTERY EMBOLECTOMY

Emboli frequently lodge at the adductor hiatus or at one of the divisions of the popliteal artery. Because these emboli often can be satisfactorily removed from the common femoral arteries as described above, our policy is to attempt removal first through this approach. However, the entire lower extremity should be prepared for surgery. If good pedal pulses are not obtained after attempted removal via the femoral arteries, the popliteal artery is exposed above the knee (Fig. 14–5, a), as described in Chapter 10 for femoral popliteal bypass. Systemic heparinization (2.0 mg/kg of body weight) is administered, and the catheter is passed proximally and distally as in the other peripheral arteries described above (Fig. 14–5, b and c). Again, if good pedal pulses are not obtained by this approach, the popliteal artery is exposed below the knee (see Chapter 10). Isolation of the anterior tibial, peroneal, and posterior tibial arteries allows direction of the catheter down each of the vessels individually under direct vision. In the presence of arteriosclerotic occlusive disease in the superficial femoral artery that prevents passage of the catheter or optimum flow, the surgeon should not hesitate to proceed with femoral popliteal bypass (see Chapter 10).

REFERENCES

1. Billig DM, Hallman GL, Cooley DA: Arterial embolism: Surgical treatment and results. Arch Surg 95:1, 1967.
2. Ssabanajeff J, quoted by Murray G: Canad Med Assoc J 35:61, 1936.
3. Danzis M: Arterial embolectomy. Ann Surg 98:249, 1933.
4. Pearse HE Jr: Embolectomy for arterial embolism of the extremities. Ann Surg 98:17, 1933.
5. Lerman J, Miller FR, Lund CC: Arterial embolism and embolectomy. JAMA 94:1128, 1930.
6. Crawford ES, DeBakey ME: The retrograde flush procedure in embolectomy and thrombectomy. Surgery 40:737, 1956.
7. Shaw RS: A method for the removal of the adherent distal thrombus. Surg Gynecol Obstet 110:255, 1960.
8. Keeley JL, Rooney JA: Retrograde milking: An adjunct in technic of embolectomy. Ann Surg 134:1002, 1951.
9. Dale WA: Endovascular suction catheters. J Thorac Cardiovasc Surg 44:557, 1962.
10. Fogarty TJ, Cranley JJ, Krause RJ, Strasser ES, Hafner CD: A method for extraction of arterial emboli and thrombi. Surg Gynecol Obstet 116:241, 1963.
11. Hardin CA, Hendren TA: Arterial embolism. Vasc Dis 2:11, 1965.
12. McCann WJ: The management of arterial emboli. Amer J Surg 108:768, 1964.
13. Cooley DA, Wukasch DC, Bennett JG, Trono R: Double velour knitted Dacron grafts for aorto-iliac vascular replacements. In *Vascular Grafts*, edited by Sawyer PN and Kaplitt MJ. Appleton-Century-Crofts, New York, 1978, pp. 197–207.
14. Lyle DP, Hall RJ, Garcia E, Cooley DA, Leachman RD, Pechacek L: Echocardiographic case presentation: Left atrial myxoma. Cardiovascular Diseases, Bulletin of the Texas Heart Institute 3(2):123, 1976.
15. Thompson JE, Sigler L, Raut PS, Austin DJ, Patman RD: Arterial embolectomy: A 20 year experience with 163 cases. Surgery 67:212, 1970.
16. Hogg GR, MacDougall JT: An accident of embolectomy associated with the use of the Fogarty catheter. Surgery 61:717, 1967.

CHAPTER 15

Sympathectomy

INTRODUCTION

Surgical removal of sympathetic ganglia (sympathectomy) was first used clinically for peripheral vascular disease in 1925 by Adson.[1] Prior to that, Leriche[2] had described and used periarterial sympathectomy by removing postganglionic fibers surrounding the femoral or brachial arteries, the effects of which were transient and unpredictable. Following Adson's report, the Leriche type of sympathectomy was discarded. Technical aspects of a properly performed sympathectomy for both the upper and lower extremities depend upon anatomic features of the autonomic nervous system and certain facts that have been gleaned from extensive clinical experience.

The principal physiologic effect that is expected from sympathectomy is release of vasomotor control and tone of the arterioles and smaller arteries having muscular elements in the vessel wall. Circulation to the skin and bone receive major improvement, while the effect upon the skeletal muscles of the arms and legs is minimal. Thus, one should hesitate to advise a patient with intermittent claudication that sympathectomy would provide relief of painful walking or motor activity of the arm. While no significant improvement in the muscular circulation is to be expected, it will not reduce muscular performance, and the benefit to the cutaneous and osseous circulation may enhance overall limb function. In addition to enhancement of circulation, the other known function is control over cutaneous sweating. Although infrequently used at present for hyperhidrosis,[3] sympathectomy may be indicated in some instances of profuse and undesirable sweating. An unusual observation is that sympathectomy and elimination of perspiration from one quadrant of the human anatomy appears to increase proportionately the perspiration elsewhere. Therefore, a patient with sympathectic denervation of both upper and lower extremities may have profuse and unacceptable perspiration in the truncal region. Accordingly, this possibility should be mentioned to a patient anticipating quadrilateral sympathectomy.

Based upon these known effects of sympathectomy, the surgeon can recommend operation for a variety of vascular disorders. The most prevalent indication for sympathectomy is the lumbar operation for arteriosclerotic peripheral vascular disease. For the patient with minor rest pain or impending cutaneous ischemia, with the presence or threat of ulceration and cutaneous gangrene, sympathectomy may be advised for either preventive or therapeutic reasons.[4] For patients with deep gangrenous ulcers or bone and tendon involvement, and for those with severe intractable pain at rest, sympathectomy offers only slightly beneficial results. Sympathectomy can be used in conjunction with the more direct revascularization techniques as described in Chapters 2 and 8. We do not, however, believe that it should be used in every patient undergoing an aortofemoral or aortoiliac bypass graft because of the threat of postsympathetic neuralgia or impotence in male patients. In patients with known arteriosclerotic occlusive disease of the popliteal and tibial arteries, concomitant removal of a single ganglion at the time of bypass grafting should enhance the result in restoring femoral pulses and improvement of circulation to the thigh muscles.

Among indications for sympathectomy may be moist ulceration of the foot or toe, the need to achieve a lower level of amputation below the knee instead of above, the need to speed up the development of collateral circulation, and for relief of acute vascular occlusion following trauma or surgical interruption of an artery. The role of sympathectomy in relieving causalgia is not understood. The results of sympathectomy in the causalgia syndrome cannot be explained completely by improved circulation to the limb. Nevertheless, sympathetic ganglionectomy is usually effective in partial and occasionally total relief of pain, in neurasthenias, in cutaneous and osseous atrophy (Sudeck-Leriche syndrome), and in the post-traumatic limb.

Few contraindications to sympathectomy are known. In our practice, we seldom recommend it for vascular disease associated with edema. Patients with diabetic neuropathy are unfavorable candidates, as are patients with the so-called "restless leg" or "aching leg" syndrome. All patients with peripheral vascular disease, particularly those with Raynaud's phenomenon involving the upper or lower extremity, should stop tobacco smoking entirely to obtain a satisfactory result of sympathectomy.[5] Surgery alone will not cure those patients who continue to use tobacco, and cigarettes appear to be more deleterious than other forms of tobacco.

COMPLICATIONS

POSTSYMPATHECTOMY NEURALGIA

Neuralgia is now well recognized as a frequent complication of sympathectomy,[6] whether of the upper or lower extremities. Reported incidence varies widely from between 2 to 3 percent to as high as 100 percent, depending upon the diagnostic criteria established by the analysis. While the exact cause of the neuralgia is not known, many observations on the usual clinical picture may be useful to the clinician. Onset of symptoms characteristically occurs on the tenth or twelfth day after operation, usually after the patient has been discharged from the hospital. Onset may be a few days earlier but, rarely, if ever, before the fourth postoperative day. However, it may occur 16 to 20 days later, or occasionally up to four weeks after operation. Patients usually first notice nocturnal symptoms, which are severely disabling and agonizing only at night. There are those, however, who develop full-blown neuralgic symptoms during the day, which extend into the night with great severity. The discomfort is usually described as "severe burning," "deep aching," or "tightness."

Following lumbar sympathectomy, the pain usually begins in the flank, lateral groin, and anterior thigh in the first two lumbar dermatomes. It persists at least two weeks, but six to eight weeks of discomfort is the usual pattern. The pain often descends into the leg, and even the foot, but this usually precedes the disappearance of symptoms, which frequently abate almost as suddenly as they appear, and the patient expresses surprise at the unexpected relief.

Postsympathectomy neuralgia in the upper extremity is less common than in the lower, and usually occurs over the shoulder and upper arm on the lateral aspect. Although the diagnosis may be readily made from the clinical history, confirmation may be obtained by various tests, including the use of instruments to study skin resistance or techniques to detect sudomotor activity. Characteristically, these tests reveal increased sympathetic activity, suggesting a "rebound" phenomenon in the nonsympathectomized adjacent dermatomes. The rebound has been attributed to regeneration of nerve fibers, degeneration of divided fibers in the rami, increased response to catecholamines, trauma to peripheral nerves, and a variety of other causes.

Treatment. No definitive treatment is known, but since the symptoms disappear in a period of less than three months, and usually in three to six weeks, palliative treatment is all that is necessary. Mild analgesics such as aspirin or codeine help to reduce the pain. Sedation, particularly at bedtime, should be administered.

Specific medications for treatment of postsympathectomy neuralgia have been recommended by Raskin at the University of California, who reported the use of phenytoin (Dilantin) or carbamazepine (Tegretol).[7] The mechanisms of action of these drugs are unclear; the former is used for control of seizures in convulsive disorders and the latter for treatment of seizures or for trigeminal neuralgia. We have not used them in our patients. When nocturnal symptoms are most severe and unrelenting, a warm sitz bath in a deep tub has relieved many patients. It is especially important to assure the patient of his ultimate recovery. An explanation of the nature of the complication and its limited duration allays his fear and worry. Most patients are reassured when told that the best results of sympathectomy have been noted in patients with the most severe symptoms. This is supported by our personal observations. Because of the relative frequency of this complication, particularly in patients with arteriosclerotic vascular disease, the surgeon should inform the patient of this potential problem before the operation. It occurs in about 20 percent of patients.

IMPOTENCE IN THE MALE

Excision of the first lumbar ganglion is frequently followed by loss of external ejaculatory function, since the internal vesicle sphincter is unable to close.[8] Consequently, when ejaculation occurs, the seminal fluid is ejected retrograde into the bladder. In years past, when removal of the lower dorsal ganglion and upper lumbar ganglion was done for arterial hypertension, many male patients also lost the ability to have a penile erection. While this complication may be less objectionable to elderly patients, in general, sympathectomy should not be done above the level of L2. Fortunately, adequate sympathetic denervation of the lower extremity can be achieved by removal of L3 and L4, thus avoiding these problems of sexual dysfunction.

PARADOXIC GANGRENE

In an occasional patient, severe ischemia and gangrene of a toe may appear after lumbar sympathectomy.[4] Theoretically, this complication could result from the sympathectomy's causing an arteriovenous shunt to open proximal to the peripheral digital capillary bed, thus reducing flow. The most likely possibility is that the ischemia is caused by embolism from an atherosclerotic aorta, iliac, or femoral artery.

INTESTINAL NECROSIS

Intestinal gangrene following lumbar sympathectomy occurs rarely, and conceivably could result from a "steal" of aortic and iliac blood from the sclerotic splanchnic bed.[9] From a logical standpoint, it seems more likely that the complication results from local trauma following forceful retraction on the mesentery during operation, embolism from the sclerotic aorta, or thrombosis due to localized vascular disease, aggravated by dehydration.

THORACIC (DORSAL) SYMPATHECTOMY

The evolution of an effective operation which is relatively free from undesirable side effects has occurred with a more accurate understanding of the anatomic features of the sympathetic system. Preganglionic sympathetic nerves derived from the spinal cord do not follow a corresponding relationship to the accompanying somatic nerves. The cervical ganglia of C1 to C4 are fused into a superior cervical ganglion, C5 and C6 into the middle cervical ganglion, and C7 and C8 into the inferior ganglion, which combines with the ganglion from T1 to form the larger stellate ganglion. Cervical ganglionectomy is not used for denervation of the upper extremity since the preganglionic sympathetic outflow from the spinal cord to the arm is usually from T2 through T9, and mostly from T2 through T4. In about 10 percent of cases, T1 preganglionic fibers also supply the upper extremity. To remove the preganglionic fibers to the upper extremity in the majority of patients, removal of paravertebral ganglia T2 and T3 is sufficient. Postganglionic fibers from these two segments often join, and branches then follow the nerves of the brachial plexus. The joined T2 and T3 fibers which bypass the stellate ganglion are known as the nerve of Kuntz.[10] To ensure that all the remaining patients who have a T1 connection through the stellate ganglion obtain adequate sympathetic denervation, the lower third or half of the stellate ganglion should also be removed, as recommended by Palumbo.[11] By confining the stellate ganglionectomy to the lower half or third, one does not interrupt the fibers from C7 and C8, and thus Horner's syndrome is avoided. Patients complain of the disfigurement of Horner's syndrome, which produces miosis, enophthalmosis, drooping of the eylids (ptosis), and flushing of the side of the face.[12] With these anatomic considerations, a logical denervation of the upper extremity may be planned.

SURGICAL TECHNIQUE OF THORACIC (DORSAL) SYMPATHECTOMY

Under general anesthesia with tracheal intubation, the patient is positioned with the left shoulder slightly elevated and the hand suspended from an intravenous standard. (The surgeon should wear a headlight or use some form of illumination other than the standard overhead operating room light. We also employ magnifying ocular loupes to enhance vision.) An 8- to 10-cm transverse incision is made in the axilla below the axillary hairline (Fig. 15–1, a). The pectoralis major anteriorly and the latissimus dorsi posteriorly define the limits of transaxillary dissection. By a combination of sharp and blunt dissection, the axillary fat pad is divided and retracted, and the third intercostal space is incised with the cautery. If the second intercostal space is entered, the intercostobrachial nerve, which supplies sensation to the medial aspect of the upper arm, should be protected from injury.

A self-retaining thoracotomy retractor or rib spreader is inserted between the second and third ribs, and the apex of the lung is retracted caudad and anteriorly to expose the dorsal paravertebral sympathetic chain (Fig. 15–1, b). Dissection of the nerve chain may be started cephalad or caudad. After incising the overlying pleurae, the ganglia are identified. The large stellate ganglion that overlies the head of the first rib should be dissected out to identify its length and upper extension. Removal of the lower third, or less than half of the ganglion, is done with scissors, usually identifying a branch that courses laterally and superiorly toward the brachial plexus (Fig. 15–1, c). The dissection of the chain caudad is continued to a point below the third or even below the fourth or fifth ganglion (Fig. 15–1, e). A metal clip is usually placed as a marker of the distal extent of the sympathectomy (Fig. 15–1, d).

Bleeding arteries and veins are carefully coagulated to obtain complete hemostasis. A number 24 French catheter is inserted at a lower interspace in the midax-

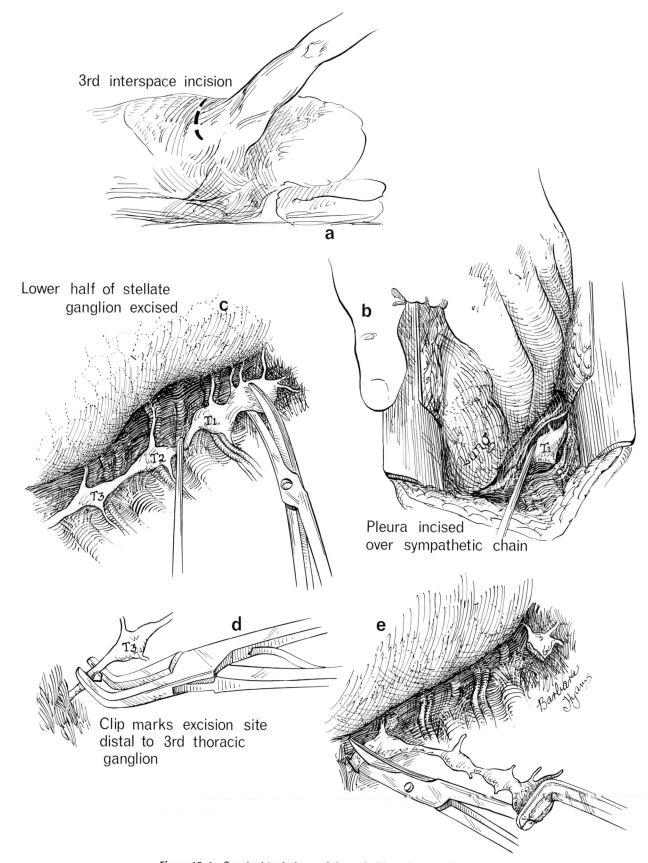

3rd interspace incision

a

b

Pleura incised
over sympathetic chain

Lower half of stellate
ganglion excised

c

T1

T2

T3

d

T3

Clip marks excision site
distal to 3rd thoracic
ganglion

e

Figure 15–1 Surgical technique of thoracic (dorsal) sympathectomy.

illary line for underwater sealed drainage for 24 hours. We do not use pericostal sutures, since they may produce radicular nerve pain, but depend upon the ribs to fall back into place normally. The subcutaneous tissues are approximated and the skin incision is closed with subcuticular absorbable sutures. For medical and possibly legal reasons, the excised chain of ganglia and nerve trunks should be sent to the pathologic laboratory for gross and microscopic study.

Comment

An immediate response to the sympathectomy should ensue, with warming and flushing of the hand. A dry, warm skin of the palm and fingers indicates a successful result. The left side of the face may be dry and free of perspiration, but none of the stigmata of Horner's syndrome should be present. While the immediate results may be striking, as mentioned before, postsympathectomy neuralgia may occur later. Also, regeneration of sympathetic fibers or the return of sympathetic activity in the upper extremity occurs much earlier (several months to a year later) and with greater frequency than after sympathectomy in the lower extremity.

LUMBAR SYMPATHECTOMY

Anatomic considerations for lumbar sympathectomy improve the expectation of a complete and lasting result as compared to dorsal sympathectomy. The anatomic features are more consistent, and the arrangement of preganglionic fibers is more favorable. Preganglionic sympathetic fibers arise from the lateral gray substance from T10 to L2 and, occasionally, L3. They emerge from the spinal cord with the anterior roots reaching the ganglia via white rami communicants and then descend in the paravertebral chain, where they meet postganglionic fibers in the lumbar ganglia. Thus, to achieve an adequate denervation of the lower extremity, removal of L3 alone would suffice in the vast majority of instances. Usually L4 should also be removed for completeness. This excision denervates the part of the lower extremity supplied by somatic nerves in the sciatic nerve, i.e., the posterior thigh and the entire extremity below the knee. A higher level of sympathectomy (L1 and L2) may be necessary in order to denervate the anterior thigh supplied by the femoral and obturator nerves. Seldom is this necessary, and to include the proximal ganglia invites additional complications, including postsympathectomy neuralgia and sexual dysfunction in the male.

SURGICAL TECHNIQUE OF LUMBAR SYMPATHECTOMY

Lumbar sympathectomy is performed with the patient lying in the supine position. Elevation of the hip or flank is not necessary in the anterior approach, which we recommend. When bilateral lumbar sympathectomy is being performed, the operating table may be tilted slightly away from the side on which the surgeon stands. General anesthesia, usually with tracheal intubation, is recommended. Muscle relaxants to the point of apnea are used to provide a completely relaxed abdominal musculature, which substantially enhances the ease and precise performance of operation.

An oblique skin incision approximately 10 cm long is made lateral to and slightly above the umbilicus medially (Fig. 15–2, *a*). Abdominal layers of muscle may be separated in line with the fibers or, in most patients, by dividing the muscles in the direction of the skin incision. After the transversal muscle is incised, an extraperiton-

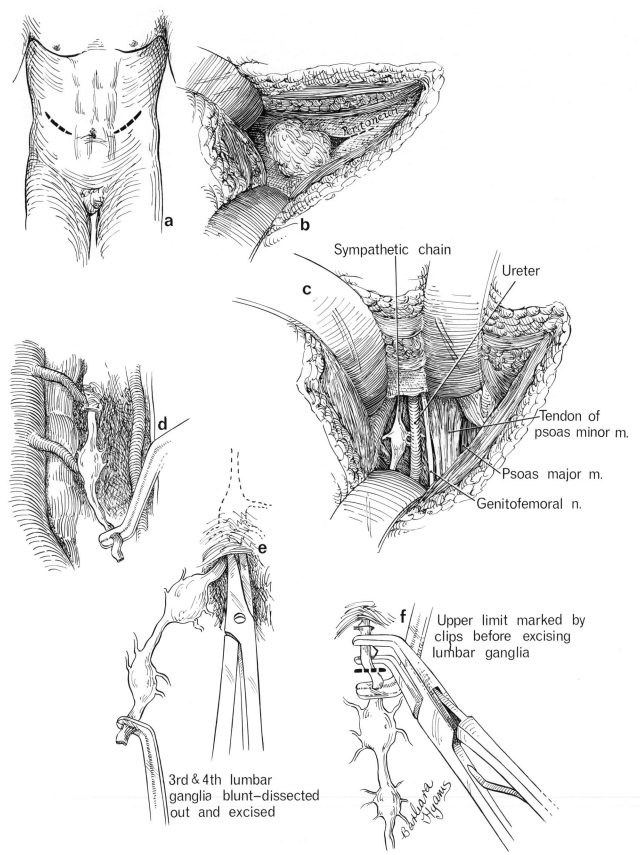

Sympathetic chain

Ureter

c

Tendon of
psoas minor m.

Psoas major m.

Genitofemoral n.

d

e

3rd & 4th lumbar
ganglia blunt–dissected
out and excised

f Upper limit marked by
clips before excising
lumbar ganglia

Figure 15–2 Surgical technique of lumbar sympathectomy.

eal plane is developed laterally, where extraperitoneal fat separates the peritoneum from the overlying fascia.

Once this plane is developed, the surgeon proceeds with blunt finger dissection until the ventral surface of the psoas muscle is identified. The ureter and gonadal vessels are swept forward until the bodies of the vertebrae are palpated (Fig. 15–2, b). In the drawing (Fig. 15–2, c), the ureter is shown separated from the tissues anteriorly, but in practice we leave the ureter attached to those structures to avoid injury. The genitofemoral nerve runs parallel to the medial margin of the psoas muscle and should not be abraded or handled roughly. Some believe that neuralgia following sympathectomy results from contusion or retraction of the genitofemoral nerve (Fig. 15–2, c). Drawings show the details of a left lumbar sympathectomy. Identification of the chain is best made by palpation of the ganglia as firm nodules, 3 to 5 mm in diameter, resting on the underlying vertebral bodies. With experience, the surgeon will never confuse these with a chain of lymphatic nodes, the ureter, or genitofemoral nerve (Fig. 15–2, d). Good visibility with magnifying ocular loupes, enhanced by a fiberoptic light source, provides optimal conditions for the ganglionectomy. With sharp and blunt dissection, L4 and L3 ganglia are identified, the former lying just above the sacral promontory, and the latter 4 to 5 cm cephalad (Fig. 15–2, e). The sympathetic chain is divided above the L3 ganglion and below the diaphragmatic fibrotic crus. The proximal extent of the excision is marked with a metal clip for future reference. Rami entering the chain do not require clips. Segmental arteries and veins that overlie the chains may be divided between metal clips, but usually careful dissection permits mobilization of the chain behind the vessels, avoiding unnecessary hemorrhage (Fig. 15–2, f).

Sympathectomy on the right side is performed in an identical manner, except that venous tributaries overlying the chain may be somewhat more troublesome. Usually, however, they can be dissected and the chain removed without injuring the vein.

The specimen of ganglionated chain should be sent to the pathologist for gross and microscopic study and confirmation for future reference and possible medicolegal reasons.

REFERENCES

1. Adson AW, Brown GE: Treatment of Raynaud's disease by lumbar ramisection and ganglionectomy and perivascular sympathetic neurectomy of the common iliacs. JAMA 84:1908, 1925.
2. Ewing M: The history of lumbar sympathectomy. Surgery 70(5):790, 1971.
3. Cullen SI: Management of hyperhydrosis. Postgrad Med 52:77, 1972.
4. Atlas LN: Lumbar sympathectomy in the treatment of peripheral arteriosclerotic disease. II. Gangrene following operation in improperly selected cases. Am Heart J 23:493, 1942.
5. de Takats G, Fowler EF: Raynaud's phenomenon. Bull Int Soc Chir 21:73, 1962.
6. Litwin MS: Postsympathectomy neuralgia. Arch Surg 84:591, 1962.
7. Raskin NH, Levinson SA, Hoffman PM, Pickett JBE III, Fields HL: Postsympathectomy neuralgia. Am J Surg 128:75, 1974.
8. Whitelaw GP, Smithwick RH: Some secondary effects of sympathectomy, with particular reference to disturbance of sexual dysfunction. N Engl J Med 245:22, 1951.
9. Kountz SL, Laub DR, Connolly JE: "Aorto-iliac steal" syndrome. Arch Surg 92:490, 1966.
10. Kuntz A: Distribution of the sympathetic rami to the brachial plexus. Arch Surg 15:871, 1927.
11. Palumbo LI: Anterior transthoracic approach for upper extremity thoracic sympathectomy. Arch Surg 72:659, 1956.
12. Palumbo LT: Upper dorsal sympathectomy without Horner's syndrome. Arch Surg 71:743, 1955.

CHAPTER 16

Fasciotomy and Amputations

FASCIOTOMY

The value of fasciotomy in relieving experimentally produced ischemic contracture in animals was demonstrated by Jepson in 1926.[1] Any alteration in the distal circulation of an extremity can result in muscle edema, progressing to restrictive muscle tamponade within the fixed fascial compartments and ischemic muscle necrosis. Elevation of pressure within the inflexible compartment to greater than arterial pressure results in further compromise of all arterial inflow and collaterals, and muscle necrosis.

The lower leg is divided into four anatomical compartments by rigid fascial layers: (1) the anterior tibial, (2) the lateral peroneal, (3) the superficial posterior, and (4) the deep posterior (Fig. 16–1, b). While any or all compartments may be affected, the anterior tibial is most frequently involved, because its blood supply is limited to end-artery branches of the anterior tibial artery, with poor collateral circulation.[2] The anterior tibial compartment is bounded by the tibia, interosseous membrane, fibula, and overlying fascia; it contains the extensor digitorum longus, tibialis anterior, extensor hallucis longus, and peroneus tertius muscles (Fig. 16–1, b). The function of these muscles is to dorsiflex the foot and extend the toes; therefore, the result of an unsatisfactorily treated anterior tibial compartment syndrome is foot drop, which may require a permanent brace. Isolated, spontaneous compression of this compartment, which may occur in the absence of a clear etiologic factor, was described by Vogt in 1943 as the anterior tibial compartment syndrome.[3] In this syndrome, swelling of the muscles in the anterior tibial compartment occurs after exercise, and apparently because of the "end-artery anatomy" of the arterial supply, spasm of the anterior tibial artery results, with further ischemia and swelling of the muscles within the compartment. This syndrome presents one of the clear-cut indications for fasciotomy, which is usually curative if performed early.[2]

The lateral compartment (Fig. 16–1, b) contains the peroneus longus and peroneus brevis muscles, used in pronation and plantar flexion of the foot. Two posterior compartments (Fig. 16–1, b), the superficial and deep, contain the posterior muscles of the leg. The superficial posterior compartment contains the gastrocnemius, soleus, and plantaris muscles, which function in plantar flexion of the foot and flexion of the leg. Within the deep posterior compartment are the popliteus, flexor hallucis longus, flexor digitorum longus, and tibialis posterior muscles, which flex the toes, foot, and leg (Fig. 16–1, b). Inability of the patient to perform foot movements specific for the compartment involved indicates the need for emergency fasciotomy in that compartment. Thus, inability to flex the foot dorsally and extend the toes signifies anterior tibial compartment compression. This compartment is usually the only one in which isolated compression occurs. Inability to pronate and plantar-flex the foot and to flex the leg indicates lateral and posterior compartment compression.

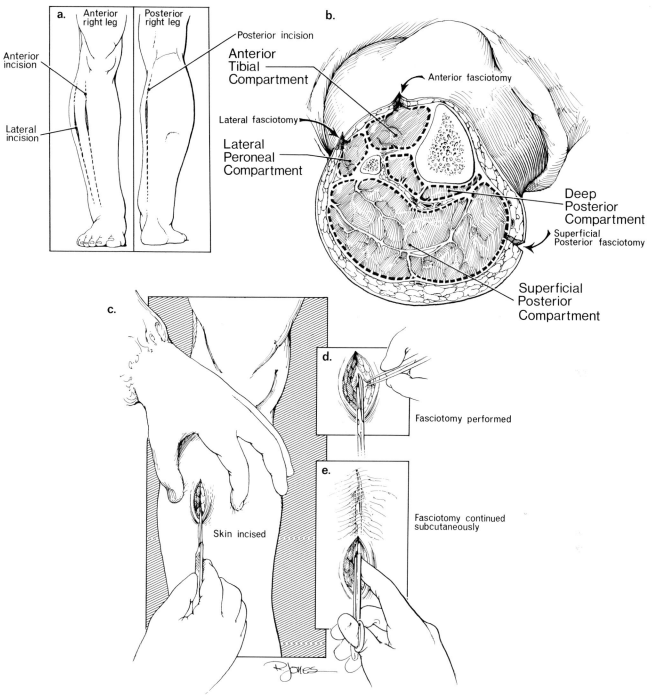

Figure 16–1   Fasciotomy.

The various conditions for which fasciotomy is indicated have been succinctly described by Patman and Thompson.[2] In their general order of frequency, these conditions are: (1) arterial injuries,[4] (2) combined arterial and venous injuries,[5] (3) massive soft tissue injuries (crush syndrome),[6] (4) circumferential extremity burns, (5) venous injuries, (6) phlegmasia cerulea dolens,[7, 8] (7) anterior tibial compartment syndrome,[9] (8) postarterial embolization, (9) wringer arm injuries, (10) postarterial reconstructive procedures, and (11) reimplantation of an extremity. Regardless of the underlying cause of ischemia, early and adequate fasciotomy is necessary to prevent ischemic necrosis of muscle and irreversible loss of function. Immediate fasciotomy is indicated by the presence of severe pain, sensory loss, and motor dysfunction. Even when extensive necrosis has already occurred, however, fasciotomy is justified in an attempt to salvage whatever viable tissue remains.

The various techniques of fasciotomy may be categorized as those using limited skin incisions, extensive skin incisions, and transfibular resection. Although all these methods are described, from a practical viewpoint, almost all situations in our experience can be satisfactorily managed by the simplest approach, namely, through limited skin incisions.[10]

LIMITED SKIN INCISIONS

In most situations, this approach is the most desirable. Light general anesthesia is preferred unless only an isolated compartment fasciotomy is required. Short skin incisions are made over each compartment (Fig. 16–1, a). The anterior tibial compartment is entered by an incision approximately 2 cm lateral to the midline of the leg. The lateral compartment is incised along the lateral aspect of the leg. The superficial posterior compartment is best entered by placement of the skin incision along the posterior-medial aspect of the leg. The deep posterior compartment may be reached by extending the posterior-medial incision through the gastrocnemius and soleus muscles into the deep fascial layer, although transfibular resection is usually required for adequate decompression of this compartment.

The skin incisions are carried through the subcutaneous tissue and fascia (Fig. 16–1, c and d). Long curved scissors are then inserted into the fascial incision and "pushed" the full length of the leg in both a cephalad and caudad direction (Fig. 16–1, e). Upon release of pressure within the fascial compartments, the muscle bellies bulge in an impressive release of pressure. If adequacy of the decompression is questionable, additional skin and fascial incisions should be made proximally and distally. The skin incisions may be closed loosely with interrupted sutures or, as is most frequently necessary, left open with delayed primary closure performed in four to five days. Occasionally, split thickness skin grafts will be necessary at a subsequent date.

EXTENSIVE SKIN INCISIONS

When the skin appears to be contributing to the compression, as in massive soft tissue injuries and circumferential burns, the skin should be incised the full length of the leg. The location of the incisions is similar to those described above (Fig. 16–1, a). This approach often presents more complicated wound healing problems, which frequently require skin grafts.

TRANSFIBULAR FASCIOTOMY OF DEEP POSTERIOR COMPARTMENT

In patients with extensive injuries and severe swelling and necrosis, adequate decompression of the deep posterior compartment is necessary.[5] This is best achieved by subperiosteal removal of the middle third of the fibula.[11] Because the fibula is not involved in weight bearing, removal of the middle third does not compromise function of the leg. The distal fibula, however, is essential in maintaining stability of the ankle joint, and must be preserved.

The fibula is approached by a long skin incision over the lateral compartment (Fig. 16–1, a). The peroneus longus and brevis muscles are separated, and the periosteum of the fibula is encountered and elevated with a periosteal elevator. Injury to the common peroneal nerve, which crosses the fibula, is avoided. The middle third of the fibula is resected. All four compartments may be decompressed through this incision by incising the periosteum anteriorly and medially, in addition to the posterior fascial wall of the lateral compartment.

This radical approach should not be used routinely but should be reserved for extreme situations: (1) cases that involve a delay of several hours between injury and treatment, (2) paralysis of plantar flexion of the foot, (3) injury to the distal popliteal artery, where repair can be facilitated by resection of the fibula, or (4) when muscle necrosis is encountered in the anterior or superficial posterior compartments.[2]

FOREARM FASCIOTOMY

Fasciotomy of the forearm may be necessary in vascular and soft tissue injuries or fractures of the elbow to prevent Volkmann's ischemic contracture. The technique is similar to that used for fasciotomy of the leg. The two compartments of the forearm are entered by dorsal and volar incisions from the elbow to the wrist. Occasionally fasciotomy of the upper arm is required, and in this event, two incisions are made medially and laterally from the shoulder to the elbow.

AMPUTATIONS

GENERAL PRINCIPLES

In the United States alone approximately 100 amputations are performed each day.[12] Because an amputation may represent failure by the surgeon to restore circulation to the patient's extremity, he frequently experiences a psychological aversion to performing the procedure, and either performs it hastily or delegates it to a junior member of the staff. The knowledge that every effort was made to save the extremity and that no one could have done anything more should allow the surgeon to accept the fact that some situations are out of his control, and allow him to proceed with a positive attitude. Thus, the candidate for amputation should receive the same degree of effort and concern that the surgeon exhibits toward more dramatic and gratifying operative procedures.

Indications for extremity amputations include (1) ischemic gangrene, (2) injury, (3) tumors, (4) inoperable occlusive disease with severe, intractable rest pain, and (5) nonresponsive infection. From a practical point of view, approximately 80 percent of lower extremity amputations are performed for occlusive disease.[12]

The major consideration in any amputation is *maximal restoration of function —* walking in most instances. Because of the obvious importance of joints in extremity function, amputation should be performed at the lowest level compatible with healing. Skin circulation is the single most important factor in determining that level.[13] Although the presence of a popliteal pulse usually indicates that below-the-knee amputation can be performed, the presence of such a pulse is not essential for healing satisfactorily at that level.[14] When in doubt, the surgeon should choose below-the-knee rather than above-the-knee amputation. Usually, nothing is lost if subsequent conversion to above-the-knee amputation is not delayed too long. In summary, a high percentage of knee joints can be saved, even in patients with arterial insufficiency.[13]

Early ambulation by using the immediate prosthesis technique described by Burgess[15, 16] offers many rehabilitative advantages. The essential aspects of this technique are stabilization of the divided muscles by suturing them to each other or to bone, and application of a plaster dressing that serves as a socket for a temporary prosthesis and allows early ambulation. This provides tremendous psychological support as well as allowing significant preservation of muscle tone and joint flexibility. Immediate prosthesis fitting should be considered for any patient who will eventually be able to use such a device. Younger patients undergoing amputation for cancer[17] or trauma are ideal candidates, and Burgess has shown that patients with arterial insufficiency may also benefit from this technique.[13] Contraindications include the presence of active infection, contractures, inadequate blood supply, or other mental or physical conditions that preclude rehabilitation and eventual ambulation. Application of the technique requires advance planning and the presence of the prosthetist in the operating room during the amputation for proper fitting of the plaster cast.[17]

BELOW-THE-KNEE AMPUTATION

The patient is placed in a supine position with the leg propped up and the knee supported by a metal basin. Although the ideal length of the stump is approximately 6 inches, prostheses can be fitted to a stump as short as 3 inches; thus, sacrificing the knee and resorting to an above-the-knee amputation for fear of making the stump too short can often be avoided. A point is measured on the anterior aspect of the leg approximately 6 inches distal to the inferior aspect of the patella, which will be the delineation of the anterior flap (Fig. 16–2, a). The skin incision is curved cephalad on both sides for approximately 2 inches, making apices one-third around the leg. The posterior flap is made by extending the incision from each apex in a caudad direction so that the posterior flap is 6 inches longer than the anterior. It must be remembered that the blood supply of the anterior aspect of the lower leg is poor and, therefore, undermining of the anterior flap should be minimal, and handling of the tissue gentle.

The incision is extended down to the tibia and fibula by incising the deep fascia and anterolateral muscles slightly proximal to the skin incision. A Gigli saw is used to transect the tibia at the level of the apex of the anterior and posterior incisions or approximately 2 inches above the level of the anterior skin incision (Fig. 16–2, b). When the tibia has been sawed about halfway through, the handles of the saw are directed cephalad to bevel the anterior aspect of the bone at a 45° angle (Fig. 16–2, c). The fibula is divided with a bone cutter 2 to 3 inches proximal to the end of the tibia. The posterior tibial, saphenous, and superficial peroneal nerves are stretched, crushed, ligated with nonabsorbable suture, transected, and allowed to retract. The posterior muscles are transected, completing the amputation (Fig. 16–2, d). The fascia, subcutaneous tissue, and skin are approximated with interrupted sutures (Fig. 16–2, e). Drains are not routinely placed.

When a plaster cast for an immediate prosthesis is not used, the stump is wrapped with a *loose* dressing of Curlex gauze. *Elastic bandages should not be used, because subsequent swelling can result in a dressing that is too tight, causing necrosis of the flap.*

ABOVE-THE-KNEE AMPUTATION

Above-the-knee amputations are of two major types: (1) ischial-bearing and (2) end-bearing. The latter results in a broad stump that bears weight on its end and distributes it through the hip in a relatively normal fashion. Although this type is popular in Great Britain and among some orthopedic surgeons in the United States, the longer stump does not provide enough room for the most functional type of knee joint prosthesis. Thus, we prefer ischial-bearing amputations at the level of the junction of the middle and distal thirds of the femur. With these, most of the weight is

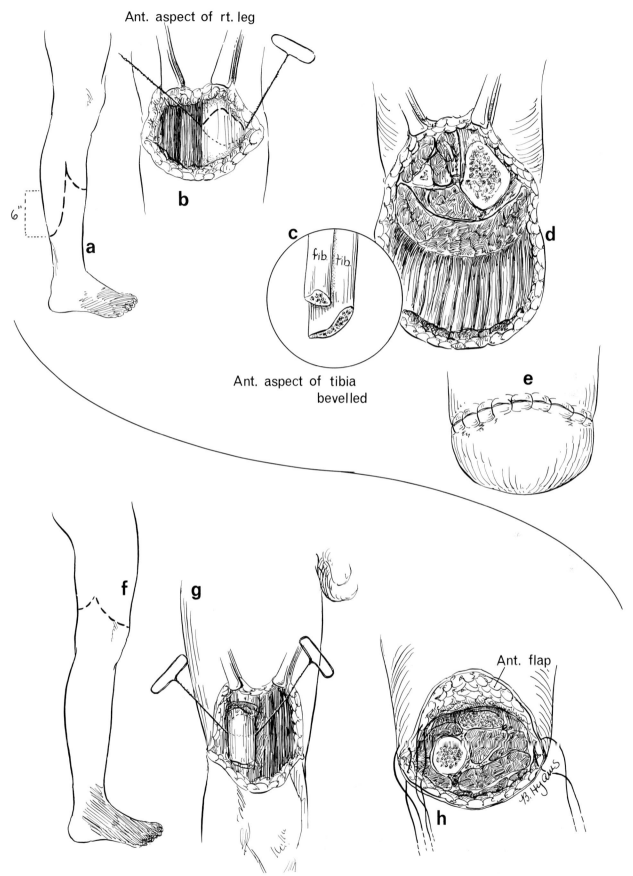

Ant. aspect of rt. leg

Ant. aspect of tibia
bevelled

Ant. flap

Figure 16–2 Below-the-knee amputation (*a-e*) and above-the-knee amputation (*f-h*).

transmitted to the ischial tuberosity, and a functional knee-joint-containing prosthesis is better accommodated.

The patient is placed in a prone position, with a roll placed beneath the thigh to be amputated. Although "dog ears" resulting from a circular incision around the thigh are not functionally detrimental to an ischial-bearing stump, we prefer a V-shaped incision that fashions anterior and posterior flaps and a more esthetic stump (Fig. 16–2, f). The anterior skin incision is made just above the superior aspect of the patella and the anterior flap is made 2 to 3 inches longer than the posterior flap, so that the final skin incision lies posteriorly. Successive layers are "coned"; that is, the fascial layer is incised approximately 1 inch cephalad to the skin edge and the femur transected 1 inch proximal to the fascial level. The femoral artery and vein are individually ligated as they transverse the adductor magnus foramen. The sciatic nerve is stretched downward, ligated, transected with a sharp knife, and allowed to retract out of the field. The tendinous attachments of the femur to the linea aspera are divided and the periosteum of the femur is elevated with a periosteal elevator. The femur is sawed transversely with either a Gigli or an amputation saw (Fig. 16–2, g). As it is being sawed, the bone is irrigated with sterile saline to cool the heat of friction and to wash away the sawdust that otherwise would remain in the wound as a foreign body.

Closure is facilitated by elevating the stump on an inverted basin. Oozing from the bone marrow is prevented by application of bone wax over the cut end of the femur. The anterior and posterior fascial layers are approximated with interrupted absorbable sutures (Fig. 16–2, h). The skin is closed with finely placed interrupted nylon sutures. Drains are not routinely placed unless there is concern regarding infection because of gangrene adjacent to the level of amputation. It is critical not to wrap the stump with an elastic bandage when dressing the wound, because a marginal blood supply to the stump may then result in pressure necrosis. For the same reason, adhesive tape should not be applied to the ischemic skin; the stump should be painted with tincture of benzoin and the dressing held in place with a stockinette rolled onto the stump. Postoperatively, the stump should not be placed on a pillow, because this position increases the risk of a flexion contracture of the hip.

TRANSMETATARSAL AMPUTATION

Transmetatarsal amputation of the foot offers a conservative alternative to below-the-knee amputation and leaves the patient a relatively functional extremity.[18] This approach is indicated for gangrene of the toes without proximal extension of the infection, as indicated by a sharp line of demarcation of the gangrene.[19] In addition to spread of infection, contraindications for transmetatarsal amputations include inadequate foot circulation manifest by dependent rubor, thin shiny skin, rest pain, and necrotic skin lesions proximal to the metatarsal-phalangeal joints. Osteomyelitis of the metatarsal bones is generally considered another contraindication.

The patient is positioned in a supine position, and the gangrenous toes are covered with a sterile rubber glove. A dorsal skin incision is made in a curved fashion across the foot at the level of transection of the metatarsals (Fig. 16–3, a). Care should be taken not to undermine the skin of the anterior flap. The incision is carried down through the tendons to the bone. The plantar incision is made at such a level as to create a posterior flap of sufficient length that it can be brought up to cover the end of the foot (Fig. 16–3, b). This line is approximately in the flexion crease between the base of the toes and the plantar aspect of the foot. To facilitate exposure for developing the plantar flap, the toes may be disarticulated at the metatarsophalangeal joints. Although it is well known to experienced surgeons, we reiterate the

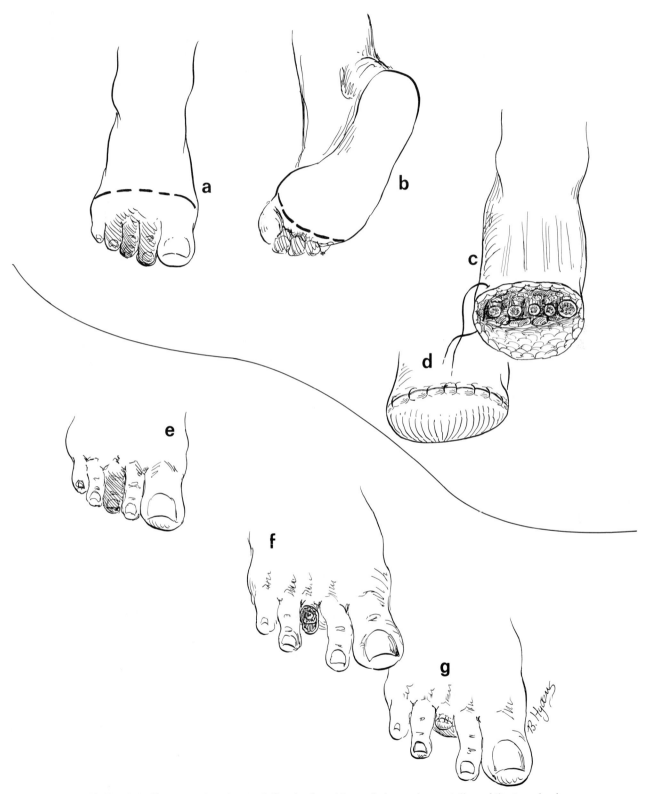

Figure 16–3 Transmetatarsal amputation (*a-d*) and transphalangeal amputation of the toes (*e-g*).

principle that an amputation is never performed by disarticulating a joint, because the articular surface is a membrane that will continue to secrete fluid. The plantar flap is then dissected proximally to the junction of the middle and distal thirds of the metatarsals. The tendinous attachments to the metatarsals are freed by sharp dissection and the metatarsal bones are transected. Although the second through the fifth metatarsals are easily cut with a bone cutter, the first metatarsal should be sawed with a Gigli saw because of the tendency for this bone to fracture when cut with a bone cutter. The wound is closed by approximating the skin only, using interrupted nylon sutures without tension (Fig. 16–3, c and d). Drains are not routinely used unless there is concern about possible osteomyelitis.

Transmetatarsal amputation may be used when either the first or fifth toe is affected by isolated gangrene. When the other toes are involved, however, a complete transmetatarsal amputation of the foot should be performed.[19] A linear incision is made over the involved metatarsal on either the medial or lateral aspect of the foot. The incision is curved around the toe, leaving as much plantar flap as possible. The metatarsal bone is transected as described above and the anterior and posterior flaps reapproximated.

TRANSPHALANGEAL AMPUTATION OF THE TOES

Toe amputation is feasible for gangrene limited to the distal or middle phalanges of a toe (Fig. 16–3, e). This conservative approach is contraindicated in the presence of an indistinct line of demarcation, with gangrene or infection extending proximal to the metatarsophalangeal joint. Toe amputation alone will usually be unsatisfactory in the presence of severe ischemia of the foot manifest by rest pain, dependent rubor, or atrophic skin changes.

An anterior semicircular incision is made over the base of the first phalanx down to the bone. A curved posterior incision is made approximately 1 cm distally to create a posterior flap (Fig. 16–3, f). The proximal phalanx is transected with a bone cutter, and the skin and subcutaneous flap are reapproximated with interrupted nylon sutures (Fig. 16–3, g).

REFERENCES

1. Jepson PN: Ischemic contracture: Experimental study. Ann Surg 84:785, 1926.
2. Patman RD, Thompson JE: Fasciotomy in peripheral vascular surgery. Report of 164 patients. Arch Surg 101:663, 1970.
3. Vogt, quoted by Horn CE: Acute ischemia of the anterior tibial muscle and the long extensor muscles of the toes. J Bone Surg 27:615, 1945.
4. Patman RD, Poulos E, Shires GT: The management of civilian arterial injuries. Surg Gynecol Obstet 118:725, 1964.
5. Chandler JG, Knapp RW: Early definitive treatment of vascular injuries in the Viet Nam conflict. JAMA 202:136, 1967.
6. Weeks RS: The crush syndrome. Surg Gynecol Obstet 127:369, 1968.
7. Snyder MA, Adams JT, Schwartz SI: Hemodynamics of phlegmasia cerulea dolens. Surg Gynecol Obstet 125:342, 1967.
8. Brockman, SK, Vasko JS: Phlegmasia cerulea dolens. Surg Gynecol Obstet 121:1347, 1965.
9. Horn CE: Acute ischemia of the anterior tibial muscle and the long extensor muscles of the toes. J Bone Joint Surg 27:615, 1945.
10. Rosato FE, Barker CF, Roberts B, Danielson GK: Subcutaneous fasciotomy — description of a new technique and instrument. Surgery 59:383, 1966.
11. Ernst CB, Kaufer H: Fibulectomy-fasciotomy. An important adjunct in the management of lower extremity arterial trauma. J Trauma 1:365, 1971.
12. Glattly HW: Aging and amputations. Artificial Limbs 10:1, 1966.
13. Burgess EM: Major lower extremity amputations following arterial reconstruction. Arch Surg 108:655, 1974.
14. Silbert S, Haimovici H: Results of midleg amputations for gangrene in diabetics. JAMA 144:454, 1950.

15. Burgess EM, Romano RL: The management of lower extremity amputees using immediate postsurgical prosthesis. Clin Orthop 57:137, 1968.
16. Burgess EM, Romano RL: New days for leg amputees. Rehabilitation Record 6:8, 1965.
17. Muilenberg AL: Prosthetic considerations for the cancer amputee. In *Rehabilitation of the Cancer Patient.* The Conference on Rehabilitation of the Cancer Patient at The University of Texas M.D. Anderson Hospital and Tumor Institute at Houston, 1970. Year Book Medical Publishers, Inc., Chicago, 1972, pp 65–73.
18. McKittrick LE, McKittrick JB, Risley TS: Transmetatarsal amputation for infection or gangrene in patients with diabetes mellitus. Ann Surg 130:826, 1949.
19. Haimovici H: Criteria for and results of transmetatarsal amputation for ischemic gangrene. Arch Surg 70:45, 1955.

CHAPTER 17

Venous Procedures

SUPERIOR VENA CAVAL OBSTRUCTION

Obstruction of the superior vena cava may be caused by trauma, infection, neoplasm, and, occasionally, iatrogenic factors. Approximately 25 percent of cases result from benign disease.[1] Many surgical techniques have been described for correcting this condition,[2-4] and inexperienced surgeons frequently undertake such procedures in the hope of relieving the obstruction. In most cases, a bypass technique is used that employs a variety of vascular prostheses.[5] These operations are generally unsuccessful and serve only to worsen the situation. *Each case of superior caval obstruction should be judiciously assessed, and enthusiasm for a dramatic cure should be tempered with carefully considered judgment.*

Removal of a substernal goiter is probably the most striking of all surgical operations to relieve caval obstruction, and may be effective immediately. The more common vena caval syndrome, which is due to invasive carcinoma of the lung, seldom lends itself to such dramatic results, but early irradiation or cobalt therapy may provide substantial relief. Schramel and Olinde[6] described a method of obtaining temporary relief of venous obstruction in a patient with terminal cancer by mobilizing and anastomosing the left greater saphenous vein to the left external jugular vein. Direct surgical attack upon such lesions is rarely justified, in our opinion, because of the terminal nature of the condition.

Operations for congenital cardiac defects such as sinus venosus atrial septal defects or complete transposition of the great vessels may lead to superior caval obstruction that, in some instances, responds to surgical correction. Relief can also occur spontaneously, however, as venous collaterals are established through the azygos, hemiazygos, and other veins that drain into the inferior vena cava.

Acute thrombosis of the superior cava and innominate veins sometimes results from trauma. A sudden blunt injury to the chest and mediastinum may cause petechial hemorrhages in the neck, supraclavicular area, and the face. This phenomenon is the result of a lack of venous valves in the jugular system. Subconjunctional hemorrhage may occur, with the patient developing a rather startling appearance. The sudden venous pulse wave undoubtedly affects intracranial veins, but permanent neurologic damage seldom results, and surgical treatment of this condition is not necessary.

Sclerosing mediastinitis with gradual onset of the superior vena caval syndrome is a rare condition that may lead to disabling symptoms, including facial and cerebral edema and exercise intolerance. Frequently, the obstruction is diffusely distributed over the superior vena cava and innominate veins and is not amenable to surgical treatment. Insertion of bypass grafts between the major venous channels and the right atrium is unsuccessful because the vascular substitute is susceptible to thrombosis and fibrosis. In all cases of superior caval syndrome, a venogram should be performed to demonstrate the actual location and extent of the caval obstruction.

We have encountered a few patients[7] in whom the obstruction was confined predominantly to the superior vena cava adjacent to the point of entry into the right atrium (Fig. 17–1, *a*). In these patients, dilation of the azygos system provides a

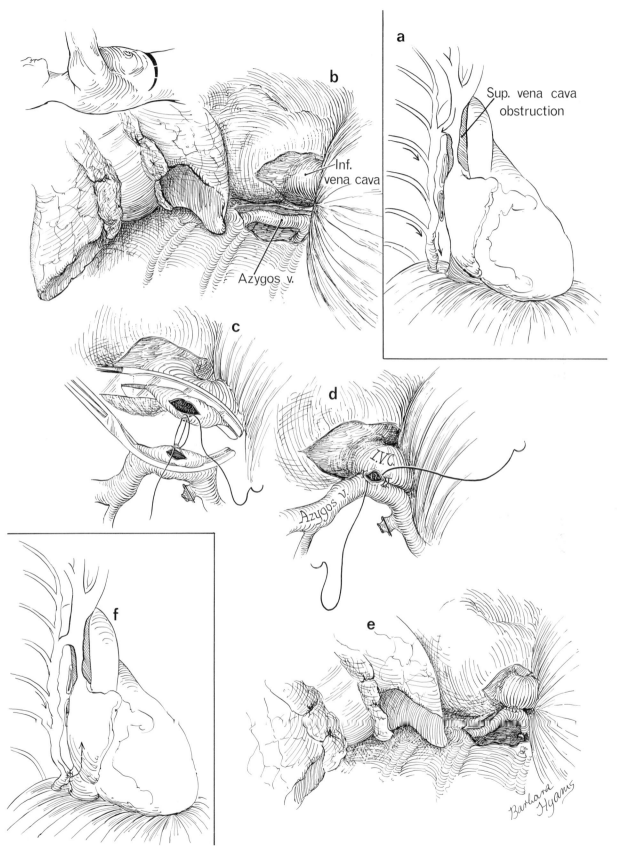

Figure 17–1 Operation for superior vena caval obstruction.

pathway for blood to enter the inferior caval system through venous collaterals. Resistance to flow through the connecting collateral system can be reduced by joining the azygos vein side to side with the inferior vena cava. This operation is performed through a right lateral thoracotomy incision in the sixth intercostal space (Fig. 17–1, b). The inferior cava is usually exposed without entering the pericardium, and the azygos vein is mobilized by dividing a segmental vein. Partial occluding clamps are applied to both vessels, and after the veins are incised longitudinally, a side-to-side anastomosis is completed (Fig. 17–1, c to f).

The results of this technique have been good, although few in number.[7] Success has been due to the absence of pathologic vein changes in this region and to the fact that prosthetic material has not been used in the repair. Miller[8] reported the use of this technique in two patients in whom the azygos vein was divided and anastomosed end to end to the extrapericardial portion of the inferior vena cava. In both patients, a significant drop in venous pressure was immediately apparent, and at the time of his report, relief of symptoms had persisted for four and a half years.

AXILLARY SUBCLAVIAN VENOUS THROMBOSIS

Axillosubclavian vein thrombus, described in the nineteenth century by Paget and von Schroetter,[9] is relatively rare, accounting for only 2 to 3 percent of all cases of deep vein thrombosis. For the patient who develops this condition, however, the symptoms can be disabling. Although most acute cases are resolved initially with conservative management, residual symptoms and recurrences persist in more than half of the affected patients,[10-12] sometimes resulting in pulmonary embolism. Despite the best possible management, some patients remain symptomatic or experience recurrent episodes, which present a difficult therapeutic problem for the surgeon.

Etiologic factors may not be apparent, and most cases occur "spontaneously," often following exercise that involves the upper extremity; hence, the term "effort thrombosis."[13] Other predisposing factors are external trauma, indwelling venous catheters, cancer, or congestive heart failure. The mechanism of axillosubclavian venous thrombosis appears to be costoclavicular compression by the clavicle and first rib at the thoracic outlet junction of the axillary and subclavian veins. (See Chapter 3: Thoracic Outlet Syndrome and Lesions in Vessels of the Upper Extremity.) An understanding of this mechanism provides the basis for the most rational form of definitive treatment, which is first rib resection.

The typical clinical pattern of the syndrome includes pain and swelling of the entire upper extremity, usually within 24 hours of strenuous exercise involving the arm. Dilated collateral venous channels are usually visible over the shoulder and anterior chest wall. A tender cord may or may not be palpable in the axilla. Exercise of the arm may aggravate the swelling and pain. Although the diagnosis is usually apparent clinically, phlebography is indicated, particularly when surgical treatment is contemplated. An upper extremity phlebogram, with contrast material injected through the antecubital vein, will typically demonstrate dilated collateral channels and obstruction of the axillary vein where it crosses the first rib.

Most patients will respond to conservative management consisting of rest, elevation, heat, and anticoagulation with systemic heparin. Because of the high incidence of recurrence and chronic symptoms, multiple methods of treatment have been advocated, either at the time of initial symptoms or for recurrent episodes.[14, 15] These include (1) emergency thrombectomy;[16] (2) division of the anterior scalene, and excision of the subclavius muscles;[17] (3) stellate ganglionectomy when vasospasm appears to be contributory; and (4) saphenous vein bypass of the obstruction, with creation of a distal arteriovenous fistula.[18] Although improvement has been reported with all these methods, long-term results continue to be disappointing.

Our approach has been basically conservative, involving the use of elevation and systemic heparinization. For patients who fail to respond to these usually successful measures within a period of three to four days, the most rational alternative appears to be emergency transthoracic first rib resection, with or without thrombectomy. In those patients who develop multiple recurrent episodes with chronic disability, saphenous vein bypass of the obstruction with creation of a distal arteriovenous fistula as described by Rabinowitz and Goldfarb[18] may be indicated.

SAPHENOUS VEIN STRIPPING FOR VARICOSE VEINS

Varicose veins (meaning swollen and dilated veins) are common, occurring in 10 to 15 percent of adults. This degenerative condition, in which the valves of the superficial veins become incompetent, is apparently the result of man's assuming an upright position, walking on two legs rather than four. The delicate valves that evolved through millions of years of ambulation on four legs are unable to withstand the increased gravitational pressure of our newly acquired upright posture.[19]

Surgical treatment of varicose veins has become less frequent in recent years, requiring more stringent indications. This is due in part to the usefulness of the greater saphenous vein as a graft material in arterial reconstructive procedures, particularly coronary artery revascularization. The vascular surgeon who has desperately needed a saphenous vein previously stripped for varicosities in a patient requiring urgent coronary artery bypass or other vascular reconstruction, is reluctant to remove this source of graft material for cosmetic reasons. When varicosities do require surgical removal, our tendency has been to strip the saphenous vein only to the level of the knee unless absolutely necessary, thus preserving the vein above the knee for possible later use.

Our indications for obliterative treatment, including either surgery or sclerotherapy, have become exceedingly selective. In general, only disability from pain unresponsive to a conscientiously followed medical program or complications of varicosities are considered valid indications for obliterative treatment. Complications include ulceration from venous stasis, recurrent attacks of superficial thrombophlebitis, and rupture of a varix. Fatal hemorrhage from ruptured varices has been reported. Unless the patient is a movie star or has some other similarly valid reason for desiring removal of varicose veins for cosmetic reasons alone, an attempt is made to dissuade him or her from seeking surgical treatment. The value of coronary artery revascularization as a life-prolonging procedure has been accepted by the general public, and therefore most intelligent patients, when given reasons for preserving their veins, will not insist on undergoing saphenous vein stripping for cosmetic purposes alone.

The treatment of choice for most varicose veins without complications is conservative management consisting of exercise, elevation, and fitted elastic stockings. Exercise should be an active, regular routine of walking, bicycling, or swimming. Standing or sitting for prolonged periods should be avoided. Elastic compression stockings* must be fitted to the individual patient by measuring the leg to provide an even distribution of pressure. It has been our experience that as much harm as good results from poorly fitting elastic stockings that produce a "garter" effect, constricting venous return.

Compression sclerotherapy, more widely used in Great Britain than in the United States, offers an alternative to surgical removal, and has reportedly produced similar improvement of symptoms, with the cosmetic advantage of less scarring.[20-22] The principle of this form of treatment is to promote adherence of the vein walls to each

---

*Jobst Institute, Inc., 653 Miami Street, Toledo, Ohio 43694.

other rather than thrombosis of the vein, which is subject to subsequent recanalization. The method involves injection of the vein with a 3 percent solution of sodium tetradecyl sulfate. Prior to injection, the patient's extremity is elevated to empty the vein, which is then collapsed by digital pressure. Collapse of the vein wall is maintained for several weeks by elastic bandage compression.

Surgical treatment is reserved for the minority of patients with distinct indications as outlined above, who have not responded to conservative management. The patient must participate in the decision regarding the disadvantage of surgical treatment in that the saphenous vein will be forever unavailable for coronary artery bypass or other arterial reconstruction. In fact, the presence of — or even a family history of — coronary artery occlusive disease, which might require future coronary artery revascularization, might be considered a relative contraindication to saphenous vein stripping. Even though the varicose saphenous vein is dilated in multiple areas, certain segments are frequently usable and may be anastomosed together to provide a more satisfactory graft than can be obtained from the upper extremity or with prosthetic materials.

Operative treatment consists of removing painful varicosities and ligating all incompetent perforating branches. These perforating branches, the removal of which is probably the most crucial aspect of obtaining a successful result,[23, 24] are identified by the Brodie-Trendelenburg test. In this test, the leg is elevated with the patient in the supine position, and a tourniquet is placed around the leg just above the area to be tested. If incompetent perforators are present, blood refluxes into the saphenous vein from the deep system when the patient stands. The normal direction of flow in the lower extremity is from superficial to deep. Multiple tourniquets can be placed around the leg at various levels to determine the exact location of incompetent perforators for planning the operative procedure.

The evening before surgery, veins to be excised are marked with a special solution that will not be washed off during the surgical preparation. One formula consists of 6 cc tincture of ferric chloride, 13 gr pyrogallol, 8 cc acetone, with ethyl alcohol 70 percent to make 15 cc. The use of this solution, which will leave marks visible for a week or more, necessitates the surgeon's ascertaining that all veins marked are excised. It is disconcerting to the patient to wake up postoperatively and see no scar over an area previously marked. In such a situation, the surgeon must have an answer ready for the inevitable "Hey, Doc, you missed one."

Surgical technique is facilitated by use of an internal flexible wire vein stripper.[25] A one-inch vertical incision is made over the anterior aspect of the medial malleolus, and the greater saphenous vein is identified and isolated. The distal vein is ligated and the stripper inserted into the vein via a transverse incision. The stripper is passed cephalad to a level just above the knee. An incision is made over the tip of the stripper at that level, the proximal vein is ligated, and an incision is made into the vein, allowing the stripper tip to exit. The acorn tip is inserted onto the distal end stripper. The proximal vein is fixed to the stripper with a ligature, and the entire segment of vein is removed by smooth, firm pulling of the stripper wire from foot to knee.

The reason for stripping the vein in a cephalad direction is that all the tributaries enter the vein obliquely from below, and the vein becomes progressively larger as it courses cephalad. Individual longitudinal incisions are made over tributaries and incompetent perforators previously identified and marked with ferric chloride–pyrogallol solution. These tributaries are meticulously dissected with scissors and excised. Performing this step prior to removal of the flexible wire stripper allows the stripper to serve as a landmark, which assists in locating the tributaries and perforating branches. Our experience with an external stripper that avulses the veins blindly has been unsatisfactory. Care is taken to avoid injury to the saphenous nerve in the area of the medial aspect of the leg.

This technique of stripping the greater saphenous vein only to the level of the knee contradicts the long-advocated principle that the entire length of saphenous vein must be removed to and including the frequently incompetent valve at the saphenofemoral junction. We believe that the advantages of preserving the greater saphenous vein in the thigh for possible later use as a graft outweigh the disadvantages of leaving the saphenofemoral junction, even if incompetent.

The short saphenous vein is often involved with varicosities, and in such cases should also be removed. This vein courses cephalad from a location posterior to the lateral malleolus, along the posterior aspect of the calf to the popliteal fossa, where it typically terminates into the saphenopopliteal junction. Care is taken to avoid injury to the sural nerve, which courses with the lesser saphenous vein from midcalf to the ankle. Stripping of the vein is best accomplished with an internal stripper as described above for the greater saphenous vein.

SUBFASCIAL LIGATION OF PERFORATING VEINS

In 1938, Linton[26] elucidated the role of incompetent perforating veins in producing postphlebitic stasis ulceration. Incompetence of the valves in the perforating veins (which normally direct flow from the superficial to the deep systems) causes the "pump mechanism" of the contracting calf muscles to propel blood from the deep venous system in a reverse direction.[27] This produces increased venous pressure in the superficial veins, which results in edema, dermatitis, and stasis ulceration. Linton in 1953[28] and Cockett in 1955[29] described the operative procedure of subfascial ligation of the perforating veins. Their original approach was through a medially placed incision through the ulcer itself. A posterior subfascial approach, which avoids making the skin incision through the stasis ulcer, was described by Felder,[30, 31] and two sizable successful series with this approach have been reported by Lim and colleagues[32] and by Blumenberg and Gelfand.[27]

Indications for subfascial ligation of perforating veins include the postphlebitic syndrome manifested by recurrent ulceration, leg edema, or severe stasis dermatitis. Blumenberg and Gelfand have extended the applicability of the procedure to severe chronic venous insufficiency manifested by recurrent and persistent stasis ulceration and dermatitis in the absence of deep venous thrombosis.[27]

The number and location of perforating veins that should be ligated has remained controversial. Cockett[29] and Dodd[33] have recognized only four significant perforating veins, all located in the lower and middle third of the calf. Harjola,[34] on the other hand, found that 43 percent of the perforating veins of the leg are located in the upper third of the calf. Others using the posterior subfascial approach have described visualizing 10 to 15 thick-walled, dilated, incompetent perforating veins.[27, 31, 32] Our own opinion is that although the distal incompetent perforators are most contributory to stasis ulcers, all incompetent perforating veins visualized by phlebography or during operation should be ligated.

Our preferred operative technique is the posterior stocking seam approach.[27] A stasis ulcer, which is our usual indication for performing the procedure, may be excised and skin grafted concomitantly (Fig. 17–2). The prone position provides optimal exposure. A long incision is made in the posterior midline from just below the popliteal crease to a point midway between the lateral malleolus and the Achilles tendon (Fig. 17–2, a). Care is taken to make the incision all the way through the skin, subcutaneous tissue, and fascia to avoid creating a flap between the fascia and subcutaneous tissue, which promotes necrosis of the skin flap. The fascial flaps are elevated, and the anterior perforating branches from the greater saphenous vein are ligated and divided (Fig. 17–2, b). Usually, two crucial large branches lie directly under the ulcer bed. However, as many as 15 to 20 perforating branches may be found during dissection of the full length of the calf. Several posterior branches from the lesser saphenous vein may also be identified and ligated (Fig. 17–2, c). The lesser saphenous vein is ligated as it enters the popliteal vein in the popliteal fossa. The

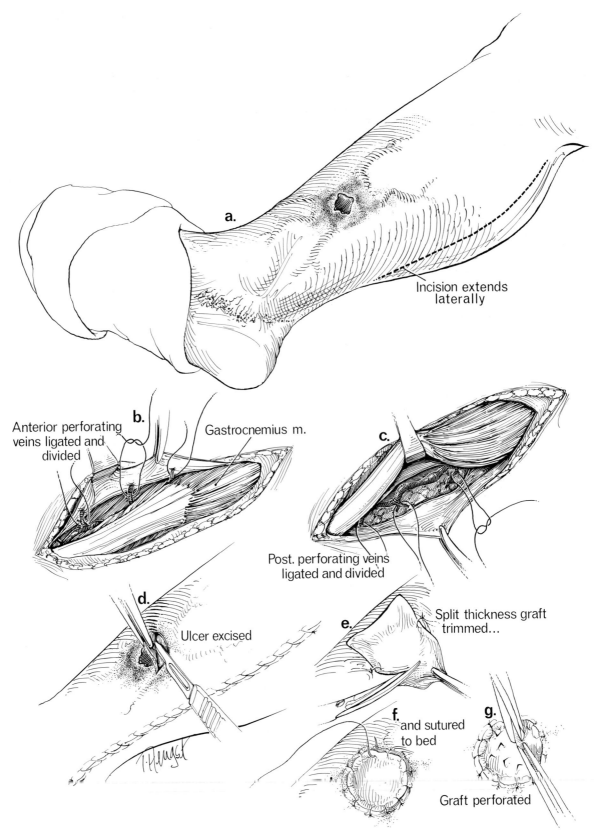

a.

Incision extends laterally

b. Anterior perforating veins ligated and divided   Gastrocnemius m.

c. Post. perforating veins ligated and divided

d. Ulcer excised

e. Split thickness graft trimmed...

f. and sutured to bed

g. Graft perforated

T. Henget

Figure 17–2   Subfascial ligation of perforating veins.

wound is closed with interrupted absorbable sutures in the fascia and with interrupted nylon skin sutures (Fig. 17–2, *d*).

Although skin grafts may be applied directly to a clean granulating ulcer base, we prefer to excise the ulcer and apply a split-thickness skin graft (Fig. 17–2, *d*). Most of these ulcers are chronic for a number of years and are subject to malignant transformation (Marjolin's ulcer). Excision precludes this possibility. The skin graft is trimmed (Fig. 17–2, *e*), sutured to the ulcer bed (Fig. 17–2, *f*), and perforated in several places to prevent serum accumulation (Fig. 17–2, *g*).

Systemic antibiotics begun preoperatively are continued for at least five days. Bed rest with elevation of the leg is recommended also for approximately five days. Because increased venous pressure is still present in the deep venous system, individually fitted elastic support hose are essential indefinitely.

INFERIOR VENA CAVA CLIPPING FOR PULMONARY ARTERY EMBOLI

Most pulmonary emboli are satisfactorily managed with intravenous heparin. An occasional patient, however, is unable to be safely heparinized because of bleeding problems or continues to experience recurrent emboli even with adequate heparinization. In such patients, interruption of the inferior vena cava (IVC) can be lifesaving. Because most fatal pulmonary emboli arise from the iliac or pelvic veins, interruption of the IVC just below the renal veins with ligation of the left ovarian vein (which enters the left renal vein) is the site of choice for interruption.

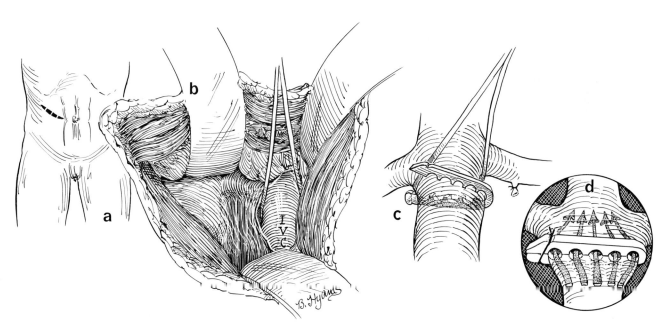

Figure 17–3   Inferior vena cava clipping for pulmonary artery emboli.

Indications for IVC interruption are (1) recurrent pulmonary emboli after adequate heparinization, (2) pulmonary emboli in patients who cannot be safely anticoagulated, and (3) circumstances necessitating pulmonary embolectomy as a prophylactic measure.

Partial interruption of the IVC with a Miles Teflon serrated clip is preferable to ligation.[35, 36] This technique lessens the incidence of chronic venous insufficiency and the formation of thrombi in the cul-de-sac between a caval ligature and the renal veins.

Operation is performed through an extraperitoneal muscle-splitting incision in the right flank at the level of the umbilicus (Fig. 17–3, a). Dissection is continued extraperitoneally, with reflection of the abdominal contents medially. The IVC is isolated just below the renal veins and a tape passed around the vein to assist in placement of the clip (Fig. 17–3, b). A Miles Teflon serrated clip is placed around the IVC and fixed in the closed position with a heavy silk ligature (Fig. 17–3, c). In women, the left ovarian vein is ligated at its juncture with the left renal vein. With proper placement of the clip immediately below the renal veins, the right ovarian vein enters the IVC below the clip and does not require ligation. After placement of the clip, blood flow through the serrations is maintained, but massive emboli are prevented from passing to the lungs (Fig. 17–3, d).

REFERENCES

1. Calkins EA: The superior vena caval syndrome: Report of 21 cases. Dis Chest 30:404, 1956.
2. Allansmith R, Richards V: Superior vena caval obstruction. Am J Surg 96:353, 1958.
3. Higginson JF: Aortic homograft substitution and bypass in superior vena caval obstruction. J Thorac Surg 32:684, 1956.
4. Scannell JG, Shaw RS: Surgical reconstruction of the superior vena cava. J Thorac Surg 28:163, 1954.
5. Botham RJ, Dracopoulos TT, Gale JW: Superior vena caval replacement with sponge Teflon prosthesis. J Thorac Cardiovasc Surg 39:202, 1960.
6. Schramel R, Olinde HDH: A new method of bypassing the obstructed vena cava. J Thorac Cardiovasc Surg 41:375, 1961.
7. Cooley DA, Hallman GL: Superior vena caval syndrome treated by azygous vein-inferior vena cava anastomosis: Report of a successful case. J Thorac Cardiovasc Surg 47:325, 1964.
8. Miller DB: Palliative surgery for benign superior vena caval syndrome. Am J Surg 129:361, 1975.
9. Hughes ESR: Venous obstruction in the upper extremity (Paget-von Schroetter syndrome). Gynecol Obstet 88:89, 1949.
10. Coon WW, Willis PW: Thrombosis of axillary and subclavian veins. Arch Surg 94:557, 1967.
11. Swinton NW Jr, Edgett JW Jr, Hall RJ: Primary subclavian-axillary vein thrombosis. Circulation 38:727, 1968.
12. Tilney NL, Griffiths HJG, Edwards EA: Natural history of major venous thrombosis of upper extremity. Arch Surg 101:792, 1970.
13. Kleinsasser LJ: "Effort" thrombosis of the axillary and subclavian veins. Arch Surg 59:258, 1949.
14. Bertelsen S, Anker W: Phlegmasia coerulea dolens: Pathophysiology, clinical features, treatment, and prognosis. Acta Chir Scandinav 134:107, 1968.
15. Mahorner H, Castleberry JW, Coleman WO: Attempts to restore function in major veins which are the site of massive thrombosis. Ann Surg 146:510, 1957.
16. DeWeese JA, Adams JT, Gaiser DL: Subclavian venous thrombectomy. Circulation 16 (Suppl 2):168, 1972.
17. McLeery RS, Kesterson JE, Kirtley JA, Love RB: Subclavius and anterior scalene muscle compression as a cause of intermittent obstruction of the subclavian vein. Ann Surg 133:588, 1951.
18. Rabinowitz R, Goldfarb D: Surgical treatment of axillosubclavian venous thrombosis: A case report. Surgery 70:703, 1971.
19. Alexander CJ: The theoretical basis of varicose vein formation. M J Australia 1:258, 1972.
20. Fegan WG: Conservative treatment of varicose veins. Progr Surg 11:27, 1973.
21. Hobbs JT: Surgery and sclerotherapy in the treatment of varicose veins: A random trial. Arch Surg 109:793, 1974.
22. Fegan WG: *Varicose Veins: Compression Sclerotherapy.* Charles C Thomas, Publisher, Springfield, Ill., 1968.
23. Larson HL, Lofgren EP, Myers TT, Lofgren KA: Long term results after vein surgery: Study of 1000 cases after 10 years. Mayo Clin Proc 49:114, 1974.

24. Lofgren EP, Lofgren KA: Recurrence of varicose veins after the stripping operation. Arch Surg 102:111, 1971.
25. Meyers TT: Results and technique of stripping operation for varicose veins. JAMA 163:87, 1957.
26. Linton R: The communicating veins of the lower leg and the operative technic for their ligation. Ann Surg 107:582, 1938.
27. Blumenberg RM, Gelfand ML: The posterior stocking seam approach to radical subfascial clipping of perforating veins. Am J Surg 136:202, 1978.
28. Linton R: The post-thrombotic ulceration of the lower extremity: Its etiology and surgical treatment. Ann Surg 138:415, 1953.
29. Cockett FB: The pathology and treatment of venous ulcers of the leg. Br J Surg 43:260, 1955.
30. Felder DA, Murphy TO, Ring DM: A posterior subfascial approach to communicating veins of the leg. Surg Gynecol Obstet 100:730, 1955.
31. Felder DA, Bernstein EF: Re-evaluation of the posterior subfascial approach for the ligation of the communicating veins in the leg. Surgery 47:349, 1960.
32. Lim RC, Blaisdell FW, Zubrin J, Stallone RJ, Hall AD: Subfascial ligation of perforating veins in recurrent stasis ulceration. Am J Surg 119:246, 1970.
33. Dodd H, Cockett FB: *The Pathology and Surgery of the Veins of the Lower Limb,* Chapter 18, p 279. Edinburgh, Churchill Livingstone, 1976.
34. Harjola P, Tala P, Ketonen P, Tolvanen E: Surgical treatment of incompetent perforating veins of the lower limb. Ann Chir Gynaecol Fenn 56:1, 1967.
35. Adams JT, Feingold BE, DeWeese JA: Comparative evaluation of ligation and partial interruption of the inferior vena cava. Arch Surg 103:272, 1971.
36. Gardner AMN, Askew AR, Harse AR, Wilmshurst CC, Turner MJ: Partial occlusion of the inferior vena cava in the prevention of pulmonary embolism. Surg Gynecol Obstet 138:17, 1974.

CHAPTER **18**

Portal Decompression Procedures for Relief of Portal Hypertension

Numerous surgical procedures for the relief of portal hypertension have been described and used extensively. Despite widespread laboratory investigations and clinical trials, no agreement has yet been reached concerning their effectiveness.[1, 2] The results of portal decompression depend largely upon selection of patients for operation. Most clinicians agree that the more extensive the liver dysfunction, the greater the risk of surgically decompressing the portal system. Ascites, icterus, reduced prothrombin activity, azotemia, and other findings of advanced liver failure increase the risk of any surgical technique.[3, 4] Once a decision to operate has been made, the surgeon may select one of several techniques for relieving portal hypertension.[5, 6] There are, however, a few facts that must be considered before making a selection, six of which are enumerated here:[7, 8]

(1) If the patient has had a previous cholecystectomy, or has had gastric or duodenal surgery in the right upper abdominal quadrant, the portal vein may be unapproachable due to adhesions and venous collaterals.

(2) If the patient has had a splenectomy or a left nephrectomy, the splenorenal anastomoses are impossible.

(3) A previous appendectomy or bowel resection may make mesenteric caval anastomosis technically difficult or impossible.

(4) The patient with advanced ascites may not tolerate a total venous bypass of the liver and therefore may develop hepatic failure and coma after operation.[9]

(5) Splenomegaly, or even hypersplenism, is not (in our opinion) an indication for splenectomy in patients with cirrhosis or congestive splenomegaly (Banti's syndrome). Preservation of the spleen with venous decompression, using splenorenal anastomosis with splenic artery ligation, is advantageous, particularly in children and young patients. By splenic preservation, the veins connected to the region of the gastroesophageal junction are preserved, thus reducing the pressure of esophageal and gastric varices.

(6) If any type of decompression procedure has been done previously, further surgery in the same anatomic region is destined for failure.

Following these rather broad considerations, the surgeon selects the technique that seems best to suit the individual patient. One must be aware, however, that consistently good results cannot be expected or guaranteed with any of the available shunt procedures.[4, 9-11]

PORTACAVAL ANASTOMOSIS

Operation is performed under general anesthesia, using agents that are least injurious to the liver. We use the midline upper abdominal incision because it provides for ample exposure with a minimal raw surface for bleeding (Fig. 18–1, *a*). A

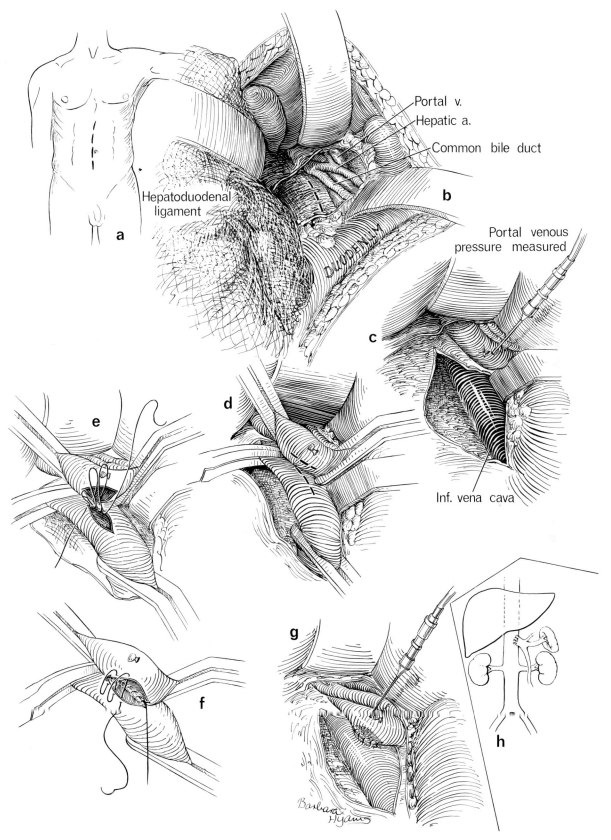

Portal v.

Hepatic a.

Common bile duct

Hepatoduodenal ligament

a

b

DUODENUM

Portal venous pressure measured

c

d

e

Inf. vena cava

f

g

h

Barbara Hyams

Figure 18–1 Surgical technique for portacaval anastomosis.

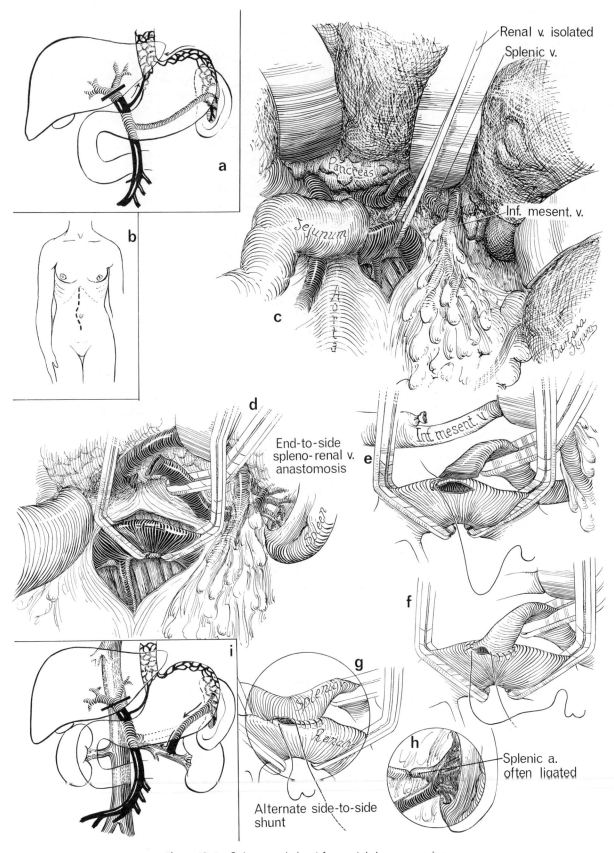

Figure 18–2 Splenorenal shunt for portal decompression.

subcostal incision, however, is sometimes preferred. After the abdomen has been explored and the ascitic fluid aspirated, an incision is made in the parietal peritoneum along the upper and outer curvature of the second portion of the duodenum, and the structures in the porta hepatis are exposed (Fig. 18–1, b). The common bile duct may be identified by aspiration with a small-gauge needle. The underlying inferior vena cava is dissected and exposed on its ventral surface.

Using a saline manometer, pressures are measured in the cava and overlying portal vein (Fig. 18–1, c). The caudate of the liver and head of the pancreas restrict the length of portal vein available for anastomosis. If sufficient length of vein is available, a side-to-side portacaval anastomosis is performed (Fig. 18–1, d). The veins may be cross-clamped as depicted in the drawing or occluded with partial-occlusion clamps, whichever provides the greatest ease of anastomosis. The longitudinal incision in the portal vein should be at least as long as the diameter of the portal vein (Fig. 18–1, d). The anastomosis is completed by a simple continuous suturing technique, using an atraumatic 5–0 or 6–0 monofilament polypropylene suture (Fig. 18–1, e and f). At the completion of the anastomosis, clamps are removed from the veins and the pressure is measured in the portal vein (Fig. 18–1, g). Formation of ascitic fluid should cease after portal decompression, and the abdomen should be closed without drainage.

End-to-side portacaval anastomosis is technically easier than side-to-side, but some clinicians believe that hepatic failure is more common with end-to-side. That point, however, remains debatable.[12-15] When the end-to-side technique is selected, the portal vein is divided close to the point of entry into the liver (Fig. 18–1, h). To gain maximum length on the vein, we apply a curved vascular clamp across the vein, adjacent to the liver, and an angled vascular clamp close to the pancreas. The hepatic end is then oversewn with a monofilament suture. Ligation of the venous stump may lead to bleeding in an inaccessible area. An end-to-side anastomosis is performed by using the same suture technique as for the side-to-side procedure.

In performing a portacaval anastomosis, the surgeon should proceed expeditiously during complete occlusion of the portal vein, since prolonged portal venous stagnation may lead to thrombosis and visceral injuries. Rather than attempting complete hemostasis during the dissection of the portal vein and vena cava, operating time must be conserved. Bleeding usually ceases once portal decompression is achieved and the portacaval shunt is opened. In our experience, the best results occur when blood transfusions are held to a minimum during the procedure. Lengthy operations with unnecessarily meticulous and tedious techniques of dissection and hemostases may jeopardize a patient's chance of recovery.[16]

SPLENORENAL SHUNT

When properly performed, this technique may effect portal decompression with the lowest patient risk and the smallest number of late hepatic complications.[6, 15, 17] Original descriptions of portal decompression by splenorenal anastomoses were mostly about proximal splenic vein anastomosis with ligation of the distal vein. These techniques provided chiefly for decompression of the gastric, intestinal and pancreatic circulation, leaving the more important proximal gastroesophageal region in the same congested condition. In a report made from this hospital in 1963,[6] the technique of side-to-side splenorenal anastomosis was described, emphasizing the importance of distal splenic vein decompression with preservation of the spleen, which is recommended, particularly in young patients. The side-to-side technique may be technically difficult, and Warren[17] has described distal decompression with the use of end-to-side anastomosis, which does not, however, effectively relieve tension in the remainder of the portal system.

Distal splenorenal shunt provides for selective decompression of the esophago-gastric region (Fig. 18–2, a) and controls bleeding from varices without altering hepatic function. Thus, it is indicated in Banti's syndrome and in all cases of extrahepatic venous obstruction. The operation is usually performed through an upper midline incision (Fig. 18–2, b). The small intestines are retracted toward the patient's right side by using an approach to retroperitoneal structures, similar to exposure of the proximal aorta for an abdominal aneurysm (Fig. 18–2, c). Reflection of the jejunum and division of the ligament of Treitz exposes the left renal vein, which is encircled with a tape. Identification of the splenic vein under the pancreas is made by isolating the easily visible inferior mesenteric vein, which is then followed proximally toward the portal vein, where it joins the splenic vein. Once the splenic vein is identified, it is gently dissected free of the pancreas, and friable tributaries to the body and tail of the pancreas are carefully ligated. When a sufficient length of the splenic vein has been developed by dissection, the vein may be divided at its junction with the inferior mesenteric vein.

After appropriate application of vascular clamps, preparations are made for an end-to-side anastomosis to the renal vein (Fig. 18–2, d). The anastomosis is performed with a 5–0 or 6–0 monofilament polypropylene suture, using a simple continuous technique (Fig. 18–2, e and f). When the clamps are released, blood flows from the gastroesophageal veins and the spleen into the inferior vena cava, thus bypassing the portal venous system. We have also used side-to-side splenorenal anastomosis (Fig. 18–2, g), a technique that provides additional partial decompression of the entire portal system without (in our experience) imposing the threat of hepatic coma. The side-to-side technique, however, results in tension on the anastomosis in some cases, and should be used only when the splenic vein and left renal vein lie closely approximated. To reduce splenic intracapsular pressure in instances of splenomegaly, particularly in patients with hematologic evidence of hypersplenism, ligation of the splenic artery may be performed (Fig. 18–2, h). Usually, the artery is easily identified as it passes along the cephalad surface of the pancreas. If it is not available after the splenic vein has been mobilized, it should be approached through the gastrohepatic omentum in the lesser sac, where it is easily identified. The splenic artery may be ligated in continuity. Viability of the spleen is maintained by circulation through short gastric arteries.

MESOCAVAL ANASTOMOSES

Alternative methods of portacaval decompression are available and may be particularly useful when more standard and time-tested techniques are not possible. The two techniques that have been used successfully are the iliac vein superior mesenteric anastomosis (Fig. 18–3, a), and the caval-mesenteric "H" graft anastomosis (Fig. 18–3, b).[17] We have used the iliac mesenteric technique infrequently, mostly in children with extrahepatic portal venous obstruction, where previous splenectomy or splenorenal shunt has failed to relieve portal obstruction. In order to reach the mesenteric vein, the right iliac vein must be dissected distally to its bifurcation into internal and external branches or beyond. The bifurcation of the inferior vena cava must be mobilized from behind the overlying aortic bifurcation. This requires that the left common iliac vein be divided. The inferior cava with iliac vein is then freed posteriorly so that the end-to-side anastomosis may be performed without tension and without kinking. This technique has the major disadvantage of interrupting venous return from the lower extremities; fortunately, the few patients in whom we have used it have shown no evidence of subsequent complications.

Cavo-mesenteric anastomosis using an "H" graft is an alternative technique that takes less time than the portacaval shunt procedure and has been useful in patients

a

b

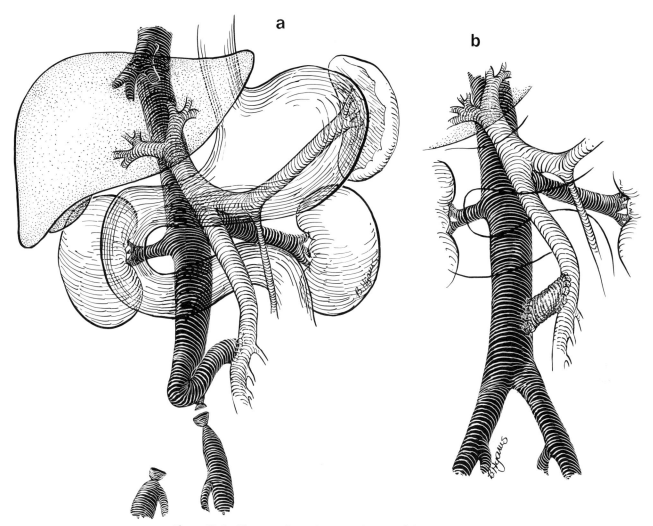

Figure 18–3 Mesocaval anastomoses for portal decompression.

with acute gastroesophageal hemorrhage due to alcoholic cirrhosis. Selection of a suitable prosthetic graft is important, because fabric grafts have a tendency to thrombose when placed in the venous system. A woven graft of Teflon is particularly resistant to the deposition of fibrin but is otherwise not much better than a graft made of woven Dacron. The recent development of fabric grafts treated with pyrolytic carbon seems to be a promising solution.[18-20]

A large diameter vascular graft, size 14 to 18 mm, should be selected, and the anastomoses performed with monofilament sutures, using the same continuous suture technique.

Some surgeons have removed the patient's right internal jugular vein for the interposition graft. The vein should be removed over the entire length, and a 10-cm graft is ideal. While removal of the vein is usually well tolerated, cerebral edema can be a complication, particularly in the acutely ill patient with reversed albumen-globulin ratio. Owing to its softness and biologic structure, subsequent collapse and fibrosis of the autograft may occur. Thus, we prefer to use a synthetic graft in spite of its known limitations.

REFERENCES

1. Voorhees AB Jr, Price JB Jr: Extrahepatic portal hypertension: Retrospective analysis of 129 cases and associated clinical implications. Arch Surg 108:338, 1974.
2. Resnick RH, Chambers TC, Ishihara AM, Garceau AJ, Callow AD, Schimmel EM, O'Hara ET: A controlled study of the prophylactic portacaval shunt: A final report. Ann Intern Med 70:675, 1969.
3. Voorhees AB Jr, Price JB Jr, Britton RC: Portasystemic shunting procedures for portal hypertension: 26-year experience in adults with cirrhosis of the liver. Am J Surg 199:501, 1970.
4. Linton RR, Ellis DS, Geary JE: Critical comparative analysis of early and late results of splenorenal and direct portacaval shunts performed in 169 patients with portal cirrhosis. Ann Surg 154:446, 1961.
5. Cooley DA: Side-to-side splenorenal anastomosis with splenic preservation for portal hypertension. Surg Gynec Obstet 116:626, 1963.
6. Warren WD, Salam AA, Hutson D, Zeppa R: Selective distal splenorenal shunt: Technic and results of operation. Arch Surg 108:306, 1974.
7. Jackson FC, Perrin EB, Felix WR, Smith AG: A clinical investigation of the portacaval shunt: V. Survival analysis of the therapeutic operation. Ann Surg 174:672, 1971.
8. Fischer JE, James HJ: Treatment of hepatic coma and hepatorenal syndrome: Mechanism of action of L-dopa and Aramine. Am J Surg 123:222, 1972.
9. Hallenbeck GA, Wollaeger EE, Adson MA, Gage RP: Results after portal-systemic shunts in 120 patients with cirrhosis of the liver. Surg Gynec Obstet 116:453, 1963.
10. Sherlock S, Hourigan K, George P: Medical complications of shunt surgery for portal hypertension. Ann NY Acad Sci 170:392, 1970.
11. Britton RC: Surgical treatment of complications of portal hypertension. Ann NY Acad Sci 170:358, 1970.
12. Liebowitz H: Splenomegaly and hypersplenism pre- and post-portacaval shunt. New York J Med 63:2631, 1963.
13. Shalimov AA, Shoos VA: Lateral splenorenal shunt with preservation of the natural portacaval anastomoses in portal hypertension. Klin Khir 5:17, 1966.
14. Orloff MJ, Chandler JG, Charters AC III, Condon JK, Grambort DE, Modafferi TR, Levin SE: Emergency portacaval shunt treatment for bleeding esophageal varices: Prospective study in unselected patients with alcoholic cirrhosis. Arch Surg 108:293, 1974.
15. Haller JD, Glick H, Hallman GL, Cooley DA: Portal decompression by side-to-side splenorenal venous anastomosis. Arch Surg 102:316, 1971.
16. Resnick RH, Iber FL, Ishihara AM, Chalmers TC, Zimmerman H, and the Boston Inter-Hospital Liver Group (Boston): Controlled Study of therapeutic portacaval shunt. Gastroenterology 67:843, 1974.
17. Warren WD, Salam AA, Smith Robert B II: Mesosplenorenal shunt procedures: Comprehensive approach to portosystemic decompression. Ann Surg 179:791, 1974.
18. Haubold AD, Norman JC: Ultra low temperature isotropically (ULTI) deposited carbon (biolyte): A promising new flexible biomaterial and blood interface. Cardiovascular Diseases, Bulletin of the Texas Heart Institute 4(#4):369, 1977.
19. Norman JC, Cooley DA, Hallman GL, Nihill MR: Left ventricular apical-abdominal aortic conduits for left ventricular outflow tract obstructions: Clinical results in eleven patients with a special composite prosthesis. Cardiovasc Surg (Suppl 2), Circulation 56(#3):II,62, 1977.
20. Bokros JC, Akins RJ, Shim HS, Haubold AD, Agarwal NK: Prostheses made of carbon. Chemtech, January 1977, pages 40–49.

CHAPTER **19**

Arteriovenous Fistulae

Arteriovenous (AV) fistulae may appear in many anatomic locations. The effectiveness of surgical therapy depends upon the etiology as well as the anatomic location and extent of the lesion.[1-4] When the lesion results from trauma, surgical repair may be practical and straightforward. In most congenital arteriovenous malformations, however, *complete* cure may be achieved only by wide excision or, when the lesion involves an extremity, by amputation. Thus, the choice of surgical approach must be based upon characteristic features of each lesion.[5, 6]

TRAUMATIC AND SPONTANEOUS AV FISTULAE

These lesions usually result from penetrating injuries such as those caused by knives, picks, and other sharp instruments, or from gunshot wounds. Spontaneous AV fistulae occur when aneurysms of the ascending thoracic aorta rupture into the adjacent vena cava, the left innominate vein, or even into the main or left pulmonary artery.[7-10] Aneurysms of the abdominal aorta may rupture into the inferior vena caval or left renal vein.[11] We have successfully repaired all of these types of fistulae.

Occasionally, AV fistulae are inadvertently caused during surgery by the combined suture ligation of an artery and vein. Simple ligation of a vascular pedicle containing an artery and vein seldom causes this complication, but penetration of the artery and vein by a needle during suture ligation may inadvertently create a communication that results in a persistent AV fistula. Before the modern era of vascular surgery, optimum surgical treatment of an AV fistula in the upper or lower extremities consisted of quadruple ligation, i.e., ligation of both the afferent and efferent arterial and venous limbs of the lesion. Emphasis is presently placed upon the restoration of normal pulsatile arterial flow distal to the lesion, and with the availability of synthetic vascular prostheses, restoration of normal circulation has become the primary goal of surgery. In most instances, continuity of the accompanying vein may also be restored. Excision or simple suture obliteration is acceptable only in smaller AV fistulae involving vessels that are not vital to an extremity or a visceral organ.

REPAIR OF TRAUMATIC ILIAC AV FISTULA

The drawing (Fig. 19–1, *a* to *h*) depicts findings in a 42-year-old patient who developed an iliac AV fistula after operation for excision of a herniated nucleus pulposus. It appears that surgical penetration of the anterior spinal ligament injured the underlying left common iliac artery and vein, resulting in an aneurysm and large fistula which caused cardiac failure (Fig. 19–1, *a*). The surgical approach was through a midline abdominal incision (Fig. 19–1, *b*). The aortic bifurcation was exposed by reflecting the small intestine to the right, revealing the course of the left ureter (Fig. 19–1, *c*). Dissection of the proximal common iliac artery and the distal

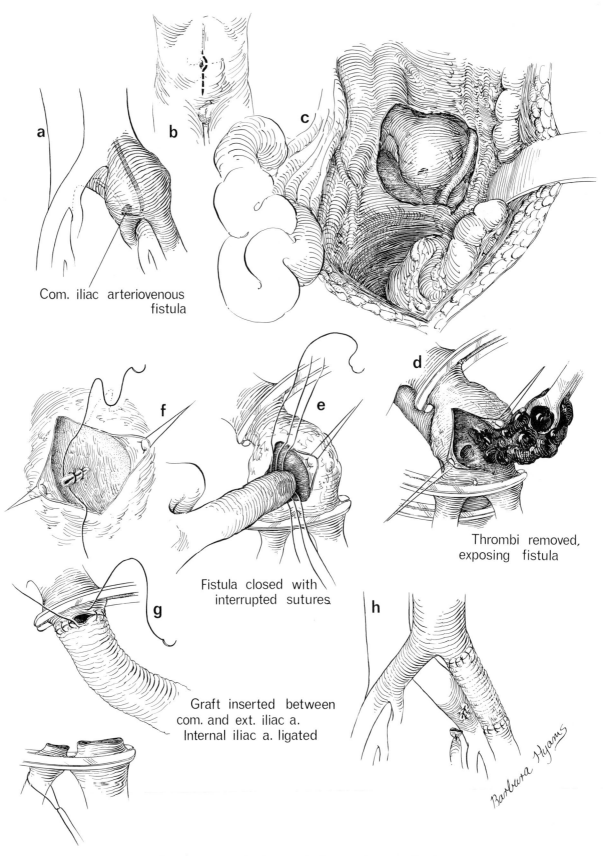

Figure 19–1 Repair of traumatic iliac arteriovenous fistula.

external and internal iliac arteries was performed first (Fig. 19–1, d). The distal iliac vein was also controlled, but encirclement of the common iliac vein was prevented by scar tissue which resulted from previous perforation of the anterior spinal ligament. After control of the arterial supply of the fistula was obtained along with occlusion of the distal limb of the venous channel, the aneurysm was incised. Bleeding from the venous circulation was controlled by an index finger placed over the fistulous opening (Fig. 19–1, e). Interrupted sutures were then inserted in the ostium and tied while the assistant provided hemostasis by maintaining traction on the remaining sutures (Fig. 19–1, f). After the fistula was sutured, arterial flow into the external iliac artery was restored with the use of a 10-mm velour knitted Dacron graft (Fig. 19–1, g and h).

The technique of using the surgeon's index finger to prevent venous bleeding has been effective in other types of acquired AV fistulae, as in cases of rupture of abdominal aortic aneurysm into the inferior vena cava. This technique allows restoration of both venous and arterial flow after surgical correction. Since restoration of venous continuity is seldom successful with synthetic fabric grafts, the fistula should be sutured without excision of venous afferent and efferent limbs.

Fistulae in the brachiocephalic circulation require that surgical exposure and control of arterial flow be achieved either by sternotomy or intercostal thoracotomy, employing clavicular excision and other means when necessary; although proximal control of arterial circulation is usually essential, control of the other limbs of an "H" type fistula may be obtained by finger pressure on the ostium or use of a balloon catheter in the distal artery. Best results are obtained when there is minimum dissection of adjacent tissues.[12]

REPAIR OF TRAUMATIC FEMORAL AV FISTULA

Gunshot wounds may produce AV fistulae; therefore, the physical examination of any penetrating wound of an extremity in the vicinity of major vessels includes auscultation for detection of a bruit. The presence or absence of pulses in the extremity is not diagnostic. A suspected AV fistula must be confirmed by arteriography.

An example of treatment for an AV fistula of the superficial femoral artery and femoral vein is depicted in Figure 19–2. Exposure of the fistula is obtained by an excision, usually best made over the site of the previous wound, which may be well healed by the time of diagnosis (Fig. 19–2, a). The femoral artery and vein are isolated and mobilized by ligating small branches adjacent to the fistula (Fig. 19–2, b). Following systemic heparinization (2 mg/kg of body weight) and occlusion of the vessels, the fistula is excised and the artery and vein repaired by end-to-end anastomosis (Fig. 19–2, c). When more extensive resection of the artery is required, a segment of autogenous saphenous vein or Dacron graft is interposed (Fig. 19–2, d). Reconstruction of the femoral vein by graft replacement is less satisfactory because of almost inevitable thrombus of the graft. However, even temporary flow through the graft and possible recanalization following thrombosis may justify autogenous saphenous vein graft reconstruction of the femoral or popliteal veins, which cannot be repaired primarily.

CONGENITAL AV FISTULAE AND AV MALFORMATIONS

While these lesions are occasionally cured by local excision, they are usually diffuse and relieved only by amputation of an extremity; thus, one must fully realize when recommending surgery that attempts to achieve a complete cure may lead to

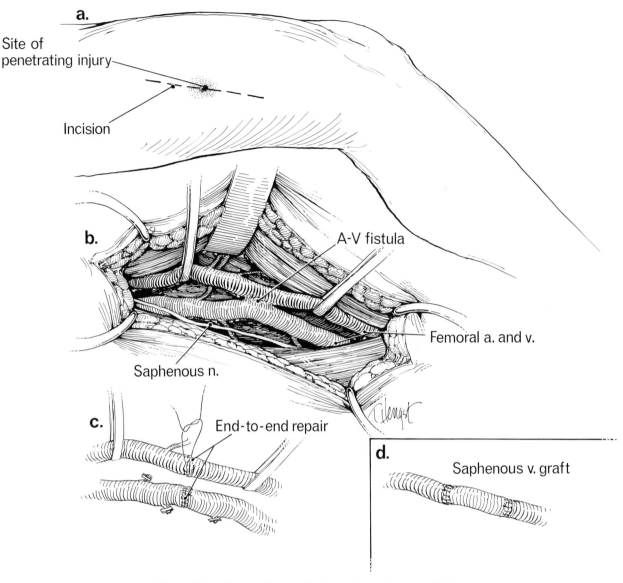

Figure 19–2 Repair of traumatic femoral arteriovenous fistula.

mutilation or serious and painful complications in the patient's extremities. Angiographic study of these lesions is mandatory,[13, 14] since physical examination alone may result in the erroneous impression that the fistula is localized, while, in fact, it may be extensive, involving the entire arm or leg. When extensive AV malformation causes discomfort, resulting from distention of the extremity (hand or foot), ligation of the afferent artery may provide symptomatic relief. Although this form of palliative therapy is often temporary, we prefer it to the more radical procedures. Subsequent palliative therapy may be required, involving additional ligation of major arterial channels that feed the malformation.

INTRA-ARTERIAL EMBOLIZATION

The technique of intra-arterial embolization (IAE) may be used successfully in treating diffuse AV malformations,[15-18] sometimes combined with ligation of the afferent artery; full angiographic assessment should be made, however, before deciding to use IAE. With a catheter inserted into the afferent artery, appropriate materials (combinations of Gelfoam, lead pellets, or macerated autogenous muscle) are injected to promote thrombosis.[17] Recently, injections of Silastic spheres of various diameters have proved to be practical and effective. A sphere diameter is selected that will most likely occlude the fistulae. Although many of the smaller spheres will pass through the AV malformation and ultimately lodge in the lung, those that collect in the malformation may significantly reduce the shunt, relieving symptoms and reducing disfigurement.

The technique is the same, regardless of which type of embolus is used. A catheter is first selectively positioned under fluoroscopic control in the arterial vessel or vessels that feed the arteriovenous malformation (AVM). Emboli are then flushed through the catheter, using either small quantities of normal saline or contrast material. Frequent radiographs are made to ascertain the effectiveness of the vascular occlusion, and the procedure is continued until adequate obliteration of the malformation is achieved. Usually an AVM cannot be completely destroyed, but a sufficient reduction of blood flow into the lesion may ameliorate symptoms.

With the introduction of Silastic spheres, the use of Gelfoam as the embolizing agent has diminished. The disadvantage in using Gelfoam is that recanalization following occlusion of a vessel is a possibility. In addition, the Silastic spheres are radiopaque, and thus easier to see on follow-up films.[19]

Gelfoam remains useful, particularly as an adjunct to surgery, and its use in preoperative embolization has been reported to decrease blood loss at surgical removal of AVMs.

Embolization in general continues to be beneficial as a primary modality of treatment for AVMs that are too large or are otherwise inaccessible to surgery. In addition, the resection of AVMs of the external carotid circulation will often require surgery that leaves unacceptable cosmetic results.

A patient in our institution was treated for an extensive AVM of the face and nasopharynx with Gelfoam embolization of the appropriate branches of the external carotid artery. The lesion was studied before embolization via injections of the vertebral artery. Under general anesthesia a catheter was surgically placed in the external carotid artery that had been previously ligated, but ineffectively so because the AVM had recurred from collateral pathways of filling from the left vertebral artery. Gelfoam emboli were then flushed into the lesion using small amounts of contrast material. Each Gelfoam embolus was approximately 2 mm in size, but compacted. When these emboli lodged in small branches of the AVM, they re-expanded, creating a secure obstruction.

The patient did well postoperatively, experiencing the usual mild swelling and tenderness of the left side of the face, which lasted three days and then completely disappeared.

A follow-up arteriogram six months later showed no change from the final check films at the time of embolization. The large, cavernous hemangioma of the face was no longer seen on angiography, and the patient's symptoms of headache and throbbing suboccipital pain had virtually disappeared.

In treating patients who have diffuse congenital AV fistulae or AV malformations the surgeon must remember that a *complete cure is seldom attained*. Thus, surgery should be limited to *symptomatic* patients, or to those in whom unattractive disfigurement or overgrowth of an extremity causes concern. Cutaneous hemangiomata or birthmarks are also common AV malformations. Consultation with a dermatologist or plastic surgeon may help in achieving the best cosmetic result. Techniques of freezing with solid carbon dioxide ("dry ice"), injection of sclerosing substances, or electrocoagulation may be effective;[20] excision of cutaneous lesions with skin grafting may also aid in cosmetic improvement.

REFERENCES

1. Ennis JT, Bateson EM, Moule NJ: Uncommon arteriovenous fistulae. Clin Radiol 23:392, 1972.
2. Nennhaus HP, Javid H: The distinct syndrome of spontaneous abdominal aortocaval fistula. Am J Med 44:464, 1968.
3. Gomes MMR, Bernatz PE: Arteriovenous fistulas: A review and ten year experience at the Mayo Clinic. Mayo Clin Proc 45:81, 1970.
4. Szilagyi DE, Elliott JP, DeRusso FJ, Smith RF: Peripheral congenital arteriovenous fistulas. Surgery 57:61, 1965.
5. Holman E: *Abnormal Arteriovenous Communications, Peripheral and Intracardiac, Acquired and Congenital.* Springfield, Ill., Charles C Thomas, 1968, 245 pp.
6. Sumner DS: Arteriovenous fistula. Physiology and pathological anatomy. In Strandness DE Jr, ed: *Collateral Circulation in Clinical Surgery.* Philadelphia, W. B. Saunders Company, 1969.
7. Mohr LL, Smith LL: Arteriovenous fistula from rupture of abdominal aortic aneurysm. Arch Surg 110:806, 1975.
8. Baker WH, Sharzer LA, Ehrenhaft JL: Aortocaval fistula as a complication of abnormal aortic aneurysms. Surgery 72:933, 1972.
9. Colley AL, Annon WT Jr: Aortic-vena caval fistula from ruptured aortic aneurysm. JAMA 194:1137, 1965.
10. Kazmier FJ, Harrison CE: Acquired aortocaval fistulas. Am J Med 55:175, 1973.
11. Shumacker HB, Jontz J: Rupture of abdominal aortic aneurysm vena cava: Successful surgical repair. Am Surg 22:1182, 1956.
12. Meyer J, Wukasch DC, Hallman GL, Cooley DA: Aneurysm and fistula of the sinus of Valsalva. Ann Thorac Surg 19:170, 1975.
13. McCoy JA, Meyer J, Cooley DA: Congenital coronary artery to main pulmonary artery fistula: A report of four cases. Cardiovascular Diseases, Bulletin of the Texas Heart Institute 1:384, 1974.
14. Meyer J, Reul GJ Jr, Mullins CE, McCoy J, Hallman GL, Cooley DA: Congenital fistulae of the coronary arteries: Clinical considerations and surgical management in 23 patients. J Cardiovasc Surg 16:506, 1975.
15. Olcott C IV, Newton TH, Stoney, RJ, Ehrenfeld WK: Intra-arterial embolization in the management of arteriovenous malformations. Surgery 79:(#1)3, 1976.
16. Bookstein JJ, Goldstein HM: Successful management of postbiopsy arteriovenous fistula with selective arterial embolization. Radiology 109:535, 1973.
17. Rizk GK, Atallah NK, Bridi GI: Renal arteriovenous fistula treated by catheter embolization. Br J Radiol 46:222, 1973.
18. Meaney TF, Chicatelli PD: Obliteration of renal arteriovenous fistula by transcatheter clot embolization. Case report and experimental observations. Cleve Clin Q 41:33, 1974.
19. Luessenhop AJ, Kachmann RJ, Shevlin W, Serrero AA: Clinical evaluation of artificial embolization in the treatment of large cerebral arteriovenous malformations. J Neurosurg 23:400, 1965.
20. Gardner AMN, Stewart IA: Treatment of arteriovenous malformation by endarterial electrocoagulation. Br J Surg 59:146, 1972.

CHAPTER 20

Complications of Vascular Surgery

INTRODUCTION

The paramount goal in vascular surgery is obviously the restoration of blood flow with alleviation of symptoms and the salvage of life or limb without complications. The nature of the circulatory system, with tissue dependence upon oxygenated blood, predisposes the patient undergoing vascular reconstructive procedures to a wide range of complications. The incidence of these complications may be minimized by an experienced surgeon applying the surgical principles described. However, the surgeon who accepts the responsibility of treating patients with various stages of vascular disease — some hopeless or with little chance for restoration to normal — must accept some incidences of complication and acquire the knowledge necessary to manage them. Although the insecure surgeon can reduce his rate of complications to near zero by means of rigid patient selection, this approach denies the possibility for improved quality of life to many patients in the higher-risk groups. The following old adage is applicable: *The surgeon who never gets a complication is one who is not operating.*

The conscientious surgeon dedicated to improving his results must spend time and effort in keeping accurate records and undergoing periodic, critical self-examination. When an undesirable trend toward a certain complication appears, he must perform a soul-searching review of what he might have done differently, also gleaning from the experience of others. It is in this spirit that our complications are described herein.*

At the Texas Heart Institute from January 16, 1970, through July 31, 1978, a total of 1864 patients underwent arterial reconstructive procedures with the use of prosthetic tube grafts.** The distribution of patients by the conditions for which the procedure was performed and as to whether operation was elective or emergency (Salvage)*** is listed in Table 20–1. Table 20–2 lists the distribution and incidence of 412 specific complications among the entire series of 1864 patients.† The risk of each complication in various disease categories is listed in Table 20–3.†† Early results and mortality are described in Appendixes 4 and 5.

---

*All vascular operative procedures are recorded on a standard protocol format, and the data are subjected to computerized analysis. The protocol form used is included as Appendix 6 and contains early and late results. Data presented here comprise only early results defined as events occurring during the period of hospitalization, with the exception of late graft infections, which (for the sake of completeness) are listed in early complications.

**Includes woven, knitted, and double-velour Dacron grafts manufactured by Meadox Medicals, Inc. This series does not include arterial reconstructions that did not utilize Dacron tube grafts, such as carotid endarterectomy or femoral popliteal bypass with autogenous saphenous vein grafts.

***The *Salvage* category implies emergency procedure, i.e., *Salvage Abdominal Aortic Aneurysm,* and indicates patients with ruptured aneurysm.

†These complications are further separated by disease categories in Appendix 2 A, B, C, and D.

††The absolute number of patients from which these percentage figures were derived is listed in Appendix 2 A, B, C, and D.

In reviewing the complications occurring in our series, it is apparent that there is a wide spectrum of problems that can occur. The prevention and management of most of these complications have been previously discussed within the appropriate chapters, unless they fall into the field of general surgical problems, the management of which is adequately described in standard general surgery texts. Three of the most complex complications that require special management[1, 2] are aortoduodenal fistula, graft infection, and microembolism ("trash foot"); these will be discussed individually.

Table 20–1 DISTRIBUTION OF 1864 PATIENTS UNDERGOING ARTERIAL RECONSTRUCTION

	Number of Patients		
	Elective	Salvage	Total
Abdominal Aortic Aneurysm	753	47	800
Aortoiliac Occlusive Disease	649	54	703
Femoropopliteal Occlusive Disease*	77	7	84
Miscellaneous Arterial Reconstructions**	260	17	277
TOTAL	1739	125	1864

*Includes only Dacron tube graft reconstructions; excludes the more numerous category of patients revascularized with the use of autogenous saphenous vein grafts.
**See Appendix 2: Distribution of 277 Miscellaneous Arterial Reconstructions by Type of Lesion.

Table 20–2A DISTRIBUTION OF EARLY COMPLICATIONS IN 1864 PATIENTS* UNDERGOING ARTERIAL RECONSTRUCTION

Early Complications	Elective	Salvage	Total
Hemorrhage	39	6	45
Graft Infection**	2	0	2
Wound Infection	16	4	20
Pulmonary Embolus	7	2	9
Early Thrombosis	56	11	67
Embolism Major Vessel	6	0	6
Microembolus ("Trash Foot")	26	5	31
Myocardial Infarction	18	4	22
Cerebrovascular Accident	12	1	13
Mesenteric Infarction	11	2	13
Pancreatitis	2	0	2
Intestinal Obstruction	25	4	29
Renal Failure	53	8	61
Pulmonary Respiratory Failure	24	7	31
Pneumonia—Not Requiring Tracheostomy	9	2	11
Pneumonia—Requiring Tracheostomy	6	2	8
Other Miscellaneous Complications	40	2	42
TOTAL	352	60	412

*Some patients experienced several complications.

Number of Patients	
Elective	1739
Salvage	125
TOTAL	1864

**Includes late graft infections.

Table 20–2B INCIDENCE OF EARLY COMPLICATIONS FOR ENTIRE SERIES OF 1864 PATIENTS UNDERGOING ARTERIAL RECONSTRUCTION (PERCENT)*

Early Complications	Elective (%)	Salvage (%)	Total (%)
Hemorrhage	2.24	4.80	2.41
Graft Infection**	0.12	—	0.11
Wound Infection	0.92	3.20	1.07
Pulmonary Embolus	0.40	1.60	0.48
Early Thrombosis	3.22	8.80	3.59
Embolism Major Vessel	0.35	—	0.32
Microembolus ("Trash Foot")	1.50	4.00	1.66
Myocardial Infarction	1.04	3.20	1.18
Cerebrovascular Accident	0.69	0.80	0.70
Mesenteric Infarction	0.63	1.60	0.70
Pancreatitis	0.12	—	0.11
Intestinal Obstruction	1.44	3.20	1.56
Renal Failure	3.05	6.40	3.27
Pulmonary Respiratory Failure	1.38	5.60	1.66
Pneumonia—Not Requiring Tracheostomy	0.52	1.60	0.59
Pneumonia—Requiring Tracheostomy	0.35	1.60	0.43
Other Miscellaneous Complications	2.30	1.60	2.25

*Some patients experienced several complications.

Number of Patients

Elective	1739
Salvage	125
TOTAL	1864

**Includes late graft infections.

TABLE 20–3 RISK (%) OF EARLY COMPLICATIONS BY TYPE OF OPERATION IN 1864 PATIENTS UNDERGOING ARTERIAL RECONSTRUCTION

Early Complications	Abdominal Aortic Aneurysm			Aortoiliac Occlusive Disease			Femoropopliteal Occlusive Disease			Miscellaneous Arterial Disease Categories		
	Elective	Salvage	Total	Elective	Salvage	Total	Elective	Salvage	Total	Elective	Salvage	Total
Hemorrhage	2.8	6.4	3.0	1.4	5.6	1.7	—	—	—	3.5	—	3.2
Graft Infection*	—	—	—	0.31	—	0.28	—	—	—	—	—	—
Wound Infection	0.53	2.1	0.63	1.7	3.7	1.8	—	14.3	1.2	0.38	—	0.36
Pulmonary Embolus	0.53	2.1	0.63	0.31	1.9	0.43	1.3	—	1.2	—	—	—
Early Thrombosis	2.3	6.4	2.5	4.2	11.1	4.7	9.1	14.3	9.5	1.9	5.9	2.2
Embolism Major Vessel	0.4	—	0.38	0.46	—	0.43	—	—	—	—	—	—
Microembolus ("Trash Foot")	1.1	2.1	1.1	2.3	7.4	2.7	1.3	—	1.2	0.77	—	0.72
Myocardial Infarction	1.7	2.1	1.75	0.62	5.6	1.0	1.3	—	1.2	—	—	—
Cerebrovascular Accident	1.1	—	1.0	0.46	1.9	0.57	—	—	—	0.38	—	0.36
Mesenteric Infarction	0.80	2.1	0.88	0.77	—	0.71	—	—	—	—	5.9	0.36
Pancreatitis	—	—	—	0.31	—	0.28	—	—	—	—	—	—
Intestinal Obstruction	1.5	8.5	1.9	1.5	—	1.4	—	—	—	1.5	—	1.4
Renal Failure	3.9	12.8	4.4	2.3	3.7	2.4	—	—	—	3.5	—	3.2
Pulmonary Respiratory Failure	1.5	8.5	1.9	1.1	5.6	1.4	1.3	—	1.2	1.9	—	1.8
Pneumonia—Not Requiring Tracheostomy	0.53	2.1	0.63	0.46	1.9	0.57	—	—	—	0.77	—	0.72
Pneumonia—Requiring Tracheostomy	0.53	2.1	0.63	0.31	1.9	0.43	—	—	—	—	—	—
Other Miscellaneous Complications	2.8	—	2.6	1.5	1.9	1.6	—	—	—	3.5	5.9	3.6

*Includes late graft infections.

AORTODUODENAL FISTULAE

Aorto-enteric fistulae occur most commonly as the result of a false aneurysm of the proximal suture line of an aortic graft, but may result from spontaneous rupture of an abdominal aortic aneurysm. Although over 80 percent of aorto-enteric fistulae occur in the third portion of the duodenum, they have been reported in the stomach and in both the large and small intestines.[3] The incidence in association with prosthetic aortic grafts is approximately 1.0 percent.[4]

The postoperative patient who has previously undergone aortic grafting and experiences gastrointestinal bleeding with or without back pain or low-grade temperature elevation should undergo aortography. The characteristic tendency of these lesions to produce recurrent, self-limited episodes of hemorrhage usually provides the surgeon time for diagnostic studies. Massive, potentially exsanguinating hemorrhage eventually occurs, and in such circumstances emergency operation should be performed.

Operation is performed through a midline incision, with reflection of the small bowel to the right. The false aneurysm of the proximal anastomosis is typically found to have eroded into the medial aspect of the third portion of the duodenum (Fig. 20–1, a). Once the diagnosis is ascertained, no further dissection of the false aneurysm is performed until systemic heparinization is instituted and proximal control of the supraceliac aorta at the diaphragm is obtained (Fig. 20–1, b). The distal aorta is clamped and the false aneurysm incised (Fig. 20–1, c). The defect in the duodenum is repaired in two layers with interrupted sutures. The disrupted proximal suture line is completely taken down and a new segment of graft anastomosed proximally to the aorta and distally to the previous graft (Fig. 20–1, d). Special attention is given to approximating the peri-aortic tissues, including the wall of the false aneurysm around the graft and a viable segment of omentum between the duodenum and graft (Fig. 20–1, e). In situations where a satisfactory new anastomosis cannot be made to the friable, scarred proximal aorta distal to the renal arteries, it is necessary to transect the renal arteries, perform the anastomosis more proximally, and reanastomose the renal arteries into the graft. Occasionally it is necessary to oversew the aorta below the renal arteries and place the proximal anastomosis of the new graft into the supraceliac aorta at the level of the diaphragm (Fig. 20–1, b).*

GRAFT INFECTIONS

Among the complications that may occur after vascular surgery, infection is perhaps the most dreaded — particularly when a synthetic vascular prosthesis is used. Morbidity from infection leads to further secondary complications such as abscess, bacteremia, chronic draining sinuses, and secondary hemorrhage. These conditions cause much pain, anxiety, prolonged hospitalization, and extra expense to the patient. Reports of mortality resulting from graft infections are truly alarming: Authorities such as Fry and associates[5] report 75 percent and Szilagyi[6] 40 to 60 percent mortality in connection with aortic and iliac vascular restoration. Although these statistics may be discouraging, appropriate and selected management of infections after vascular surgery should produce favorable results.

Infection after vascular surgery occurs mostly after operations that involve the femoral and popliteal arteries. Less frequently, an abdominal synthetic graft replacing an abdominal aneurysm or occluded bifurcation will become infected, but this usually occurs only when an injury was inadvertently made into the bowel. When the distal limbs of a bifurcation graft are brought below the inguinal ligament into the femoral artery, infection may occur distally, and contamination of the entire graft ensues. The type of fabric in the vascular substitute plays an important role in the development of infection. Our studies[7, 8] have revealed that fabrics with knitted velour surfaces heal more securely than woven fabrics and become an integral part of the surrounding tissues. Therefore, whenever a fabric graft is to be placed in the groin or below, we prefer a knitted velour graft. For femoropopliteal bypass procedures, autogenous veins have a low rate of infection, and for this and other reasons

*See also: Chapter 8, Lesions of the Visceral Arteries, and Chapter 9, Aortoiliac Occlusive Disease.

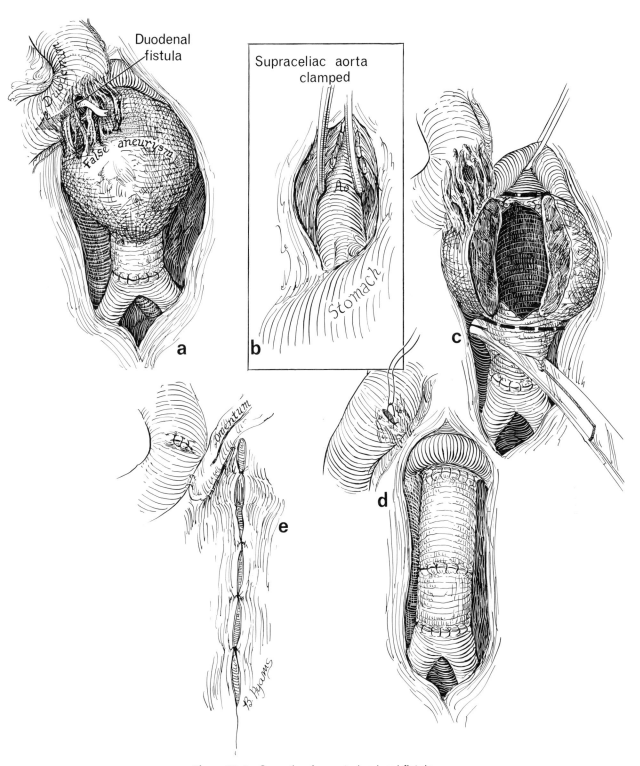

Figure 20–1 Operation for aortoduodenal fistula.

they remain the most satisfactory arterial substitute. Another factor that influences the incidence of graft infection is the presence of a hematoma around the graft, especially in the groin or thigh. Prolonged operations of several hours or more in duration invite infection. Extensive dissection in incisions of the lower extremity also predispose to the accumulation of serum, lymph, and blood. The elimination of dead space, use of interrupted sutures, and meticulous expeditious surgery should lower the incidence of infection. Excessive handling of the skin by the surgeon or placing the graft in contact with the skin may lead to wound and graft contamination. It seems unnecessary to state that application of the established principles of surgery will prevent most complications caused by infection.

Infections may become manifest at almost any time after implantation of a vascular prosthesis or foreign body. Indeed, some patients may enjoy a completely benign and uncomplicated early recovery and be dismissed from the hospital only to manifest the presence of infection several weeks later. An occasional patient may develop a suture line disruption several years later, when a low-grade infection caused by mildly pathogenic bacteria has been present since operation. Erosion of a fabric graft into an adjacent section of duodenum or jejunum will produce extensive graft contamination and often a massive intestinal hemorrhage. Secondary or late contamination may also occur, particularly if the patient has developed cellulitis of the toes or foot, or bacteremia from some unrelated illness. Therefore, the onset of infection is not constant or predictable. Some patients may have fever within a few hours or days of surgery. Fortunately, such fever is infrequently due to an infected graft or wound infection. Pulmonary, respiratory, and urinary complications are much more likely causes of early fever.

The question of whether and how to use prophylactic antibiotic therapy before, during, and after operation remains unsettled. After much consideration of the subject, we have adopted the use of a broad-spectrum antibiotic for "coverage," beginning 12 hours before vascular surgery and continuing 48 to 72 hours after operation. Intraoperative antibiotics are seldom used on our service unless some contamination or unexpected break in sterile technique has occurred.

TREATMENT OF GRAFT INFECTIONS

When wound infection is suspected after operation, the prime objective is to identify the anatomic site and obtain a culture of the offending bacteria. Blood cultures should be made for a spiking fever to identify the organism and employ the specific antibiotic. Sometimes, however, the surgeon may act prematurely and increase the possibility of graft contamination and more serious consequences. Not infrequently a mass develops in the groin after aortofemoral or femoropopliteal bypass. Simple evacuation of the fluid, which is basically lymph, should be done. A more radical approach with extensive wound exploration may lead to deep contamination of the underlying graft, which had not been previously involved. One should remember that most properly fabricated and selected vascular grafts resist rather than encourage infection. Give nature a chance — drain, culture, and treat with antibiotics. Most early wound infections respond favorably, and the patient suffers no late ill effects.

Chronic or persistent infections provide the true surgical dilemma, since the surgeon must grapple with the problem of whether to concentrate on radical elimination of the infection or to select a compromise position, prolonging the patient's life — or at least improving or maintaining its quality. Thus, the consideration of loss of life and limb arises. Ideally, the optimum treatment of an infected fabric graft would be to remove the graft entirely and wait for complete wound healing. Then, when conditions become favorable and all infection has been eliminated, a new graft

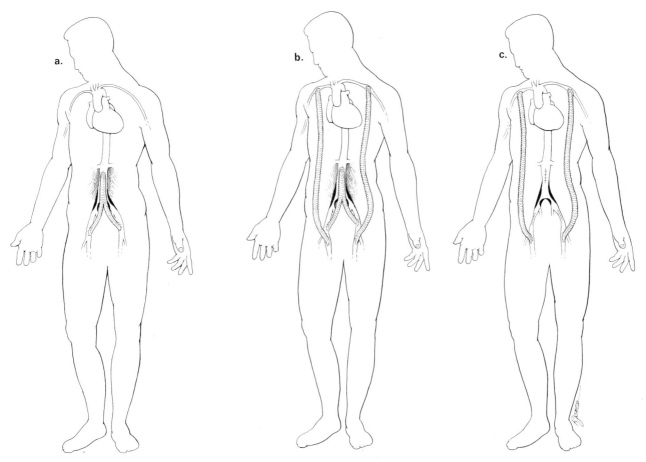

Figure 20–2   Techniques applicable for infected fabric grafts involving the area of the aortic bifurcation (*a*). Axillofemoral bypass grafts are tunneled subcutaneously along the anterolateral aspect of the trunk (*b*). After the bypass grafts have been completed and distal circulation restored, the fabric graft is removed at the same time or subsequent operation (*c*). Such grafts are subject to thrombosis if the patient lies on them while asleep. This technique has provided salvage in some serious problems with distal aortic occlusion.

can be implanted. Rarely does the clinical situation permit such rational treatment. Removal of the infected foreign body from the abdomen or lower extremity frequently results in severe ischemia of distal parts, requiring extensive amputation, or causing death. Therefore, a compromise with the ideal is usually necessary, and experienced judgment must be exercised.

Aggressive treatment of an infected aortic bifurcation graft with distal iliac anastomoses may be effected by performing an axillofemoral bypass graft using vascular prostheses with subsequent removal of the infected graft (Fig. 20–2, *a* to *c*). However well planned such procedures may be, emergency circumstances and clinical considerations often result in cross contamination of the new grafts, leading to late graft infection. Moreover, subsequent thrombosis of such extensive bypass grafts is highly probable, and the subcutaneously placed tubes are disfiguring to the patient. Other types of bypass procedures that may offer advantages in special circumstances are available (Figs. 20–3 and 20–4). We have used bypass grafts from the ascending aorta to the femoral artery (Fig. 20–3, *a*), or from the supraceliac portion of the proximal abdominal aorta (Fig. 20–3, *b* and *c*) in some instances with satisfactory results.[9] For the most part, however, such procedures are temporizing and may only delay the inevitable.

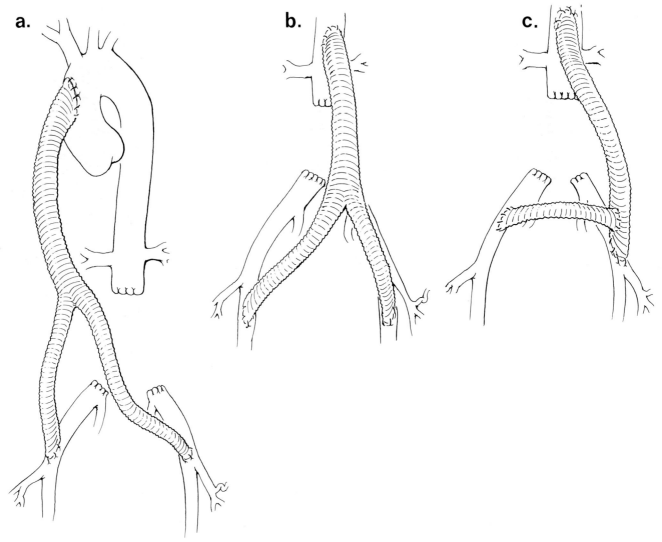

Figure 20–3 Depiction of other methods of bypassing infected grafts of the upper abdominal aorta: (*a*) ascending thoracic aorta to femoral arteries, (*b*) supraceliac abdominal aorta to both femoral arteries, and (*c*) supraceliac abdominal aorta to left femoral artery and femoral-femoral bypass to right femoral artery. The surgeon must select the most appropriate technique to suit the particular infected case.

SECONDARY HEMORRHAGE

Of all the problems that confront the vascular surgeon, that of secondary hemorrhage from an infected, previously placed prosthesis may be the most challenging, and consultation with another, perhaps more experienced, senior vascular surgeon is usually advisable. When hemorrhage occurs, procrastination or temporizing with antibiotic therapy is of no avail. Thus, the surgeon must select a course to save the life of his patient, fully cognizant of the fact that life after amputation of the lower extremities may be undesirable or intolerable. If the hemorrhage is from proximal aortic anastomosis, emergency celiotomy is necessary. Proximal control of the aorta must be the first objective, and exposure of the supraceliac aorta should be the initial step. Once the aorta is cross-clamped at this proximal level, the aortic anastomosis may be exposed. Disruption of the suture line is demonstrated, and direct repair should be performed. In our experience, the upper end of the fabric graft should be excised and an entirely new segment of graft inserted to provide a secure anastomosis without tension on the suture lines. If the infection appears to be localized,

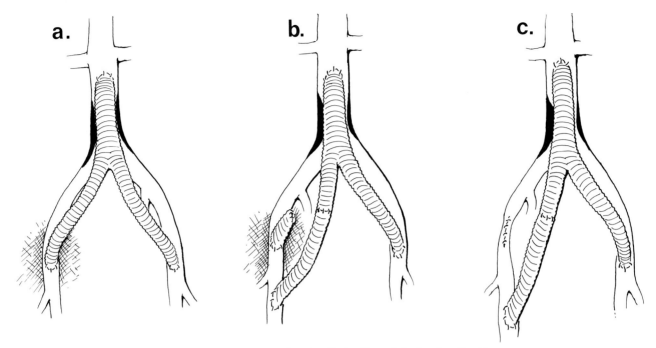

Figure 20–4 Technique that may be used in an occasional patient with an infection localized to one limb of an aortoiliac bypass graft. The area of infection is avoided during the dissection and bypass to the more distal femoral artery. The infected area may be isolated so that the infected segment is excised as a separate step without contaminating the newly implanted graft segment.

removal of the entire abdominal graft should be avoided. Direct control of hemorrhage and restoration of distal vascular continuity are the vital objectives, and at that time the persistence of the foreign body and infection are of secondary importance. *Eliminate the bleeding and save the life.*

Secondary hemorrhage from a femoral or popliteal anastomosis does not cause such a critical situation from the surgeon's standpoint, since usually the patient's life is not immediately at stake. Proximal control of the patent artery, whether at the iliac, femoral, or popliteal level for cross-clamping, permits exploration of the infected anastomosis. Local control of collateral bleeding from distal or proximal orifices may be achieved by using inflatable balloon catheters, thus avoiding extensive and tedious dissections. Once the bleeding has been controlled, the disrupted anastomosis may be explored. In such situations, the surgeon may elect simply to repair the anastomosis with interrupted sutures, while in others, the graft is locally excised and the entire anastomosis redone. After vascular continuity is restored, it may be advisable to drain the wound or even leave tubes for irrigation with antibiotic solutions. Unfortunately, the final solution for controlling hemorrhage and restoring vascular continuity usually represents a compromise with the ideal solution, which would eliminate the presence of bacterial infection.

Comment

Not all chronic infections are best approached by a radical surgical plan of graft excision and extra-anatomical bypass. The surgeon should equate the quality and length of life to the best advantage of the patient. Temporizing or conservatism may actually be the most desirable course for the individual patient in the full realization that the ultimate outcome is probably inevitable.

The following example describes the prolonged course of a patient managed more conservatively than recommended by other surgeons:

On May 27, 1955, a 63-year-old attorney underwent insertion of a lyophilized aortic homograft bypass for aortoiliac occlusive disease. On June 8, 1955, a left femoral popliteal bypass with the use of a lyophilized equine carotid artery was performed for treatment of an occlusion of the left superficial femoral artery. This graft subsequently became thrombosed. Eighteen months after the initial operation, the aortic homograft became thrombosed, and a bypass graft from the abdominal aorta to the left common femoral and right external iliac arteries was performed with a woven nylon Edwards-Tapp tube graft. Following this procedure, a superficial wound infection developed in the left inguinal area. It was incised and drained, at which time it was apparent that the left limb of the graft was infected. The infection was treated conservatively, and a chronic draining sinus developed that persisted for the next 16 years.

The patient returned in 1963, and at that time he had developed pseudoaneurysms of both distal anastomoses. These were resected and the distal anastomoses revised by inserting segments of knitted Dacron tube grafts. The chronic draining sinus persisted in the left groin without further complication for the next seven years, until the patient returned in 1970 and required incision and drainage of an abscess of the left groin. He was discharged after several days. Approximately six months later, in August 1970, he returned and underwent resection of a false aneurysm on the left femoral graft with revision of the anastomosis.

The patient continued to do satisfactorily until 1972, when he was readmitted to undergo exploration and debridement of the chronic draining sinus tract from the left inguinal region. Six months later in September 1972, he was readmitted for bleeding from the chronic draining sinus. He had developed fistulae between the left colon and duodenum in connection with the Dacron graft. Closure of the duodenal and colonic fistulae was performed. However, the patient developed hepatorenal failure and expired on October 5, 1972. During the entire 16-year period, while this patient had an established graft infection, he was active as a federal judge and, among other things, enjoyed golf several times a week. Although the graft infection did contribute to his death at the age of 80, he was able to enjoy 16 years of active life despite the handicap of persistent graft infection. It is doubtful whether radical surgery would have improved his clinical course.

In many instances, the patient would accept the circumstances of a chronic draining sinus from an infected prosthesis if the consequences of radical surgery were explained by the surgeon. Long-term oral antibiotic regimens with a daily dressing change may be much more practical and acceptable than the alternatives of extensive surgery, prolonged hospitalization, and the very real possibility of a fatal outcome.

PERIPHERAL MICROEMBOLISM ("TRASH FOOT")

Development of gangrene of the toes in the presence of bounding pedal pulses after an otherwise successful aortic reconstructive procedure is discouraging to both patient and surgeon. This complication, which results from the dislodgment of microemboli at the time of clamping or unclamping of the aorta, has been termed "trash foot." Once it has occurred, little can be done in the way of treatment; therefore, prevention during the operative procedure is a major consideration.

We have developed a technique of "internal flushing" that, when applied as described in Chapter 3 (Fig. 3–1, a to c), has proved successful in reducing the occurrence of this complication to a minimum. By means of this technique, loose debris in the proximal aorta is flushed into the internal iliac or profunda femoris arteries, where it is tolerated without adverse effects except for occasional mottling of the thighs — a location which is far better than in the toes. Proximal external flushing is avoided to prevent unnecessary blood loss and also multiple clamping and unclamping of the aorta, which dislodges more atheromatous material than a single episode of clamping. With this technique, the proximal clamp is applied only once during the procedure and is not released until the graft is in place and all anastomoses are completed. Prior to completion of the distal anastomoses, the distal clamps are removed to effect forceful retrograde flushing, which should result in visible debris on the first attempt at least 50 percent of the time.[10] Following completion of both proximal and distal anastomoses of a tube or aortoiliac bifurcation graft, one of the distal clamps is moved from the common iliac to the external iliac artery. The proximal aortic clamp is then gradually released, directing the blood flow and any debris from the proximal aorta into the internal iliac artery. In case of an aorto–common femoral artery bypass, the proximal femoral clamps are first removed, and, with release of the aortic clamp, flow and debris are directed retrograde up the common femoral arteries into the internal iliac arteries. The profunda femoris artery clamps are then removed, directing blood and debris into the thighs. The superficial femoral artery clamps are the last to be released (see Chapter 3, Fig. 3–1, a to c). One additional maneuver to prevent microembolization when clamping an abdominal aortic aneurysm is to apply the distal clamps first, thus trapping debris within the aneurysm. Debris dislodged by application of the distal clamps can be evacuated by retrograde flushing prior to completion of the distal anastomosis.

Once microembolization has occurred, little can be done to treat it. The use of low molecular weight dextran has been advocated;[11] although we have used this on occasion, we doubt its efficacy. When the toes become discolored postoperatively, the surgeon must be patient to allow final demarcation before proceeding to amputation. Often, only the outer layers will demarcate and slough over a period of weeks, whereas the toes will remain viable and will eventually heal.

Again, as in many other situations in surgery, *prevention is the best cure.*

REFERENCES

1. Javid H, Julian OC, Dye WS, Hunter JA: Complications of abdominal aortic grafts. Arch Surg 85:142, 1962.
2. Mannick JA: Complications of peripheral arterial surgery and their management. Am J Surg 116:387, 1968.
3. Reckless JPD, McColl I, Taylor GW: Aorto-enteric fistulae: An uncommon complication of abdominal aortic aneurysms. Br J Surg 50:458, 1972.
4. Pinkerton JA Jr: Aortoduodenal fistula. JAMA 225:1196, 1973.
5. Fry WJ, Lindenauer SM: Infection complicating the use of plastic arterial implants. Arch Surg 94:600, 1967.
6. Szilagyi DE, Smith RF, Elliott JP, Vrandecic MP: Infection in arterial reconstruction with synthetic grafts. Ann Surg 176:321, 1972.
7. Cooley DA, Wukasch DC, Bennett JG, Trono R: Double velour knitted Dacron grafts for aortoiliac vascular replacements. In *Vascular Grafts* (Phillip N. Sawyer and Martin J. Kaplitt, editors). New York City, Appleton-Century-Crofts, 1978, pp. 197–208.
8. Wukasch DC, Cooley DA, Bennett JG, Trono R: Results of a new Meadox-Cooley double velour Dacron graft for arterial reconstruction. J Cardiovasc Surg (Torino), 1979 (in press).
9. Wukasch DC, Cooley DA, Sandiford FM, Nappi G, Reul GJ Jr: Ascending aorta-abdominal aorta bypass: Indications, techniques and report of 12 patients. Ann Thorac Surg 23:442, 1977.
10. Imparato AM, Berman IR, Bracco A, Kim GE, Beaudet R: Avoidance of shock and peripheral embolism during surgery of the abdominal aorta. Surgery 73:68, 1973.
11. Foster JH, Killen DA, Jolly PC, Kirtley JH: Low molecular weight dextran in vascular surgery: Prevention of early thrombosis following arterial reconstruction in 85 cases. Ann Surg 163:764, 1966.

Distribution of Early Complications in 800 Patients
Undergoing Resection of Abdominal Aortic Aneurysm*

Early Complications	Elective	Salvage (Ruptured)	Total
Hemorrhage	21	3	24
Graft Infection**	0	0	0
Wound Infection	4	1	5
Pulmonary Embolus	4	1	5
Early Thrombosis	17	3	20
Embolism Major Vessel	3	0	3
Microembolus ("Trash Foot")	8	1	9
Myocardial Infarction	13	1	14
Cerebrovascular Accident	8	0	8
Mesenteric Infarction	6	1	7
Pancreatitis	0	0	0
Intestinal Obstruction	11	4	15
Renal Failure	29	6	35
Pulmonary Respiratory Failure	11	4	15
Pneumonia—Not Requiring Tracheostomy	4	1	5
Pneumonia—Requiring Tracheostomy	4	1	5
Other Miscellaneous Complications	21	0	21
TOTAL	164	27	191

*Includes 753 elective and 47 salvage (ruptured)
**Includes late graft infections

APPENDIX 1B

**Distribution of Early Complications in 703 Patients
Undergoing Revascularization for Aortoiliac Occlusive Disease***

Early Complications	Elective	Salvage	Total
Hemorrhage	9	3	12
Graft Infection**	2	0	2
Wound Infection	11	2	13
Pulmonary Embolus	2	1	3
Early Thrombosis	27	6	33
Embolism Major Vessel	3	0	3
Microembolus ("Trash Foot")	15	4	19
Myocardial Infarction	4	3	7
Cerebrovascular Accident	3	1	4
Mesenteric Infarction	5	0	5
Pancreatitis	2	0	2
Intestinal Obstruction	10	0	10
Renal Failure	15	2	17
Pulmonary Respiratory Failure	7	3	10
Pneumonia—Not Requiring Tracheostomy	3	1	4
Pneumonia—Requiring Tracheostomy	2	1	3
Other Miscellaneous Complications	10	1	11
TOTAL	130	28	158

*Includes 649 elective and 54 salvage
**Includes late graft infections

APPENDIX 1C

**Distribution of Early Complications in 84 Patients Undergoing
Revascularization with Dacron Grafts for Femoropopliteal Occlusive Disease***

Early Complications	Elective	Salvage	Total
Hemorrhage			
Graft Infection**			
Wound Infection		1	1
Pulmonary Embolus	1		1
Early Thrombosis	7	1	8
Embolism Major Vessel			
Microembolus ("Trash Foot")	1		1
Myocardial Infarction	1		1
Cerebrovascular Accident			
Mesenteric Infarction			
Pancreatitis			
Intestinal Obstruction			
Renal Failure			
Pulmonary Respiratory Failure	1		1
Pneumonia—Not Requiring Tracheostomy			
Pneumonia—Requiring Tracheostomy			
Other Miscellaneous Complications			
TOTAL	11	2	13

*Includes 77 elective and 7 salvage
**Includes late graft infections

APPENDIX 1D

**Distribution of Early Complications in 277 Patients
Undergoing Miscellaneous Arterial Reconstructions*†**

Early Complications	Elective	Salvage	Total
Hemorrhage	9		9
Graft Infection**			
Wound Infection	1		1
Pulmonary Embolus			
Early Thrombosis	5	1	6
Embolism Major Vessel			
Microembolus ("Trash Foot")	2		2
Myocardial Infarction			
Cerebrovascular Accident	1		1
Mesenteric Infarction		1	1
Pancreatitis			
Intestinal Obstruction	4		4
Renal Failure	9		9
Pulmonary Respiratory Failure	5		5
Pneumonia—Not Requiring Tracheostomy	2		2
Pneumonia—Requiring Tracheostomy			
Other Miscellaneous Complications	9	1	10
TOTAL	47	3	50

*Includes 260 elective and 17 salvage
**Includes late graft infections
†See Appendix 2 for Distribution of Miscellaneous Arterial Reconstructions

**Distribution of 277 Miscellaneous Arterial Reconstructions
by Type of Lesion**

Primary	Number
Ascending Thoracic Aortic Aneurysm	89
Descending Thoracic Aortic Aneurysm	65
Carotid Artery Occlusive Disease	24
Iliofemoral Occlusive Disease	24
Generalized Arteriosclerotic Occlusive Disease	22
Innominate Artery Occlusive Disease	14
Thoraco-Abdominal Aortic Aneurysm	10
Femoral Artery Aneurysm	9
Popliteal Artery Aneurysm	7
Thoracic Aortic Arch Aneurysm	2
Aortic Valve Stenosis (Left Ventricle to Abdominal Aorta Conduit)	3
Aortic Transection (Traumatic)	2
False Aneurysm Any Vessel	2
Coarctation of Thoracic Aorta	1
Supravalvular Aortic Stenosis	1
Profunda Femoral Artery Occlusive Disease	1
Other Arterial Aneurysm	1
TOTAL	277

APPENDIX 3A

Early Results in 1864 Patients Undergoing Arterial Reconstruction
(Number of Patients)

Type of Lesion		Improved	Unchanged	Worse	Amputation	Expired
Abdominal Aortic	Elective	687	—	18	3	45
Aneurysm	Salvage	36	—	1	2	8
	TOTAL	723	—	19	5	53
Aortoiliac	Elective	603	3	21	8	14
Occlusive Disease	Salvage	35	—	5	6	8
	TOTAL	638	3	26	14	22
Femoropopliteal	Elective	74	—	1	1	1
Occlusive Disease	Salvage	5	—	1	1	—
	TOTAL	79	—	2	2	1
Other	Elective	242	3	3	1	11
Miscellaneous Arterial Reconstructions	Salvage	14	1	—	1	1
	TOTAL	256	4	3	2	12

APPENDIX 3B

Early Results in 1864 Patients Undergoing Arterial Reconstruction
(Percent)

Type of Lesion		Improved	Unchanged	Worse	Amputation	Expired
Abdominal Aortic	Elective	91.2	—	2.39	0.40	5.98
Aneurysm	Salvage	76.6	—	2.13	4.26	17.0
	TOTAL	90.4	—	2.38	0.62	6.63
Aortoiliac	Elective	92.9	0.46	3.24	1.23	2.16
Occlusive Disease	Salvage	64.8	—	9.26	11.1	14.8
	TOTAL	90.8	0.43	3.70	1.99	3.13
Femoropopliteal	Elective	96.1	—	1.30	1.30	1.30
Occlusive Disease	Salvage	71.4	—	14.3	14.3	—
	TOTAL	94.0	—	2.38	2.38	1.19
Other	Elective	93.1	1.15	1.15	0.38	4.23
Miscellaneous	Salvage	82.4	5.88	—	5.88	5.88
Arterial						
Reconstructions						
	TOTAL	92.4	1.44	1.08	0.72	4.33

APPENDIX 4

Early Mortality in 1864 Patients Undergoing Arterial Reconstruction*

Type of Lesion		No. of Deaths	Percent Mortality (%)
Abdominal Aortic	Elective	45	5.98
Aneurysm	Salvage	8	17.02
	TOTAL	53	6.63
Aortoiliac Occlusive	Elective	14	2.16
Disease	Salvage	8	14.81
	TOTAL	22	3.13
Femoropopliteal	Elective	1	1.30
Occlusive Disease	Salvage	—	—
	TOTAL	1	1.19
Other Miscellaneous	Elective	11	4.23
Arterial Reconstructions	Salvage	1	5.88
	TOTAL	12	4.33

*Total No. of Deaths............ 88
Total No. of Patients 1864
Mortality for Entire Group... 4.72%

APPENDIX 5A

**Causes of Death in 800 Patients Undergoing
Abdominal Aortic Aneurysm Resection**

Cause of Death	Number of Patients
Cardiac Arrest—Cause Undetermined	15
Myocardial Infarction	14
Respiratory Insufficiency	5
Renal Failure	4
Hemorrhage	4
Cardiac Arrhythmia	3
Mesenteric Infarction	2
Congestive Heart Failure	1
Infection	1
Ruptured Anastomotic Aneurysm	1
Pulmonary Embolus	1
Cerebral Vascular Insufficiency	1
Cerebrovascular Accident	1
TOTAL	53

APPENDIX 5B

Causes of Death in 703 Patients Undergoing Arterial Reconstruction for Aortoiliac Occlusive Disease

Cause of Death	Number of Patients
Myocardial Infarction	10
Cardiac Arrest — Cause Undetermined	3
Respiratory Insufficiency	2
Hemorrhage	2
Renal Failure	1
Mesenteric Infarction	1
Cerebrovascular Accident	1
Infection	1
Congestive Heart Failure	1
TOTAL	22

APPENDIX 5C

Causes of Death in 84 Patients Undergoing Arterial Reconstruction for Femoropopliteal Procedures

Cause of Death	Number of Patients
Myocardial Infarction	1

APPENDIX 5D

Causes of Death in 277 Patients Undergoing Miscellaneous Arterial Reconstruction

Primary Cause of Death	Number of Patients
Cardiac Arrest—Cause Undetermined	4
Hemorrhage	3
Renal Failure	2
Infection	1
Ruptured Anastomotic Aneurysm	1
Trauma	1
TOTAL	12

APPENDIX 6

MEDICAL RECORD KEEPING FOR DATA ANALYSIS

GRAFT EVALUATION

Med. Record No. 1_____

Card ID   7_____

Name 12_____

Age (00-99)	40 ____	
Circle Appropriate Codes		
Sex: Male	42	M
Female......	43	F

Diabetes Mellitus (Circle if Yes)   44   Y

Pre-Operative Data

Aorto-Iliac Occlusive Disease...	45	A
Abdominal Aortic Aneurysm	46	B
Femoral-Popliteal Occlusive Disease	47	C
Coarctation of Aorta	48	D
Renal Artery Stenosis	49	E
Celiac Artery Stenosis	50	F
Superior Mesentery Artery Stenosis..	51	G
Inferior Mesentery Artery Stenosis...	52	H
Subclavian Artery Stenosis	53	I
Other_____(Enter Code.	54	J
_____J must be circled)	55	

Principal Procedure

Elective	59	E
Salvage or Ruptured	60	S

Date of Operation..(MMDDYY)   61

Card 1.

CARD 2 (Duplicate First 6 Columns)

CARD ID   7_____

Keypunch three lines of address only
DO NOT punch name (1st line on label)

12-
34-
56-

Card 2.

CARD 3 (Duplicate First 6 Columns)

CARD ID   7_____

Reconstruction ....Circle Appropriate Code(s)

Aorto-Common Iliac	12	A
Aorto-External Iliac	13	B
Aorto-Ilio-Femoral	14	C
Aorto-Common Femoral..	15	D
Aorto-Superficial Femoral	16	E
Aorto Profundis Femoral	17	F
Femoral-Popliteal (AK)	18	G
Femoral-Popliteal (BK)	19	H
Femoral-Distal to Popliteal	20	I
Resection AAA	21	J
Repair of Coarctation	22	K
Aorto-Renal Bypass...	23	L
Aorto-Coeliac Bypass	24	M
Aorto-Superior Mesentery Bypass	25	N
Aorto-Inferior Mesentery Bypass	26	O
Subclavian Bypass	27	P
Other_____(Enter Code.	28	Q
_____Q must be circled)	29	_|_|_|_

FOR EACH RECONSTRUCTION CIRCLED ABOVE, COMPLETE ONE LINE OF THE FOLLOWING:

	Reconstruction Code	Graft Material	Graft Configuration	Graft Size
34	_____	_____	_____	_|_|_
41	_____	_____	_____	_|_|_
48	_____	_____	_____	_|_|_

LEGEND:

Reconstruction Code   See Reconstruction Above

Graft Material
K   Knitted
L   Woven-low porosity
W   Woven-standard porosity
D   Double velour
B   Bovine Heterografts
V   Vien biograft
G   Graft to graft
S   Soft weave
O   Other_____

Graft Configuration
T   Tube
B   Bifurcation
P   Patch
O   Other_____

Graft Size   Actual size in mm x mm, except with umbilical cord grafts which are mm x cm. Record all as two digits.
EXAMPLE. Write 0 mm as 00.

Card 3.

CARD 4 (Duplicate First 6 Columns)

CARD ID   7_____.

Circle Appropriate Codes
Right .... 12 R
Sympathectomy   Left .... 13 L

Early Complication
  Hemorrhage.. 14 A
      Graft.. 15 B
      Suture Line.................................. 16 C
      Other Non-Related to Graft .... 17 D
  Graft Infection.. 18 E
  Wound Infection... 19 F
  Pulmonary Embolus .... 20 G
  Early Thrombosis .... 21 H
  Embolism Major Vessel .... 22 I
  Microembolus (Trash Foot) .... 23 J
  Myocardial Infarction.................................... 24 K
  CVA (Stroke) .... 25 L
  Mesenteric Infarction.................................... 26 M
  Pancreatitis .... 27 N
  Intestinal Obstruction .... 28 O
  Renal Failure .... 29 P
  Pulmonary Respiratory Failure........................ 30 Q
  Pneumonia .... 31 R
  Required Tracheostomy .... 32 S
  Other_____(Enter Code. 33 T
  _____T must be circled) 34

Re-Operative for—Early Complication ....Yes .... 38 Y
    (Non-Graft Related)

Re-Operative Date—Secondary Operation.................(MMDDYY) 39

Condition Necessitating—Secondary Re-Operation
  Hemorrhage.. 45 A
      Graft.. 46 B
      Suture Line.................................. 47 C
      Other Non-Related to Graft .... 48 D
  Early Thrombosis .... 49 E
  Graft Infection.. 50 F
  Other_____(Enter Code. 51 G
  _____G must be circled) 52

(Fill in specifics.)

Card 4.

Card 4. (*Continued*)

Blood Lost During Primary Operation   (0000-9999)   56 _ | | _ |_
     Recorded or Not Recorded   (R/N)   60 _____

Total Number of Graft Related   (00-99)   61 ___|___
     Operation(s) Performed

Early Results (Hospital stay) .... Enter Code From Legend Below
     Primary Operation .... 63 _____
     Secondary Operation.. 64 _____
     If more than two graft operations were performed give the results   65 _____
        for the last graft related operation

   LEGEND:
     E   Excellent—Asymptomatic
     G   Good
     I   Improved
     U   Unchanged
     W   Worse
     A   Amputation
     D   Expired

History   (Y/N)
     Had the patient undergone a previous graft implant?   66 _____
     Had the patient undergone a previous graft implant, which was   67 _____
     replaced either completely or partially at the time of the primary surgery?

Card 4. *(Continued)*

CARD 5 (Duplicate First 6 Columns)

CARD ID   7 _____

Death
     Date ....(MMDDYY)   12 _| _|_ | _|_|_
     Cause of Death ....(See Code Sheets)   18 __|_ | _|_
        Cause of Death Modifier .... 22 ___ |
     Secondary Cause of Death .... 24 _|_ _| _|
        Secondary Cause of Death Modifier .... 28 ___|__

Card 5

Index

Page numbers in *italics* indicate illustrations; (t) indicates Table.